MEDICAL CARE *of the* Cancer Patient

Second Edition

Susan Rosenthal, M.D.
Professor of Oncology in Medicine
University of Rochester School of Medicine and Dentistry and
University of Rochester Cancer Center
Rochester, New York

Joanne R. Carignan, M.D.
Associate Professor of Oncology in Medicine
University of Rochester School of Medicine and Dentistry and
University of Rochester Cancer Center
Rochester, New York

Brian D. Smith, M.D.
Associate Professor of Medicine
University of Rochester School of Medicine and Dentistry
Rochester, New York

W. B. SAUNDERS COMPANY
Harcourt Brace Jovanovich, Inc.
Philadelphia London Toronto Montreal Sydney Tokyo

W. B. SAUNDERS COMPANY
Harcourt Brace Jovanovich, Inc.

The Curtis Center
Independence Square West
Philadelphia, Pennsylvania 19106

Library of Congress Cataloging-in-Publication Data

Medical care of the cancer patient / [edited by] Susan Rosenthal, Joanne R. Carignan, Brian D. Smith.—2nd ed.

p. cm.

Includes bibliographical references and index.

ISBN 0-7216-3959-3

1. Cancer. I. Rosenthal, Susan N. II. Carignan, Joanne R. III. Smith, Brian D. (Brian Drew) [DNLM: 1. Neoplasms—therapy. WZ 266 M4875]

RC262.M4 1993

616.99′4—dc20

DNLM/DLC 92-49938

MEDICAL CARE OF THE CANCER PATIENT ISBN 0–7216–3959–3

Printed in the United States of America.

Last digit is the print number: 9 8 7 6 5 4 3 2 1

NOTICE

The editors, authors, and the publisher of this book have made every effort to ensure that all therapeutic modalities that are recommended are in accordance with accepted standards at the time of publication, and that all drug dosages and regimens are correct. Nevertheless, anyone not familiar with cancer treatment should carefully check other sources and preferably consult an oncologic specialist before administering or prescribing any form of cancer treatment. Furthermore, several of the drugs and other therapeutic regimens described in this book are experimental and are only available to approved qualified investigators or through cancer centers or cooperative groups.

THE EDITORS

The following chapters are based in part on work by contributors to the previous edition: Chapter 3, Diagnostic Imaging in Oncology, Theodore F. Van Zandt; Chapter 4, Principles of Radiation Oncology, Charles L. Lewis; Chapter 9, Hodgkin's Disease, Richard F. Bakemeier; Chapter 15, Genitourinary Malignancies, Brian D. Smith; Chapter 16, Gynecologic Oncology, Jackson B. Beecham and Cynthia Angel; Chapter 21, Endocrine Malignancies, Susan Rosenthal; and Chapter 22, Cancer of Unknown Primary Origin, Brian D. Smith.

CONTRIBUTORS

George R. Abbott, M.D.
Clinical Assistant Professor of Pathology, University of Rochester School of Medicine and Dentistry, Rochester, New York
Pathology of Malignant Disease

John M. Bennett, M.D.
Professor of Oncology in Medicine, Pathology and Laboratory Medicine, University of Rochester School of Medicine and Dentistry and University of Rochester Cancer Center, Rochester, New York
The Chronic Leukemias

Martin Brower, M.D.
Associate Professor of Oncology in Medicine, University of Rochester School of Medicine and Dentistry and University of Rochester Cancer Center, Rochester, New York
Lung Cancer; Genitourinary Malignancies

Joanne R. Carignan, M.D.
Associate Professor of Oncology in Medicine, University of Rochester School of Medicine and Dentistry and University of Rochester Cancer Center, Rochester, New York
Cancer Biology: Carcinogenesis, Oncogenes, and Epidemiology; Gynecologic Oncology

Alex Yuang-Chi Chang, M.D.
Associate Professor of Oncology in Medicine, University of Rochester School of Medicine and Dentistry and University of Rochester Cancer Center, Rochester, New York
Biotherapy of Cancer

Elizabeth M. Cyran, M.D.
Assistant Professor of Oncology in Medicine, University of Rochester School of Medicine and Dentistry and University of Rochester Cancer Center, Rochester, New York
Hematopoietic Growth Factors

Kathleen S. Doerner, B.S.N.
Nurse Manager, Rochester General Hospital Cancer Center, Rochester, New York
Oncologic Nursing

Deborah J. Dudgeon, R.N., M.D., FRCP(C)
Assistant Professor of Medicine, University of Manitoba, Winnipeg, Manitoba
Psychosocial Care of the Cancer Patient

Zachary B. Kramer, M.D.
Assistant Professor of Oncology in Medicine, University of Rochester School of Medicine and Dentistry and University of Rochester Cancer Center, Rochester, New York
Non-Hodgkin's Lymphomas

Robert M. Lerner, M.D., Ph.D.
Associate Professor of Diagnostic Radiology, University of Rochester School of Medicine and Dentistry, Rochester, New York
Diagnostic Imaging in Oncology

Jane L. Liesveld, M.D.
Assistant Professor of Medicine, University of Rochester School of Medicine and Dentistry, Rochester, New York
Bone Marrow Transplantation

John E. Loughner, Pharm. D.
Assistant Professor of Oncology in Health Services, University of Rochester School of Medicine and Dentistry and University of Rochester Cancer Center, Rochester, New York
Clinical Pharmacology of Antineoplastic Agents; Management of Pain in the Cancer Patient

H. Reid Mattison, M.D.
Infectious Disease Consultant, Infectious Diseases of Indianapolis, Indianapolis, Indiana
Infections in the Cancer Patient

Craig S. McCune, M.D.
Associate Professor of Oncology in Medicine, University of Rochester School of Medicine and Dentistry and University of Rochester Cancer Center, Rochester, New York
Malignant Melanoma

Gary R. Morrow, Ph.D., M.S.
Associate Professor of Oncology in Psychiatry (Psychology), University of Rochester School of Medicine and Dentistry and University of Rochester Cancer Center, Rochester, New York
Management of Nausea in the Cancer Patient

John P. Olson, M.D.
Professor of Medicine, University of Rochester School of Medicine and Dentistry, Rochester, New York
Multiple Myeloma

Kishan J. Pandya, M.D.
Associate Professor of Oncology in Medicine, University of Rochester School of Medicine and Dentistry and University of Rochester Cancer Center, Rochester, New York
Cancers of the Head and Neck

Richard B. Patt, M.D.
Assistant Professor of Anesthesiology, Psychiatry and Oncology, University of Rochester School of Medicine and Dentistry and University of Rochester Cancer Center, Rochester, New York
Management of Pain in the Cancer Patient

Pradyumna D. Phatak, M.D.
Assistant Professor of Medicine, University of Rochester School of Medicine and Dentistry, Rochester, New York
Hodgkin's Disease

Susan Rosenthal, M.D.
Professor of Oncology in Medicine, University of Rochester School of Medicine and Dentistry and University of Rochester Cancer Center, Rochester, New York
Breast Cancer; Gastrointestinal Cancers

Jacob M. Rowe, M.D.
Professor of Medicine, University of Rochester School of Medicine and Dentistry, Rochester, New York
Acute Leukemias

Deepak Sahasrabudhe, M.D.
Associate Professor of Oncology in Medicine, University of Rochester School of Medicine and Dentistry and University of Rochester Cancer Center, Rochester, New York
Sarcomas of Soft Tissue and Bone; AIDS-Associated Malignancies

Duncan E. Savage, M.D.
Assistant Professor of Radiation Oncology, Albany Medical College, Albany, New York
Principles of Radiation Oncology

Brian D. Smith, M.D.
Associate Professor of Medicine, University of Rochester School of Medicine and Dentistry, Rochester, New York
Malignant Brain Tumors; Endocrine Malignancies

Julia L. Smith, M.D.
Assistant Professor of Oncology in Medicine, University of Rochester School of Medicine and Dentistry and University of Rochester Cancer Center, Rochester, New York
Cancer of Unknown Primary Origin; Hospice Care

Timothy J. Woodlock, M.D.
Assistant Professor of Oncology in Medicine, University of Rochester School of Medicine and Dentistry and University of Rochester Cancer Center, Rochester, New York
Clinical Pharmacology of Antineoplastic Agents; Oncologic Emergencies

PREFACE

The medical care of the cancer patient encompasses a wide range of diagnostic and therapeutic programs for a host of different tumor types and patient problems. While many oncology textbooks are currently available, most are so large and detailed that a practical but complete approach to an individual patient can be hard to extract. *Medical Care of the Cancer Patient* is designed for internists, family physicians, residents, medical students, and oncology nurses who require a succinct but thorough and readable review of clinical oncology.

The scope of this book is wide, even though the presentation is compact. From carcinogenesis and oncogenes to recent trends in immunotherapy and bone marrow transplantation, this book serves as an introduction to the rapidly evolving field of oncology. Initial chapters review the basic principles of oncologic pathology, radiology, radiation therapy, and pharmacology of antineoplastic agents. The specialized disciplines of gynecologic, psychosocial, and nursing oncology are presented, along with up-to-date reviews of pain management, nausea and vomiting, hospice care, growth factors, and infections in the immunocompromised host. Specific cancers are also individually considered, with pertinent details of diagnosis, staging, treatment, and prognosis.

Cancer represents a challenge as well as a threat. Cancer medicine has made great advances and looks forward to more in the very near future. We hope that this book will provide our colleagues and students with a pragmatic, comprehensive, and affordable guide to the current state-of-the-art in oncology and to the prospects for future advances.

SUSAN ROSENTHAL, M.D.
JOANNE R. CARIGNAN, M.D.
BRIAN D. SMITH, M.D.

CONTENTS

1
CANCER BIOLOGY: CARCINOGENESIS, ONCOGENES, AND EPIDEMIOLOGY

Joanne R. Carignan

From the time of Hippocrates, patients have reacted with fear and despair to a diagnosis of cancer, yet with current therapy half of newly diagnosed cancer patients are alive 5 years after diagnosis. As researchers learn more about cancer biology, further improvements in therapy will occur that will benefit the one-third of Americans destined to develop cancer in their lifetimes. It is unlikely that any single revolutionary discovery will lead to the cure of cancer; rather, as in the past, our understanding of cancer will gradually evolve, and clinicians will slowly translate scientific advances into clinical successes.

CANCER BIOLOGY

A cancer is a tumor that can infiltrate through normal tissue barriers into adjacent structures and spread to distant sites, eventually leading to death. Most cancers originate from a single altered cell. This "single cell of origin" theory is supported by several lines of evidence:

- A single malignant cell injected into an animal can initiate cancer in some models.
- Many tumors are clonal–that is, the tumor cells are homozygous for certain markers for which the host is heterozygous (e.g., G6PD in chronic myelogenous leukemia).

As tumors grow and metastasize, subclones emerge, imparting heterogeneity to the malignant cell population. Genetic instability and tumor progression are basic characteristics of cancer. By the time a tumor can be detected clinically, subpopulations of cancer cells may have already acquired such properties as resistance to chemotherapeutic drugs.

Both normal and malignant cells pass through the phases of the cell cycle (Fig. 1–1). The G1 phase is a variable period before synthesis of DNA, and in general, more slowly growing cells have longer G1 periods than more rapidly growing cells. The G1 phase may even be skipped by cells that grow very rapidly. Cells synthesize DNA in S phase, and G2 represents the stage prior to mitosis. The growth of a population of cells depends on the cell cycle time (the time between two successive mitoses), the growth fraction (the percentage of cells actively cycling), and the rate of cell loss. There is considerable variability and overlap among normal and abnormal tissues in all three of these factors. For instance, normal colonic mucosa may have a shorter cell cycle time and higher growth fraction than certain malignancies. The basic difference between normal and malignant tissues is that in an adult, in whom growth has stopped, the number of normal cells produced equals the number lost, whereas malignant cells lose the ability to differentiate into properly functioning nonproliferating endstage cells, and immature undifferentiated cells consequently accumulate. In malignant tissues, the number of new cells produced exceeds the number lost. One promising approach to cancer treatment uses agents that induce differentiation of malignant cells into the proper functional nonproliferating phenotype.

Once growth is established, tumors spread by local invasion and metastasis. As cancer progresses, tumor cells break through the epithelial basement membrane (Fig. 1–2). Cancer cells travel through the extracellular matrix by both mechanical and chemical processes. Membrane receptors act as sites of attachment for tumor cells, and the tumor cells in turn alter and degrade the matrix by the secretion of a variety of proteinases. Pharmacologic inhibition of these proteases is under active investigation in an attempt to control the metastatic process. Once through the matrix, tumor cells have access to lymphatic and venous channels, allowing distant metastases to occur.

Neoplastic cells enter the circulation in enormous numbers, in part as a result of the abnormal nature of tumor vasculature, where wide gaps between endothelial cells and discontinuity in the basement membrane allow easier vascular access. However, despite

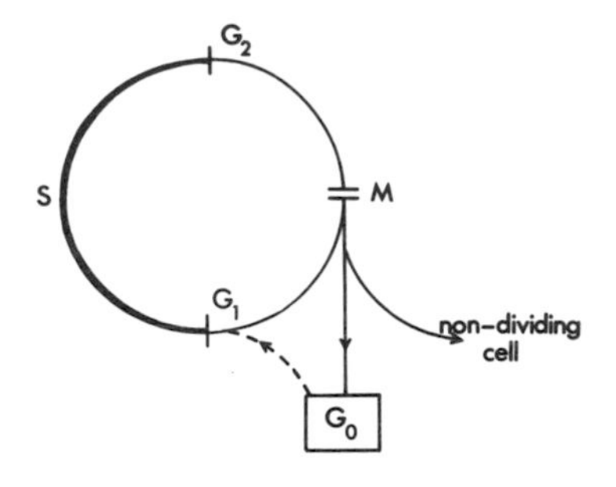

Figure 1–1. The cell cycle. Continuously dividing cells go around the cycle from one mitosis (M) to the next. Nondividing cells will die without dividing again. Quiescent G_0 cells can be induced to reenter the cycle by an appropriate stimulus. (*From* Baserga R: The cell cycle. Reprinted by permission of the New England Journal of Medicine 304:453–459, 1981.)

the large number of neoplastic cells that circulate, the number of metastases established is relatively small. A successful metastasis requires that the tumor cell survive the hostile environment of the circulation, either grow in or pass through the first capillary bed (often the liver or lung), bind preferentially to the site of metastasis, and establish a locally favorable environment for metastatic development. This is a complex and specialized process, so it is not surprising that most cancer cells do not succeed. Only a small subset of the total tumor cell population is functionally able to metastasize; this is an important manifestation of tumor cell heterogeneity. The recent identification of a metastasis suppressor gene, nm 23, whose expression is markedly reduced in tumors with a high metastatic potential, may help in understanding this process.

CARCINOGENESIS

The causes of cancer appear to be nearly as diverse as the cancers themselves. Even food, sunshine, air, and heredity are among the villains. Carcinogenesis probably represents a "multiple-hit" process. In theory, cancer occurs in patients with an inherited or induced genetic predisposition who have been exposed to secondary cofactors (often environmental or perhaps viral). After an extremely variable latent period, the precancerous lesion overcomes bodily defenses and becomes an invasive malignancy.

ONCOGENES

The most stimulating development in cancer research in the past decade has been the discovery of the oncogenes. The transforming oncogenes of RNA viruses (v-oncs) represent

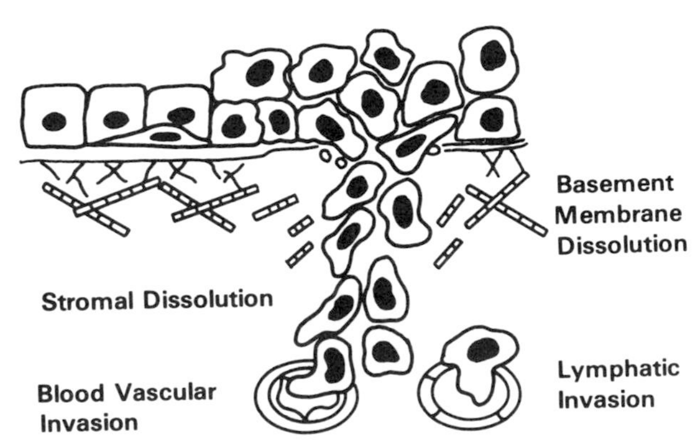

Figure 1–2. The mechanism of tumor invasion. As in situ carcinoma cells penetrate the basement membrane, local invasion precedes distant metastases. Systemic dissemination results from entry into the vascular and lymphatic systems. (*From* Liotta L: Mechanism of cancer invasion and metastasis. *In* DeVita VT, Hellman S, Rosenberg SA (eds): Important Advances in Oncology 1985. Philadelphia, JB Lippincott, 1985, p. 32.)

Table 1–1. **PROPERTIES OF SELECTED CELLULAR ONCOGENES IMPLICATED IN HUMAN TUMORS**

PROPERTY	EXAMPLE	ACTIVITY
Growth factor	c-*sis*	B chain PDGF (platelet-derived growth factor)
Transmembrane growth factor receptor	c-*erb* B	Truncated EGF (epidermal growth factor) receptor
Signaling proteins	*src, ras*	Tyrosine kinase or GTP-binding proteins involved in intracellular signaling
Nuclear proteins	*myc, myb, fos, jun*	Regulation of DNA replication

highly conserved homologs of the cellular proto-oncogenes (c-oncs) found in most species of animal and humans. These cellular homologs of the retroviral oncogenes are usually present as single copies in the human genome. This remarkable discovery suggests that retroviruses acquired their transforming capacity as a consequence of their ability to incorporate cellular oncogenes into their genomes. It appears likely that the gene products of the oncogenes have important functions in normal cell growth and differentiation. They are expressed at increased levels during embryogenesis, for instance. The DNA sequences of some of the proto-oncogenes and the amino acid sequences of their protein products have been determined; many appear to be related to or identical to cellular growth factors, growth factor receptors, cellular signaling proteins, or nuclear regulatory proteins (Table 1–1; Fig. 1–3). Oncogene activation may result in overproduction of these products or in production at an unsuitable time or place.

Proto-oncogenes can be activated by nonviral and viral means, but in humans three nonviral mechanisms are most common: point mutation, chromosome rearrangement, and gene amplification.

Point Mutations. A lesion as small as a point mutation can change the proto-oncogene sufficiently so that the altered protein product can induce the altered cellular behavior characteristic of cancer. Point mutations in the *ras* oncogene family were noted in bladder

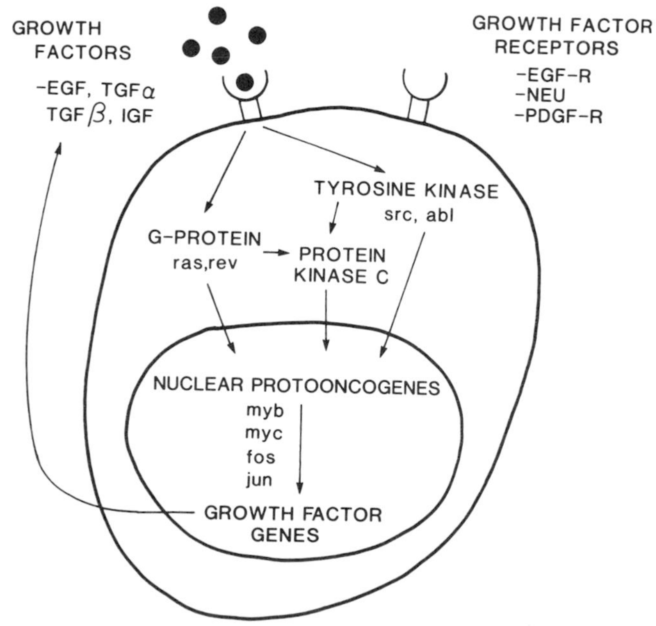

Figure 1–3. Oncogene products and growth regulation in human cells. (*From* Miller DM, Blume S, Borst M, et al: Oncogenes, malignant transformation, and modern medicine. Am J Med Sci 300:59–69, 1990.)

tumor cell lines as early as 1981, and similar point mutations involving these oncogenes occur commonly in human colorectal, pancreatic, and non–small cell lung cancers.

Chromosomal Rearrangements. These occur during translocations of deoxyribonucleic acid (DNA), and DNA translocations are well described in several malignancies. The oncogene c-*myc* normally resides on chromosome 8, but in Burkitt's lymphoma c-*myc* sequences have been found on chromosomes 2, 14, and 22, suggesting that the c-*myc* oncogene has been translocated in the malignant cells. The areas to which c-*myc* is translocated are known to regulate immunoglobulin synthesis (mu, kappa, and lambda on chromosomes 2, 14, and 22, respectively). These translocations result in significantly increased c-*myc* expression, which may be important in the neoplastic process.

The Philadelphia chromosome of chronic myelogenous leukemia (CML) involves a reciprocal translocation between chromosomes 9 and 22. The c-*abl* proto-oncogene is translocated from chromosome 9 to an area on chromosome 22 called the breakpoint cluster region (bcr). The result is a novel *bcr/abl* gene product with high levels of tyrosine kinase activity that acts as a growth signal transducer important to the etiology of CML.

In acute promyelocytic leukemia (APL), translocations between chromosomes 15 and 17 include the gene on chromosome 17 that encodes retinoic acid receptor alpha. Administration of all-*trans* retinoic acid, a ligand for retinoic acid receptor alpha, can induce dramatic remissions in APL. Response correlates with the presence of this particular translocation. Interestingly, this oncogene appears to participate in the pathogenesis of APL, while also contributing to its sensitivity to a specific treatment.

Gene Amplification. Amplification of oncogenes has been well described in pediatric neuroblastomas in which amplification of the N-*myc* oncogene leads to overexpression of the oncogene product (up to 250 times normal levels). Amplification of *myc* family oncogenes also occurs in small cell lung cancer, and amplification of c-*erb* B family oncogenes is common in glioblastomas and breast and ovarian cancers.

In summary, oncogenes represent highly conserved genetic sequences present in most species that frequently encode information for the production of growth factors or growth factor receptors. Oncogenes begin to function in an abnormal or enhanced fashion when their genetic sequence or that of a nearby regulatory neighbor is disturbed. Only rarely will a change in a single oncogene transform a normal cell into a malignant cell; in most instances, 10 to 20 genetic changes accumulating over years are necessary to accomplish malignant transformation.

TUMOR SUPPRESSOR GENES

The classic oncogene acts in a dominant fashion contributing to a cascade of events resulting in carcinogenesis. Studies of hereditary tumors, particularly retinoblastoma, reveal the existence of recessive oncogenes or tumor suppressor genes. The presence of one normal allele of these tumor suppressor genes adequately protects against the initiation of a particular tumor. In the inherited form of retinoblastoma, one copy of the retinoblastoma (RB) gene is inactivated in the germ line, and then the second is inactivated in the somatic line; the absence of the RB gene product removes a negative control on cancer origination. The sporadic form of retinoblastoma requires the two events to occur in the somatic line, a much less likely occurrence. Chromosomal studies reveal characteristic abnormalities of chromosome 13q14, the site of the RB gene. Homozygosity for the inactive RB gene also occurs in the secondary malignancies, most frequently osteosarcomas, commonly described in familial retinoblastoma survivors. Perhaps the most common genetic abnormality in human malignancies is the deletion of the portion of chromosome 17 that codes for the p53 protein, a potent growth-suppressing agent.

Inactivation of tumor suppressor genes has been found in an increasing number of human cancers, and the loss of certain chromosomal loci is characteristic of the location of the tumor suppressor genes (Table 1–2). Carcinogenesis in vivo may require a sequence of activations of oncogenes and inactivations of tumor suppressor genes. One proposed model for colon cancer carcinogenesis graphically describes this interaction (Fig. 1–4). Additional research indicates possible participation of certain oncogenes and their gene products at specific stages in the development, proliferation, and maintenance of both primary and metastatic tumors.

Table 1–2. **CHROMOSOMAL DELETIONS ASSOCIATED WITH CANCER**

CHROMOSOMAL DELETION	ASSOCIATED TUMOR SUPPRESSOR GENE	TYPE OF CANCER
1p		Melanoma, neuroblastoma, medullary thyroid carcinoma, pheochromocytoma, MEN-2, ductal breast carcinoma
1q		Breast carcinoma
3p		Small cell lung carcinoma, renal cell carcinoma, cervical carcinoma
5q		Familial adenomatous polyposis, sporadic colorectal carcinoma
6q		Melanoma
11p	WT1	Wilms' tumor, breast carcinoma, rhabdomyosarcoma, hepatoblastoma, transitional cell bladder carcinoma
11q		MEN-1*
13q	RB1	Retinoblastoma, osteosarcoma, small cell lung carcinoma, ductal breast carcinoma
17p	p53	Small cell lung carcinoma, colorectal carcinoma, breast carcinoma, osteosarcoma
17q	NF1	Neurofibroma
18q	DCC	Colorectal carcinoma
22		Meningioma, acoustic neuroma, pheochromocytoma

From Hollingsworth RE, Lee HW: Tumor suppressor genes: New prospects for cancer research. J Natl Cancer Inst 83:91–96, 1991.
*MEN: Multiple endocrine neoplasia.

VIRAL CARCINOGENESIS

Viruses cause cancers in animals. The most convincing evidence that they cause cancer in humans is derived from work with human T-cell leukemia-lymphoma virus (HTLV-I). A characteristic clinical pattern occurs in patients infected with this RNA retrovirus: onset during adulthood, rapid progression, lymphadenopathy, hepatosplenomegaly, hypercalcemia, and skin changes. Retroviral particles have been seen budding from cell membranes in this unusual and aggressive T-cell lymphoma. The affected T cells are OKT4 positive (helper lymphocytes). Epidemiologic studies reveal geographic pockets of increased incidence (Japan and the Caribbean), and antibodies to HTLV-I have been found in increased numbers in patients and the local populations. Virus isolated from each area is identical to the original HTLV-I. T cells infected with HTLV-I produce both interleukin-2 (T-cell growth factor) and interleukin-2 receptors. The result is autostimulation and consequent uncontrolled proliferation.

Other viruses have also been implicated in the causation of human cancers. Epstein-Barr virus, associated with African Burkitt's lymphoma, is thought to promote or precipitate the genetic rearrangement causing c-*myc* activation, but other cofactors such as chronic antigenic stimulation by malaria may also be involved. Epstein-Barr virus is also associated with nasopharyngeal carcinoma and with non-Hodgkin's lymphomas in immunosuppressed hosts. Hepatitis B virus is linked to hepatoma. Specific types of human papillomaviruses have been convincingly implicated in the causation of cervical cancer. Human immunodeficiency virus (HIV) is clearly associated with certain malignancies (lymphomas, Kaposi's sarcoma) in acquired immune deficiency syndrome (AIDS) patients; whether HIV causes the Kaposi's sarcoma directly or it occurs as a consequence of the profound immunodeficiency state produced by infection with HIV remains to be determined.

CHEMICAL CARCINOGENESIS

One-third of cancers worldwide result from the use of cigarettes and other tobacco products. In addition, a wide variety of chemicals, medicines, and environmental contaminants is strongly suspected to play a role in cancer causation (Table 1–3). In many cases, these chemicals are transformed into "electrophilic reactants" that can cause DNA damage. Whether a cancer arises or not depends in turn on the body's ability to "detoxify" the carcinogen and repair the DNA damage. Chemical carcinogenesis consists of a multiple-phase phenomenon in which chemicals initially damage DNA (initiation) and then other

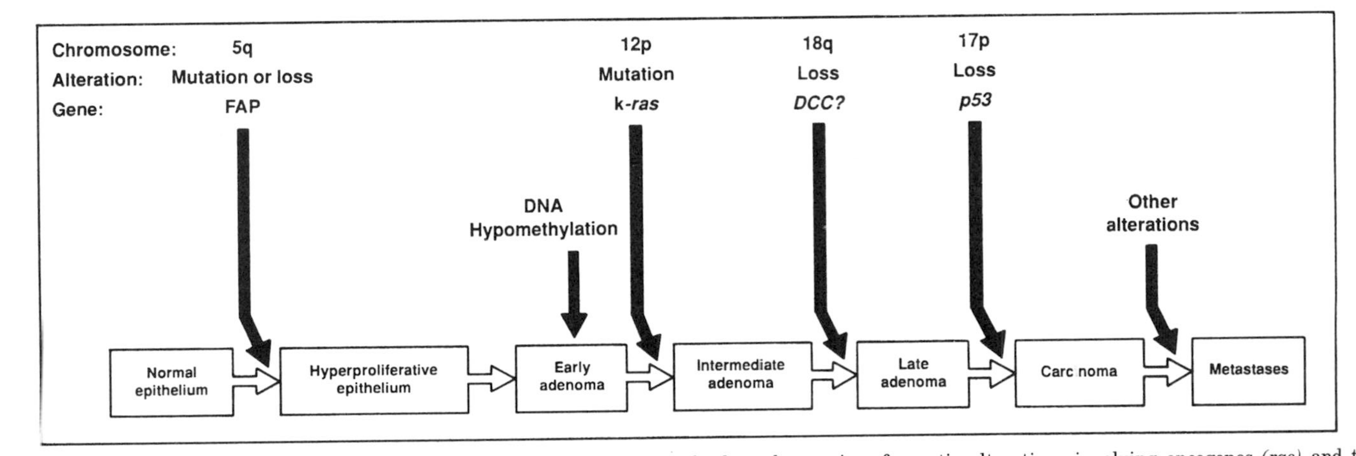

Figure 1–4. A genetic model for colorectal carcinogenesis. Tumorigenesis proceeds through a series of genetic alterations involving oncogenes *(ras)* and tumor suppressor genes (particularly on chromosomes 5q, 17p, and 18q). However, the order of these changes is not invariant, and accumulation of these changes, rather than their order with respect to one another, seems most important. (*From* Fearon ER, Vogelstein B: A genetic model for colorectal tumorigenesis. Cell 61:759–767, 1990.)

Table 1–3. **CHEMICALS KNOWN OR STRONGLY SUSPECTED TO BE CARCINOGENIC FOR HUMAN BEINGS**

CHEMICAL	SITE OF CANCER
Occupational Contacts	
Aromatic amines	Bladder
Arsenic	Skin and bronchus
Asbestos	Bronchus, pleura, and peritoneum
Benzene	Marrow
Bis(chloromethyl)ether	Bronchus
Bis(chloroethyl)sulfide	Respiratory tract
Cadmium	Prostate
Chrome ores	Bronchus
Coke ovens	Bronchus
Nickel ores	Bronchus and nasal sinus
Soots, tars, and oils	Skin and lungs
Wood dust	Nasal sinuses
Vinyl chloride	Liver
Medical Agents	
Alkylating agents (e.g., melphalan and cyclophosphamide)	Hematopoietic tissue and bladder
Anabolic steroids	Liver
Arsenic	Skin
Chlornaphazine	Bladder
Diethylstilbestrol	Vagina
Immunosuppressive drugs	Lymphoid tissue
Phenacetin (acetophenetidin)	Renal pelvis
Others	
Aflatoxins	Liver
Tobacco smoke	Bronchus, mouth, pharynx, larynx, esophagus, bladder, and pancreas
Oral contraceptives	Liver
Betel nut and lime	Mouth

From Farber E: Chemical carcinogenesis. Reprinted, by permission, from the New England Journal of Medicine 305:1379–1389, 1981.

chemicals or environmental cofactors cause the abnormal cell to proliferate (promotion). The ability of vitamin A and retinoids to reverse this progression is currently under study.

Dietary factors (including alcohol) and deficiencies have also been implicated in cancer causation. Since vitamin A promotes cellular differentiation, epidemiologists have studied cancer incidence in relation to vitamin A intake. Lung, bladder, gastrointestinal, and breast cancers are all less common among individuals with high vitamin A intake. Little evidence supports a role for vitamins C and E in cancer protection. Selenium is an antioxidant; epidemiologic studies indicate higher cancer rates in areas with low selenium levels in the soil. High dietary fat content accompanies an increased risk for breast and colon cancers in some populations, and obesity seems to be a risk factor for endometrial and possibly breast cancer. All of these dietary factors remain only presumptive cofactors in carcinogenesis. The inability to study large populations of human subjects with manipulated diets and constant environments over extended periods of time will make confirmation of the role of diet in human cancer causation and protection very difficult.

In theory, alcohol promotes the efficacy of other ingested or inhaled carcinogens. Esophageal and head and neck cancers are particularly common among those who abuse both alcohol and tobacco. Whether alcohol increases the risk for gastric, lung, and colorectal carcinoma remains controversial.

RADIATION CARCINOGENESIS

Diagnostic x-rays represent the most common exposure to carcinogenic ionizing radiation. Fortunately, radiogenic cancer is uncommon and is estimated to account for less than 30 cancers per million persons per year. Sensitivity to radiation-induced carcinogenesis varies; radiation exposures in utero, in childhood, or in young women result in higher rates of hematologic, thyroid, and breast malignancies. New technology and scrupulous quality control have considerably decreased radiation exposure from diagnostic studies.

Environmental exposure to ionizing radiation may occur from radon, a gaseous decay product of uranium. While the impact of radon carcinogenesis is small, concern exists because of the widely variable levels of radon present in different homes. In recent studies, up to 2% of U.S. homes had radon levels that were eight times normal. The corresponding risk of lung cancer is estimated to increase fourfold, with a marked susceptibility in smokers and to a lesser degree in nonsmokers.

The carcinogenic effect of electromagnetic fields due to common household appliances and high-power lines remains speculative and controversial. The existing studies are flawed and have conflicting results. Occupational studies suggest an increased risk for acute myeloid leukemia in electrical workers, but the results are not conclusive.

CANCER STATISTICS

Figure 1–5 shows the 1991 estimate of cancer mortality by the National Cancer Institute. This group estimated 1.1 million new cases of cancer and 514,000 deaths from cancer would occur in the United States in 1991. Of children born in 1985, the probability at birth of eventually developing cancer of a major site is 36.9% for white males, 35.2% for black males, 36.1% for white females, and 31.5% for black females. The probability at birth of eventually dying of cancer of a major site is 23.2% for white males, 24.6% for black males, 20.0% for white females, and 19.5% for black females. As mortality from infection and cardiovascular diseases decreases, the National Cancer Institute data indicate a continuing but small increase in the probability of developing cancer and succumbing to it.

Age-adjusted cancer death rates shown in Figures 1–6 and 1–7 reveal how cancer as a public health problem has changed over the past 50 years. Encouragingly, stomach cancer mortality has decreased markedly for males and females. This has been attributed to improvements in food storage and preparation. Uterine cancer mortality figures also reveal dramatic improvement, largely due to decreased cervical cancer mortality because of improved screening and early detection. Lung cancer mortality remains a national health disaster. Age-adjusted death rates for men have increased by 75% and for women by 175% over the past 25 years. In 1987, lung cancer deaths (42,748) surpassed breast cancer deaths (40,899) in women. This is largely attributable to tobacco use and as such is evidence of the disappointing failure of measures to curtail cigarette smoking.

Incidence data indicate substantial increases in rates of breast cancer, prostate cancer, and melanoma. Mortality figures remain stable for these cancer types. Changes in diagnostic practices and improved and earlier treatment may account for this statistical

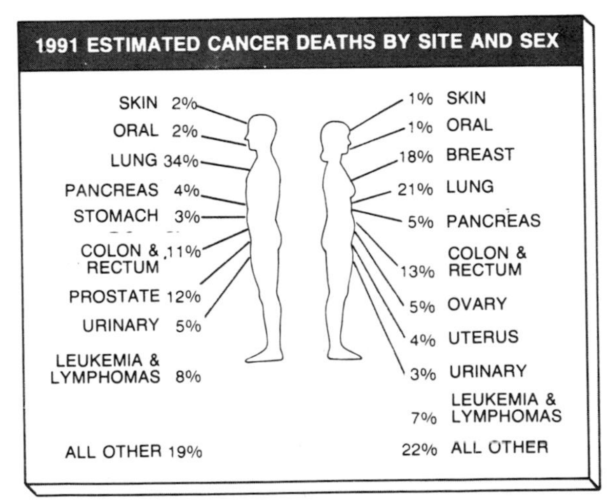

Figure 1–5. 1991 Estimated cancer deaths by site and sex. (*From* Boring CC, Squires TS, Tong T: Cancer statistics, 1991. CA 41:19–39, 1991.)

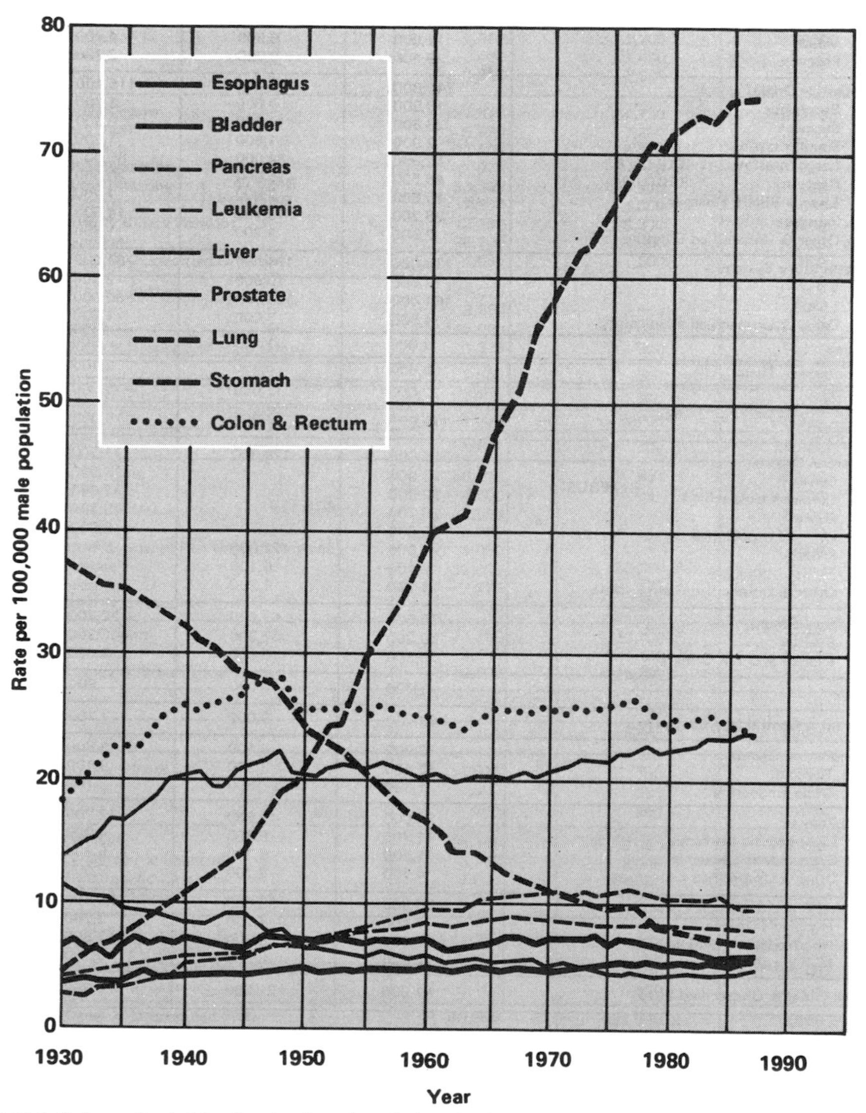

Figure 1–6. Age-adjusted death rates for selected sites (males), United States, 1930–1987. (*From* Boring CC, Squires TS, Tong T: Cancer statistics, 1991. CA 41:19–39, 1991.)

divergence. The increased incidence of melanoma may be due to increased surveillance and may also represent increased recreational sun exposure. The virulence of advanced melanoma and lack of effective treatment after primary surgery make the increased incidence of this cancer particularly ominous.

CANCER PREVENTION

The single most effective way to prevent cancer and to decrease cancer mortality is to avoid tobacco products. Cigarette smoking is associated with a marked increased risk for cancers of the lung, larynx, oral cavity, esophagus, bladder, and pancreas as well as possibly contributing to the risk of stomach and cervical cancer. Recent estimates implicate

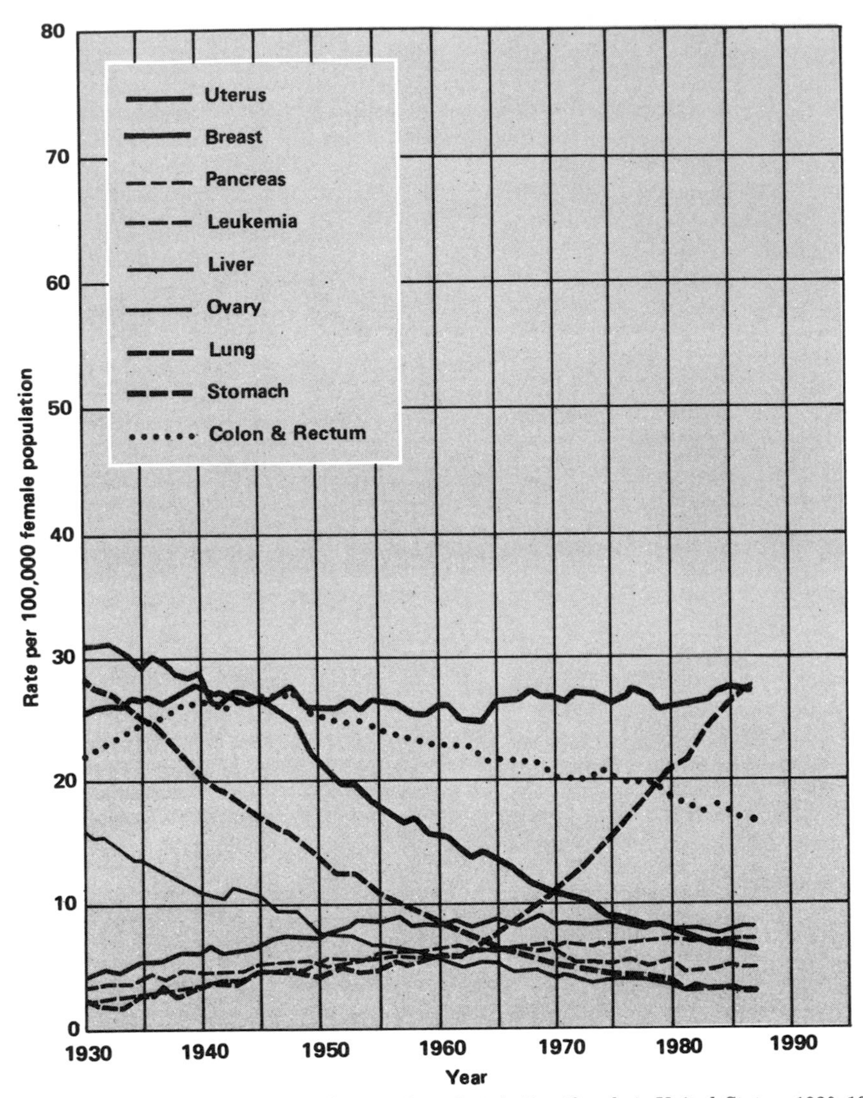

Figure 1–7. Age-adjusted cancer death rates for selected sites (females), United States, 1930–1987. (*From* Boring CC, Squires TS, Tong T: Cancer statistics, 1991. CA 41:19–39, 1991.)

cigarette smoking as a cause of 30% of cancer deaths and 85% of lung cancers in the United States. Low-tar brands of cigarettes can decrease lung cancer mortality by 26%; however, overall, lung cancer mortality of low-tar cigarette smokers remains much higher than that of nonsmokers. The number of carcinogens and cocarcinogens in tobacco smoke is appalling, and yet the tobacco industry refuses to acknowledge the danger of its product. "Smokeless" oral tobacco products may avoid the risk of lung cancer but drastically increase the risk of oral cavity cancers. "Passive smoking" by individuals who live with heavy smokers increases the risk of lung cancer by 30% when compared with inhabitants of nonsmoking households. Additional studies on the risk of involuntary smoking support current efforts to provide nonsmokers with a smokefree environment.

Despite the overwhelming evidence that tobacco is directly related to cancer causation, 26% to 30% of the American population continue to smoke. Demographics reveal alarming frequencies of smoking among teenagers, especially girls, with highest frequencies among the lower socioeconomic groups and some ethnic minorities. The tobacco industry's aggressive marketing policies linking smoking with glamour, sports, and leisure represent callous disregard of the hazards of smoking. The increasing emphasis on tobacco exports to Third World populations is a national disgrace. Intensive educational and smoking cessation projects should be implemented vigorously.

Other measures to decrease cancer incidence may also be difficult to implement. In a "sun-worshipping" population, sun avoidance is difficult to promote. However, moderation in sun exposure and the use of sun-screening products are advisable, especially for patients with light hair and fair complexions. Sensible dietary recommendations for good health include decreased fat, increased fiber, and the avoidance of extreme obesity or excessive alcohol ingestion. Interventional studies with beta-carotene and alpha-tocopherol are under way. A very large breast cancer prevention trial with tamoxifen (an antiestrogen) versus placebo for "high-risk" patients has recently begun.

REFERENCES

Cancer Biology

Cohen PS, Israel MA: Basic molecular biology for the pediatric hematologist/oncologist. Am J Pediatr Hematol Oncol 11:467–480, 1989.

Fearon ER, Vogelstein B: A genetic model of colorectal tumorigenesis. Cell 61:759–767, 1990.

Heppner GH, Miller BE: Therapeutic implications of tumor heterogeneity. Semin Oncol 16:91–105, 1989.

Killion JJ, Fidler IJ: The biology of tumor metastasis. Semin Oncol 16:106–115, 1989.

Oncogenes and Tumor Suppressor Genes

Druker BJ, Mamon HJ, Roberts TM: Oncogenes, growth factors, and signal transduction. N Engl J Med 321:1383–1391, 1989.

Hollingsworth RE, Lee WH: Tumor suppressor genes: New prospects for cancer research. J Natl Cancer Inst 83:91–96, 1991.

Miller DM, Blume S, Borst M, et al: Oncogenes, malignant transformation, and modern medicine. Am J Med Sci 300:59–69, 1990.

Weinberg RA: Oncogenes, antioncogenes, and the molecular bases of multistep carcinogenesis. Cancer Res 49:3713–3721, 1989.

Carcinogenesis

Lazo PA, Tsichlis PN: Biology and pathogenesis of retroviruses. Semin Oncol 17:269–294, 1990.

Mackowiak PA: Microbial oncogenesis. Am J Med 82:79–97, 1987.

Shopland DR, Pechacek TF, Cullen JW: Toward a tobacco-free society. Semin Oncol 17:402–412, 1990.

Shore RE: Electromagnetic radiations and cancer. Cause and prevention. Cancer 62:1747–1754, 1988.

Cancer Epidemiology and Statistics

Byar DP, Freedman LS: The importance and nature of cancer prevention trials. Semin Oncol 17:413–424, 1990.

Greenwald P, Cullen JW, Weed D: Introduction: Cancer prevention and control. Semin Oncol 17:383–390, 1990.

Menck HR, Garfinkel L, Dodd GD: Preliminary report of the National Cancer Data Base. CA 41:7–18, 1991.

2
PATHOLOGY OF MALIGNANT DISEASE

George R. Abbott

Establishing a tissue diagnosis is the key first step in the medical care of a cancer patient. Generally, a careful microscopic examination of an adequate biopsy establishes the presence and type of malignant cells as well as the grade of the neoplasm. Not infrequently, however, poorly differentiated malignancies may be difficult to classify in spite of special stains and other techniques. Study of a surgical specimen is most productive when facts are freely interchanged between the clinician and the pathologist. Such communication is essential prior to biopsy if special studies such as imprints, immunohistochemistry, electron microscopy, or cultures are likely to be needed.

CLASSIFICATION

Classification of a specimen begins with characterization of its gross appearance. Microscopic study systematically evaluates tissue architecture, supporting tissue structure, and invasion of surrounding tissues or vessels. Individual cells are scrutinized for size, shape, degree of pleomorphism, and mitotic activity. Histochemical and immunohistochemical stains identify specific cellular products such as intermediate filaments (keratins in carcinomas, desmin and vimentin in sarcomas, glial fibrillary acidic protein or neurofilaments in central nervous system neoplasms), mucin in adenocarcinomas, melanin in melanoma, and glycogen in Ewing's tumors and in renal, adrenal, and germ cell tumors.

TUMOR GRADE

The grade of a neoplasm is a label denoting the pathologist's assessment of its malignant potential. Grade is based on the degree of differentiation (resemblance to the normal tissue elements) and the growth rate as evidenced by the numbers of mitoses. In certain lesions, malignancy appears to correlate with the number of mitoses per unit area regardless of the degree of differentiation. The grade of the cancer is stated in such terms as well, moderately, or poorly differentiated, or by numerical designations of grades I to III or I to IV, from most differentiated to least differentiated. The significance of grading rests on the assumption that a well-differentiated or low-grade neoplasm will behave less aggressively than a poorly differentiated or high-grade one. It cannot be emphasized too strongly that many other factors influence the biologic behavior of cancers. For example, a well-differentiated squamous cell carcinoma arising in sun-damaged skin has minimal potential for metastasis, whereas a virtually identical lesion arising in the oral mucosa may metastasize widely while yet clinically inapparent. Furthermore, the stage of a neoplasm is usually a more important determinant of prognosis than is its grade. To some extent, the apparent lack of predictive significance of tumor grade may reflect the subjective nature of some of the assessments upon which grading is based. Also, observed mitotic rates may be inaccurate. Recently, more objective approaches to the estimation of biologic potential have involved DNA measurements by flow or static cytometry to determine the growth fraction (proportion of cells in S phase) and to detect aneuploid cell lines. Studies have demonstrated that in several types of neoplasms poor prognosis may be predicted by high growth fractions or by the presence of aneuploidy or both. Interestingly, aneuploidy frequently correlates with the histologic finding of abnormal mitoses.

PATHOLOGY REPORT

The surgical pathology report embodies the result of study of the specimen. Generally, the essentials are stated succinctly in the "final pathologic diagnosis." The gross description and microscopic notes contain important data for accurate pathologic staging: exact size of the lesion, anatomic relations to adjacent structures, and proximity to resection margins. In cases in which the diagnosis is less than explicit, the pathologist usually comments regarding the degree of (un)certainty of the diagnosis and includes a differential diagnosis in the microscopic description or in a separate note. If such explanatory notes fail to elucidate an obscure diagnosis, the clinician must question the pathologist to clarify the situation.

LIGHT MICROSCOPY

ROUTINE PROCESSING

Small specimens are usually placed in fixative upon removal from the patient and sent to the surgical pathology laboratory for gross examination and processing for microscopic study. Certain special procedures require examination prior to routine fixation. Larger specimens, e.g., mammary, uterine, pulmonary, or gastrointestinal resections, are usually examined fresh and should be refrigerated if they are not dissected promptly. Most laboratories employ buffered 10% neutral formalin as a routine fixative but may use other solutions for particular specimens, e.g., B5 or Zenker's fixative for hematologic and lymphoid specimens.

As it arrives in the laboratory, each specimen is assigned its unique number. As samples (blocks) are taken for histologic study, they are placed in fixative in small cassettes identified with the specimen number. At the completion of the day's specimens, the cassettes are placed in an automatic processing machine, and by the next morning the tissues are ready to be embedded in paraffin, sectioned, and stained. Certain specimens, such as bowel resections, are difficult to section in the unfixed state and are usually opened, examined, pinned to boards or other supports, and fixed overnight before sections are taken. Bone and other heavily mineralized specimens require decalcification after fixation before they may be embedded and sectioned.

In some laboratories, paraffin sections of small specimens can be obtained in a few hours. This requires special equipment affording rapid fixation aided by controlled heating and followed by paraffin embedding in a vacuum device to speed infiltration of the tissue by the paraffin.

FROZEN SECTIONS

With this technique, freezing the specimen provides the support normally given by paraffin embedding in routine processing. Employed in intraoperative consultations, frozen sections usually permit immediate assessment of histologic sections and in most instances allow definitive diagnosis. Frozen sections are often used as a guide to what additional surgery may be indicated, as in a mastectomy immediately following breast biopsy. They may be used to confirm that the removed tissue contains diagnostic material before termination of the procedure, even though definitive diagnosis may not be possible. They also are used to evaluate the adequacy of surgical resection margins. Specimens for study by frozen section should be submitted unfixed because even brief exposure to fixative interferes with adherence of the sections to glass slides, resulting in their loss in staining. The histologic quality of frozen sections is usually significantly inferior to that of paraffin sections; thus, the pathologist may defer making a diagnosis until the paraffin sections can be studied. Another inherent disadvantage of frozen sections is the risk of losing small but crucial portions of a section as it is cut because it is not contained within a supporting matrix of paraffin. Because some diagnoses may require study of serial sections of paraffin-embedded tissue, many pathologists decline to use frozen sections in the evaluation of certain specimens; e.g., cervical conization biopsies of suspected microinvasive carcinoma.

IMPRINTS

All lymph nodes suspected of containing a lymphoproliferative process should be submitted promptly and without fixative so that imprints, or "touch preps," may be made and an aliquot for flow cytometry obtained. The freshly incised cut surface of the node is blotted and a series of imprints made by gently touching the tissue to clean glass slides. The best technique is to hold the node with the incised surface up and to make the imprint by a smooth rocking motion of the slide held in the other hand. Some of the air-dried imprints are Wright stained, and others can be used for cytochemistry or immunochemistry.

Imprints of other neoplasms prepared as described, but fixed immediately in Papanicolaou fixative, may be stained with hematoxylin and eosin or Papanicolaou stain.

HISTOLOGIC STAINS

The standard stain in nearly all pathology departments is hematoxylin and eosin (H and E), which stains nuclei dark blue and cytoplasm (and most extracellular substances) shades of pink. All sections are routinely stained with H and E, which demonstrates the histologic and cytologic features so well that all other staining procedures are designated "special" stains.

Connective Tissues. Trichrome stains distinguish between collagen and muscle fibers. Reticulin, the smallest collagen fiber, is demonstrated by silver impregnation techniques. Elastic fibers are most commonly stained by orcein followed by a van Gieson (picric acid and fuchsin) counterstain, which also distinguishes collagen from smooth muscle. The phosphotungstic acid–hematoxylin (PTAH) procedure stains fibrin and glial fibers and is sometimes employed to accentuate the cross striations of skeletal muscle, as in rhabdomyosarcomas.

Carbohydrates. A bewildering array of stains is used for demonstration of various carbohydrates. The periodic acid–Schiff (PAS) stain, with many modifications, is used to stain carbohydrates such as glycogen and components of basement membranes, mucosubstances, fungi, and a variety of glycolipids. The PAS reaction following controlled hydrolysis identifies deoxyribonucleic acid (DNA) in the Feulgen technique by staining the carbohydrate moiety of DNA.

Mucins. Stains for mucosubstances, a special class of carbohydrates, include the colloidal iron, Alcian blue, and iron diamine stains. With control of pH, these stains can distinguish among neutral, acidic, and sulfated mucopolysaccharides. The mucicarmine stain is commonly used as a stain for epithelial mucin, but it also stains the mucoid capsule of cryptococcal yeast forms.

Lipids. Oil red O and Sudan stains demonstrate neutral fats. These techniques require frozen sections because processing for paraffin embedding removes lipids from tissues. Glycolipids are commonly identified by modifications of the PAS reaction and may utilize paraffin sections. The Schultz stain identifies cholesterol in frozen sections, but cholesterol may be presumptively identified in paraffin sections by the acicular clefts left in the tissue after the lipid is removed in processing.

Microorganisms. Modifications of the Gram and Ziehl-Neelsen methods are used to stain organisms in sections. *Legionella* organisms require silver impregnation for demonstration in tissue or specific fluorescent antibodies in smears or imprints. Methenamine silver stains fungal and *Pneumocystis* organisms. The Giemsa stain demonstrates *Pneumocystis* sporozoites as well as numerous other protozoa. Immunohistochemical reagents for *Pneumocystis* are also available. Spirochetes are demonstrated by silver impregnation in the Warthin-Starry procedure.

Secretory Granules. Stains for most hormone-producing tissues utilize immunohistochemical procedures specific for the hormones involved. Neurosecretory granules may be demonstrated by argyrophil and argentaffin procedures. Argentaffin cells can be identified by autofluorescence in formalin-fixed unstained sections.

Miscellaneous. Glial fibers in gliomas may be demonstrated by immunohistochemical stains for glial fibrillary acidic protein or the older PTAH and trichrome stains. Amyloid stains metachromatically with crystal violet; i.e., amyloid is red, whereas everything else stains purple. With Congo red stain, deposits of amyloid exhibit apple-green dichroism when viewed by polarized light. Mast cell granules stain metachromatically with toluidine blue and are also well stained with Giemsa. Melanin gives a positive argentaffin reaction with the Fontana-Masson or Warthin-Starry stains. Hemosiderin gives a positive reaction in stains for iron. The Leder chloroacetate esterase stain is invaluable for marking cells of the neutrophil series, monocytes, and mast cells in formalin-fixed paraffin sections of suspected hematologic neoplasms.

IMMUNOCYTOCHEMISTRY

Over the past 2 decades, this technique has become widely used to demonstrate the presence and histologic localization of a variety of antigenic substances, including hormones, enzymes, oncofetal antigens, and other tumor markers in tissues. Immunoperoxidase methods utilizing enzyme-labeled antibodies may be performed on standard paraffin sections. The antibodies, which are raised in animals injected with purified antigen, are polyclonal. Thus, rigorous positive and negative controls are required to confirm the validity of the stains. Monoclonal antibodies, made by hybridoma techniques, have greater specificity and are rapidly replacing polyclonal reagents for this purpose.

Examples of tumor product identification in serum or tissue utilizing labeled antibody-antigen reactions include human chorionic gonadotropin (HCG) and alpha-fetoprotein (AFP) in germ cell tumors; prostate-specific antigen (PSA) to identify metastatic prostate carcinoma; and specific hormones produced by functional endocrine tumors.

SPECIAL STUDIES

Microbiologic cultures are best obtained under the sterile conditions of the operating room. The surgeon should confer with the pathologist to determine what cultures are indicated based on the clinical data and operative findings. Radiologic study of some specimens may be valuable, particularly in the study of bone lesions, but its widest use is in the localization in breast specimens of small lesions discovered by mammography. In some cases, mammographically directed fine wires inserted percutaneously under local anesthesia may aid the surgeon in localizing the abnormal area in a large breast. The wire, left in situ, also serves to guide the pathologist, ensuring that the appropriate tissue is examined microscopically.

ELECTRON MICROSCOPY

The transmission electron microscope significantly increases resolution compared with light microscopy. Thus, this technique may rescue the pathologist from a diagnosis of "undifferentiated malignant neoplasm" by demonstrating subcellular features that identify the lesion. For example, squamous carcinomas and adenocarcinomas have distinctly different cell surface characteristics. Squamous cells typically are joined by desmosomes that attach to tonofilaments, whereas adenocarcinoma cells generally surround acinar spaces, are united by tight junctions, and have microvilli projecting from apical surfaces. Additional features for cellular identification include cytoplasmic organelles such as electron-dense secretory granules, premelanosomes in melanoma, and skeletal muscle myofilaments in rhabdomyosarcoma.

If the need for electron microscopy is anticipated by the clinician, the pathologist should be alerted prior to surgery so that the specimen may be treated appropriately. Often it is the pathologist who first identifies the need for electron microscopy when he or she is presented with a baffling frozen section. Specimens for electron microscopy should be placed in glutaraldehyde-containing fixative as soon as possible to preserve ultrastructural features. Tissue initially fixed in formalin or tissue retrieved from paraffin blocks may be subsequently postfixed in glutaraldehyde, but electron micrographic quality is severely degraded.

BIOPSY TECHNIQUES

The biopsy is the cornerstone of diagnosis of neoplastic disease. Planning is essential to ensure that the biopsy produces the optimal contribution to management. For one lesion, an excisional biopsy may constitute definitive therapy, whereas for another lesion, the biopsy is merely a preliminary step in a complex therapeutic exercise. When the biopsy is small, utmost attention must be devoted to its correct handling. Small specimens, if crushed or not properly fixed, may be valueless for diagnosis.

FINE NEEDLE ASPIRATION

The principles developed for the evaluation of exfoliative cytology are applicable to cytologic material obtained by means of a fine needle from sites otherwise inaccessible without surgery. The simplicity of fine needle aspiration (FNA) allows its application in the outpatient evaluation of many sites; e.g., thyroid nodules or enlarged lymph nodes suspected of harboring metastatic disease. With radiologic or ultrasonographic guidance, diagnostic material may be obtained from most internal sites. Early resistance to this technique based on fear of "seeding" a cancer along the track of the needle has been dispelled by experience. However, some surgical oncologists insist that the fine needle track be located so that it can be included in the resection if the aspiration demonstrates malignancy.

SKIN BIOPSY

Most skin lesions suspected of malignancy are small enough to be completely excised with a margin of a few millimeters of normal-appearing skin. The deep line of the excision extends into the subcutaneous fat but usually does not include the fascia of the underlying muscle. Primary closure of the resulting elliptical wound, oriented along the natural lines of tension, produces satisfactory cosmetic results. If the lesion is thought to be an invasive malignant melanoma, the long axis of the ellipse should be parallel to the major lymphatic channels because of possible involvement of lymphatics by the neoplasm. Shave or saucerization techniques, while satisfactory for removal of superficial or benign lesions, should not be used for possible malignant tumors because of the likelihood of failure to remove the deep, and often diagnostically crucial, portion of such a lesion.

Some lesions are too large for primary closure after complete excision; here an incisional biopsy is preferred prior to definitive excision and reconstruction. This approach is superior to sampling large lesions by multiple punch biopsies, which often fail to preserve architectural features essential to diagnosis. Such architectural features, critical for distinguishing malignant melanoma from its benign counterparts, are equally important in differentiating squamous cell carcinomas from keratoacanthomas, which usually behave as benign and self-limited cutaneous tumors sometimes called self-healing squamous cell carcinomas.

The small fragments of neoplasm and adjacent dermis resulting from ablation of a basal cell carcinoma by curettage are usually satisfactory for confirming the diagnosis but not for evaluating completeness of removal. A 4-mm punch biopsy usually provides an adequate specimen from a basal cell carcinoma when definitive radiation therapy is planned. The Mohs technique achieves complete removal of cutaneous tumors with minimal sacrifice of adjacent tissue by a series of stepwise excisions, each evaluated by frozen section. This is a time-consuming process, and only a few dermatologic surgeons are trained in its use. Conventional excisions can be evaluated by a series of intraoperative frozen sections to ensure clear margins and permit immediate reconstruction or direct closure.

Some cutaneous malignancies, especially early in their course, may simulate inflammatory dermatoses. This is particularly true of the cutaneous T-cell lymphomas, which include mycosis fungoides and its variant, the Sézary syndrome. A series of 4-mm punch biopsies may be satisfactory for diagnosis, but larger excisional biopsies are preferable. In atypical cases, specimens for T-cell markers may be indicated. Other cutaneous lymphoma-like lesions may present great difficulty in diagnosis. Reactions to drugs, ultraviolet radiation (in susceptible individuals), and insect bites may simulate cutaneous lymphoma and confound the pathologist. Whenever possible, material from such lesions should be saved for cell marker studies.

BREAST BIOPSY

Mammography and cytologic study of fine needle aspiration smears have greatly improved routine screening for breast cancer. Concurrent therapeutic developments have greatly expanded the decision tree in the management of cancer of the breast. Since the days of Halsted, the standard approach to mammary carcinoma consisted of a biopsy under general anesthesia with an intraoperative frozen section followed by mastectomy if the frozen section demonstrated carcinoma. Today, many women desire therapy that conserves the affected breast if at all possible, and this, plus the requirements of various adjuvant measures, has added several details to the pathologic evaluation of mammary biopsies. The biopsies should be taken unfixed to the laboratory immediately and, if gross examination demonstrates a suspicious lesion, appropriate specimens for estrogen and progesterone receptor assays should be selected. As a result of greater emphasis on surveillance, mammary neoplasms are being detected and removed while too small to provide adequate tissue for hormonal receptor assays by conventional biochemical methods. Fortunately, immunohistochemical methods for estrogen receptor and progesterone receptor proteins employing paraffin sections are now available.

If breast conservation surgery (segmentectomy, quadrantectomy) is planned, the surgeon should submit the specimen without incising it to avoid distortion of the relations of the lesion to the tissues surrounding it. The pathologist should mark the periphery of the specimen with ink to allow evaluation of the adequacy of excisional margins. If indicated, a frozen section may be done for immediate confirmation of the diagnosis. Fine needle aspiration or cutting needle biopsy can confirm the diagnosis of carcinoma prior to initiation of palliative therapy in cases in which clinical evaluation demonstrates inoperability; hormonal receptors can be studied in such material by immunohistologic methods.

The clinician should be particularly wary of two special clinical presentations of breast cancer: (1) any eczematous lesion of the nipple should be biopsied to exclude Paget's disease; and (2) a cellulitis-like process involving the breast should arouse suspicion of "inflammatory" carcinoma, generally considered inoperable. The diagnosis of inflammatory carcinoma requires demonstration of permeation of dermal lymphatics by carcinoma cells.

LUNG BIOPSY

A variety of techniques permit evaluation of pulmonary masses prior to definitive therapy. The rigid bronchoscope obtains optimal biopsy material from endobronchial lesions within its reach. More distant endobronchial lesions require fiberoptic bronchoscopy for biopsy, brushings, and washings. It is frequently possible to obtain diagnostic material from peribronchial parenchymal lesions by taking transbronchial biopsies through the fiberoptic bronchoscope. Diagnostic cytologic material, and sometimes core specimens, can be obtained by transthoracic fine needle aspiration from peripheral masses inaccessible to bronchoscopic approach. Cytologic study of blood obtained from wedged pulmonary arteries can confirm the presence of lymphangitic carcinomatosis. When such techniques are nondiagnostic, open biopsy through a limited thoracotomy may yield diagnostic specimens without significantly increasing morbidity. Open biopsies may be preferable to transbronchial biopsies in some critically ill patients, e.g., those with severe thrombocytopenia, because of the greater control of bleeding possible in open procedures.

Pulmonary lesions in immunocompromised cancer patients present a differential diagnosis that includes involvement of the lung(s) by the underlying disease process; pulmonary toxicity of chemotherapy; radiation pneumonitis; infection by a variety of bacterial, fungal, or viral agents; a second neoplasm; or a combination of these. The complexity of the problem requires close cooperation among the medical oncologist, pulmonary physician, infectious disease specialist, thoracic surgeon, and pathologist. Because of the ease with which it can be obtained, sputum is usually the first specimen submitted from such patients; diagnostic results are dependent upon the quality of the material, and good deep cough specimens are essential. Bronchoalveolar lavage has become the gold standard for the diagnosis of pulmonary infections in immunocompromised patients. It is incumbent upon the physician responsible for the patient's management to oversee the handling of the specimens to ensure that the appropriate microbiologic and pathologic studies are obtained.

LYMPH NODE BIOPSY

Although clinical evaluation may leave little doubt as to the diagnosis of malignant lymphoma in many cases of Hodgkin's disease and the non-Hodgkin's lymphomas, histologic examination of an appropriate lymph node is essential to confirm the diagnosis and to determine the type of lymphoma. If enlarged nodes are inaccessible, needle aspiration may obtain material adequate to demonstrate carcinoma or other nonlymphomatous causes of lymphadenopathy, but it cannot be expected to obtain material adequate for evaluation of a lymphoma.

Care must be taken to select the appropriate node for excision. The clinically most abnormal node usually provides the best material for pathologic study. In many instances, smaller nodes superficial to a large one show only nonspecific hyperplastic changes. Unless no other nodes are involved, inguinal lymph nodes are best avoided because of the frequency with which they contain reactive or inflammatory changes that may obscure any lymphomatous involvement.

The intact node should be promptly submitted for imprints and other indicated studies. Cell marker analysis by flow cytometry is often valuable. Fortunately for hospitals that do not have flow cytometry, this procedure is offered by many reference laboratories. Numerous enzyme-labeled immunohistochemical reagents are available to supplement routine histopathologic findings. These include anti-Leu M 1, which stains granulocytes, monocytes, and Sternberg-Reed cells and numerous antibodies reacting with subsets of B and T lymphocytes. Unfortunately, monoclonality in T-cell proliferations cannot be established by immunohistologic techniques, unlike the information provided by kappa and lambda light chain analysis in B-cell lesions. Such T-cell clonality, however, can be demonstrated by molecular biologic methods: namely, detecting T-cell receptor gene rearrangements with DNA probes utilizing fresh, frozen, or formalin-fixed paraffin-embedded tissue.

BONE MARROW BIOPSY

Bone marrow biopsies are usually performed by the hematology-oncology service. A core biopsy should always be obtained. H and E-stained paraffin sections may demonstrate focal disease—lymphomatous, granulomatous, or metastatic—that is not detectable on aspirate smears. The core specimen can also confirm the presence of myelofibrosis or a packed marrow when an aspirate cannot be obtained. Thin sections from plastic-embedded material provide superior demonstration of cytologic features but require more time for preparation than paraffin-embedded tissue and are not available in all laboratories.

Chromosomal studies are often helpful in lymphomas and leukemias, many of which are associated with translocations such as the t(8;14) of Burkitt's lymphoma and some other B-cell lymphomas, the t(9;22) responsible for the Philadelphia chromosome, and the t(15;17) of acute promyelocytic leukemia. Sometimes oncogenes activated by the translocations can also be identified.

FEMALE GENITAL TRACT BIOPSY

Cervix. Colposcopically directed biopsy is the most efficient method of obtaining histologic evaluation of lesions detected by cytologic screening. Optimal sectioning requires accurate orientation of the biopsies for embedding. The coloscopists at our institution enclose their specimens in "sandwiches" of two single layers of paper towel secured by staples to preserve vertical orientation of the mucosal surfaces. Our histologic technicians maintain this orientation when embedding the biopsies so that they are sectioned perpendicularly through the epithelium.

Conization specimens are serially sectioned, usually following fixation, and embedded in a systematic fashion, most often by clockwise blocks or by quadrants. This requires anatomic orientation by the gynecologist, customarily by a stitch at the 12 o'clock position. In cases of hysterectomy for cervical neoplasia, the cervix is amputated and sectioned as described above for conization specimens.

Endometrium. Tissues from endometrial curettage or biopsy, and endocervical specimens if a fractional is done, are embedded in toto. For endometrial carcinoma, intraoperative examination of the uterus by gross inspection and possible frozen section is imperative. This allows evaluation of the extent of myometrial invasion or the possibility of cervical involvement and may provide valuable guidance regarding the necessity to extend the operation to pelvic lymph nodes. Possible occult serosal extension in such cases should be evaluated by submitting peritoneal biopsies and washings.

Ovary. Preoperative evaluation of possible ovarian tumors by routine physical examination, medical imaging scans, laparoscopy, and cytologic examination of ascitic or cul-de-sac fluid often provides staging information for ovarian carcinoma. At laparotomy, peritoneal washings and biopsies, including blind biopsies of diaphragm, together with multiple sections of omentum, obtain material for further assessment of disease extent. DNA studies by flow cytometry may provide useful information on the diagnosis and behavior of borderline ovarian tumors.

UROLOGIC TRACT BIOPSY

Endoscopic procedures obtain the most satisfactory biopsy material from the urinary bladder, and the concomitant fulguration is often adequate therapy for lower-grade urothelial neoplasms. For some tumors, brushings are the most effective means of obtaining cytologic material. Urinary cytology may serve to confirm a radiologic diagnosis of ureteral or renal pelvic lesions, but localization of the lesion requires specimens obtained by ureteral catheterization. Occasionally, inflammatory processes are associated with reactive urothelial changes that may simulate carcinoma and lead to false-positive results. Evaluation of urinary tract cytology by flow cytometry shows promise as a screening procedure for urothelial malignancies.

The educated finger of the experienced examiner remains the mainstay of detection of prostatic cancer. Office ultrasound units afford the urologist a simple means for preliminary staging of prostatic tumors and for confirming their nature by needle biopsies. Immunohistologic procedures for prostate-specific antigen and prostatic acid phosphatase are helpful in identifying poorly differentiated or undifferentiated metastases of prostatic carcinoma.

Tumors of the testis are discovered by physical examination and diagnosed histologically after orchiectomy. Biopsy or fine needle aspiration is not used because of the possibility of contamination of scrotal contents and subsequent spread to inguinal lymph nodes.

GASTROINTESTINAL TRACT BIOPSY

Advances in fiberoptic technology have revolutionized pathologic investigation of gastrointestinal neoplasia. Gastroscopic and colonoscopic biopsies are processed routinely but require careful handling because of their small size. Surveillance of patients with inflammatory bowel disease by periodic colonoscopy permits the early detection of premalignant mucosal changes. Diagnostic cytologic material may often be obtained from pancreatic and other retroperitoneal masses by fine needle aspiration, guided by ultrasonography or computed tomography. Endoscopic retrograde cholangiopancreatography produces cytologic material from pancreatic and biliary ductal lesions. The recent application of fiberoptic devices to intra-abdominal surgery has broadened their utility.

HEAD AND NECK BIOPSY

Pathologists receive biopsy material from head and neck areas submitted by oral, plastic, maxillofacial, otorhinolaryngologic, and general surgeons, as well as dermatologists. Most are handled routinely. Occasionally, excisions of facial neoplasms by the plastic surgeon may be handled by a modification of the Mohs fresh tissue technique with repeated frozen sections to evaluate margins. Fine needle aspiration cytology is most helpful in the evaluation of thyroid nodules and lymph nodes suspected of harboring metastases.

NERVOUS SYSTEM BIOPSY

The usual biopsy obtained at craniotomy from a suspected glioma consists of a few small pieces of soft grayish tan material submitted on a square of moistened cottonoid. Its exact source—meningeal or intracerebral or central or peripheral—should be stated. If the patient has a history of malignancy, advance consultation with the pathologist allows comparison of the specimen with previous pathologic material to rule out metastatic disease. Necrosis in brain tumors is a major determinant in grading, and additional material for histologic evaluation (often obtainable from the operating room suction trap) may be invaluable for demonstrating this feature.

Computerized stereotactic guidance enables the surgeon to place the biopsy forceps precisely within an intracerebral lesion, maximizing the diagnostic value of minuscule biopsies and minimizing surgical morbidity. Following histologic diagnosis, the stereotactic apparatus can be used to implant radioactive seeds, again minimizing morbidity by delivering maximal radiation to the neoplasm while sparing the surrounding normal brain.

MUSCULOSKELETAL SYSTEM BIOPSY

Conventional radiographic, angiographic, and scintigraphic studies can provide a diagnosis of a malignant tumor of bone with a high degree of probability and of many tumors of soft tissue with somewhat lesser accuracy. When the best treatment available for these malignant neoplasms was amputation and postoperative adjuvant therapy, a confirmatory biopsy was an appropriate next step. However, with the advent of limb-sparing surgery, the situation has changed. Meticulous preoperative staging and precise diagnosis are crucial in choosing the correct operation. Such staging requires high-resolution scintigraphic and computed tomography or magnetic resonance imaging scans, and accurate diagnosis may demand specialized techniques available only in a few oncologic centers. Moreover, the biopsy technique assumes a much greater importance; if improperly performed, it may condemn a limb-sparing procedure to failure.

Aggressive neoplasms of musculoskeletal tissues are not encapsulated but are surrounded by a pseudocapsule consisting of a reactive proliferation of connective tissue cells and capillaries in the adjacent tissue. The pseudocapsule so often contains peripheral extension of the sarcoma that incisions through it must be regarded as contaminated. Attempts to shell out a sarcoma and most attempts at excisional biopsies of such lesions are sure to leave remnants of the neoplasm behind to widely contaminate adjacent tissue planes. Aspiration techniques often fail to obtain adequate diagnostic material. If employed, the needle or trocar track must be placed so that it can be excised in the definitive procedure.

An incisional biopsy including representative portions of the lesion, its pseudocapsule, and adjacent normal-appearing tissue constitutes the optimal specimen for diagnosis and is less traumatic and less likely to contaminate the adjacent tissues. Diagnostic tissue can usually be obtained from extraosseous extension from a malignant bone tumor. Hemostasis following a biopsy must be complete to avoid widespread dissemination of malignant cells by postbiopsy hematoma. The cutaneous incision should be located so that its excision in the course of the subsequent definitive operation does not interfere with the necessary flaps. Subcutaneous closure minimizes contamination of adjacent tissues.

Because the proper performance of the biopsy of musculoskeletal malignancies is such an important factor in their management, there is a growing consensus that the patient should have the biopsy done in the same referral center where definitive surgery will follow.

REFERENCES

Anastasi J: Interphase cytogenetic analysis in the diagnosis and study of neoplastic disorders. Am J Clin Pathol 95(suppl 1):522–528, 1991.

Bartow SA: Diagnostic and prognostic applications of oncogenes in surgical pathology. Am J Surg Pathol 14(suppl 1):5–15, 1990.

Berrey BH Jr: The treacherous biopsy. Military Med 154:171–174, 1989.

Blocking A: Cytological versus histological evaluation of percutaneous biopsies. Cardiovasc Interven Radiol 14:5–12, 1991.

Carr I, Pettigrew N: How malignant is malignant? A brief review of the microscopic assessment of human neoplasms and the prediction of whether they will metastasize and kill. Clin Exp Metast 9:127–137, 1991.

Koss LG, Czerniac B, Herz F, Wertso RP: Flow cytometric measurements of DNA and other cell components in human tumors: A critical appraisal. Hum Pathol 20:528–548, 1989.

Linder J: Immunohistochemistry in surgical pathology. The case of the undifferentiated malignant neoplasm. Clin Lab Med 10:59–76, 1990.

Rosenow EC III,Wilson WR, Cockerill FR III: Pulmonary disease in the immunocompromised host, Part 1. Mayo Clin Proc 60:473–487, 1985.

Saccani Jotti G, Bonadonna G: The pathologist and the clinical oncologist: A new effective partnership in assessing tumor prognosis. Eur J Cancer Clin Oncol 25:585–598, 1989.

Wilson WR, Cockerill FR III, Rosenow EC III: Pulmonary disease in the immunocompromised host, Part 2. Mayo Clin Proc 60:610–631, 1985.

Woosley JT: Measuring cell proliferation. Arch Pathol Lab Med 115:555–557, 1991.

3
DIAGNOSTIC IMAGING IN ONCOLOGY

Robert M. Lerner

During the past two decades a technologic revolution has taken place in diagnostic radiology. The development of computed tomography (CT), major improvements in gray-scale ultrasound (US) and in radionuclide (NM) imaging techniques, and the recent addition of magnetic resonance imaging (MRI) have combined to make the radiology department of today unrecognizable to the physician of yesterday. All of these developments have led to improvements in the diagnosis, staging, and follow-up of cancer patients. In addition, however, they have resulted in confusion over selection of the optimal imaging modality for a variety of situations.

For these reasons, particularly in the evaluation and management of cancer patients, the radiologist has taken on a new role—that of imaging consultant. Familiar with the strengths and weaknesses of each modality and the appearance and likely routes of spread of the major malignancies, the radiologist can recommend to the clinician the examination with the greatest chance of yielding the required information. This process of consultation is most effectively carried out in person, in front of a view box, with all previous imaging studies available for review and discussion.

Although in rare instances a definite diagnosis can be made on the basis of a given image, most often the x-ray report lists a differential diagnosis. The radiologist, in personal communication with the clinician, can expand on the report, assigning rough degrees of certainty to each of the possible diagnoses and suggesting additional useful examinations. If all imaging studies on a given patient are stored in a single location and kept in the same envelope, opportunity exists for a thorough review of all studies simultaneously. The practice of filing images in separate departments—nuclear scans in the nuclear medicine department, CT scans in the CT department, and so forth—impedes communication, encourages unnecessary duplication, and prevents derivation of maximum information from each study. Only by examining all the studies together and discovering correlations and contradictions among them can a complicated case be fully understood.

THE IMAGING REPORT

Ideally, the imaging report should consist of five distinct components:

1. A statement of the examination performed. Examples:
   XR (x-ray) Erect frontal and lateral chest
   CT Upper abdomen with oral and intravenous contrast
   US Lower abdomen, including pelvis
   NM (nuclear medicine) Liver and spleen scan, technetium sulfur colloid
2. A description of the objective findings. Examples:
   XR Abnormal density right lower lobe, with volume loss
   CT Sharply defined low-density, 3-cm spherical mass, right kidney
   US Hypoechoic 4-cm area, left lobe of liver
   NM Photon-deficient areas, multiple, 2 to 5 cm, throughout liver
3. A conclusion, where appropriate, as to the fundamental abnormality. Examples:
   XR Atelectasis, right lower lobe
   CT Water density mass, right kidney
   US (no further statement)
   NM (no further statement)
4. A summary, impression, diagnosis, or final conclusion. This must be very carefully worded to avoid misleading as to degree of certainty. Both overstatement and equivocation should be avoided. Examples:
   XR Endobronchial carcinoma to be excluded
   CT Benign right renal cyst
   US Metastasis left lobe of liver (this report is overstated)

NM Multiple metastases throughout liver most likely; multiple hemangiomas or abscesses possible but less likely

5. A recommended course of further action, where appropriate. Examples:
   XR Bronchoscopy recommended
   CT No further investigation required
   US Percutaneous biopsy under US or CT guidance recommended
   NM Angiography would be helpful to exclude hemangiomas, if clinically appropriate

Additional information derived from clinical history, physical findings, laboratory data, and other imaging modalities may greatly influence the diagnostic impression and the recommendations of the radiologist. It is therefore imperative that the physician personally review the imaging studies performed on his or her patients and consult with the radiologist. In this way, all the clinically relevant material can be used to formulate the best diagnosis and most efficient therapeutic plan.

SELECTION OF THE IMAGING PROCEDURE

Clearly, no procedure should be performed unless its results will influence decisions about patient management. Ordering a study simply to satisfy one's curiosity is unacceptable. Often (perhaps too often) medical texts recommend particular procedures for all patients with a certain condition; in many cases, proof of the value of these studies is lacking.

When several modalities can be brought to bear on the same problem, the selection of the most useful study is difficult. Each modality has its own advantages and disadvantages, and in a particular setting one may be more reliable than another. In general, it is best to begin with the least expensive examination that is likely to demonstrate the abnormality. In most cases, this is conventional radiography, with or without iodinated contrast. Barium studies are often next, but the need for subsequent US, NM, and CT studies should be considered, since residual barium in the gastrointestinal tract can interfere with these examinations. The diagnostic radiologist can often suggest the most efficient sequence of examinations and which studies can be combined or eliminated in the evaluation of a given problem.

SPECIFIC IMAGING PROBLEMS

PULMONARY NODULES

The lungs are among the most common sites of distant metastasis, and pulmonary evaluation is necessary in the work-up of all patients with newly diagnosed malignant disease. The detection of pulmonary metastases may alter the management of the cancer patient, particularly if therapy with curative intent had been anticipated.

Imaging modalities employed in assessing the lungs for metastases include plain x-ray films, conventional whole lung tomography, and CT. High-quality plain films often suffice to exclude pulmonary metastases. A small increment in sensitivity can be added with tomography; this may be desirable under certain circumstances. Computed tomography is clearly superior to plain film tomography for this purpose.

Evaluation of a solitary pulmonary nodule detected as an incidental finding on a chest x-ray performed for another purpose represents a challenging problem. If the lesion was not present on previous films or if no previous films are available for comparison, the most expeditious course is to proceed directly to surgical excision (after a several-week delay to make certain that the lesion does not mysteriously "evaporate"—a phenomenon known to, but not explained by, every experienced imager). Percutaneous biopsy makes little sense: if the lesion is malignant, it should be removed surgically with curative intent, and if the biopsy does not yield malignant cells, surgical excision is necessary in any case since falsely negative biopsies are common. Presurgical CT scanning, although considered controversial in some places, is frequently done to detect mediastinal lymphadenopathy or additional pulmonary nodules.

The appearance of a solitary pulmonary nodule in a patient with a previous primary malignancy represents another problem. Although metastatic disease would seem the most likely diagnosis, most patients who undergo thoracotomy in this setting are found to have primary cancer of the lung. Therefore, tissue diagnosis in this setting is mandatory; the assumption of metastatic disease is unwarranted. The patient's first malignancy may be cured, and resection of the lung nodule may be curative of the second.

Obviously, the appearance of multiple pulmonary nodules in a patient with a known malignancy almost certainly represents metastatic disease. Multiple pulmonary nodules in a patient without known prior malignancy require tissue diagnosis for identification. Bronchoscopy with transbronchial biopsy is the procedure of choice for obtaining tissue when innumerable tiny pulmonary nodules are present. If the nodules are large, percutaneous transthoracic needle biopsy under fluoroscopic guidance is the best approach. This technique is very accurate, yielding only extremely rare false-positive diagnoses. False-negative results occur in 10 to 20% of cases in experienced hands. Pneumothorax follows the procedure in 5 to 30% of cases, depending on needle gauge, but rarely (<5%) requires chest tube placement. Pulmonary hemorrhage and hemoptysis are rare if normal clotting studies are documented prior to biopsy.

MEDIASTINAL LYMPH NODES

Mediastinal lymph nodes may be involved by metastatic spread from a variety of malignancies. Lymphomas frequently involve superior mediastinal and paratracheal lymph nodes. Primary lung cancers, usually following extension to ipsilateral hilar nodes, may invade mediastinal nodes. The right pretracheal (azygous) and left aortopulmonary (ductus) nodes are the most common sites. Breast cancer often metastasizes to internal mammary, subcarinal, and anterior mediastinal nodes. Esophageal cancer, testicular carcinoma, and others involve mediastinal nodes frequently.

Imaging modalities available for evaluation of the mediastinum include: (1) plain films, often employing oblique (55°) projections and barium swallow; (2) conventional tomography; (3) CT; (4) gallium scanning; and (5) MRI.

Plain films suffice for detection of bulky mediastinal disease. CT scanning is a more sensitive method and can identify lymph nodes 1 to 2 cm in diameter. However, not all enlarged lymph nodes detected on CT represent tumor; when knowledge regarding mediastinal involvement is essential for therapeutic decision making, tissue diagnosis obtained via mediastinotomy (Chamberlain procedure) or mediastinoscopy is required. This situation often arises in determining resectability of carcinoma of the lung (Chapter 13). In some cases, mediastinal nodes can be biopsied percutaneously with a needle as well.

Gallium scanning can detect occult mediastinal involvement with lung cancer or lymphoma. The specificity of this modality is low, and false-positive results are encountered with inflammatory reactions and other nonmalignant conditions. In most cases, CT provides more reliable information.

MRI is useful for presurgical evaluation of superior sulcus tumors, especially to assess for invasion through the lung apex and into the lower neck.

LIVER METASTASES

Like the lungs, the liver is a common site of metastatic spread of many malignancies. Four imaging modalities are available for evaluation of the liver: MRI, NM, US, and CT. MRI is approximately twice as expensive as CT, which in most locales is again twice as expensive as NM or US. At present, CT and MRI are the most sensitive, with CT favored for greater availability and lower cost. Hepatic metastases on CT may be hypodense, isodense, or hyperdense as compared with normal hepatic parenchyma, but hypodense metastases are most common. Metastases that are isodense with contrast (and thus not recognizable) but visible without contrast are unusual, but optimal examination requires scanning both with and without contrast. Most busy imaging departments cannot afford this generous time expenditure and perform the scan with contrast only, running the risk of missing some isodense metastases. Hemangiomas, cysts, fatty change, artifacts (secondary to partial voluming and cardiac motion, especially in the left lobe), and hepatic abscesses can mimic the appearance of metastases; tissue diagnosis is advisable under some clinical circumstances.

Ultrasonography is inexpensive and does not require contrast. It reliably distinguishes cystic from solid lesions, a distinction the other modalities cannot make. It is also not hampered by cardiac motion or partial voluming associated with CT and MRI. Although US is the most suitable modality for frequent follow-up examinations for assessment of changes over time, precise serial measurements of lesions may be seriously hampered, since their ultrasonic appearance may change considerably (i.e., central necrosis and irregular growth with confluence of boundaries). Protocols requiring precise size assessments ideally would have an MRI baseline and MRI follow-up to provide the most reliable indication of response to treatment.

MRI and NM are performed less frequently today owing to competition from the other two modalities. MRI or NM may be employed when findings from US and CT are contradictory or equivocal. Radionuclide blood pool imaging is adequate for confirming that a large lesion (>4 cm) is a hemangioma. If smaller lesions are suspected to be hemangiomas, MRI is recommended.

Regardless of which procedure is chosen, it is wise to employ the same modality for follow-up examinations. It is very difficult to assess changes in disease when comparing successive images obtained by different techniques.

When the presence of metastatic involvement of the liver will significantly alter the therapeutic plan, tissue confirmation may be necessary. Currently, percutaneous fine needle aspiration biopsy (22-gauge) under CT or US guidance is the preferred method for obtaining tissue. If this is unsuccessful, automated small-bore 18- to 20-gauge histology biopsy needles have recently been introduced and provide improved tissue recovery at a marginally increased risk.

OBSTRUCTIVE JAUNDICE

Jaundice is common among cancer patients, arising either as a consequence of hepatic metastases or extrahepatic biliary obstruction. Extrahepatic obstruction may occur as a result of primary cancers of the pancreas, bile ducts, duodenum, and ampulla of Vater. Less often, metastatic involvement of porta hepatis nodes with lymphoma or carcinomas of the breast, lung, and gastrointestinal tract may produce biliary obstruction by compression of the common bile duct.

Initial evaluation of the jaundiced patient must distinguish obstructive from non-obstructive jaundice. In the patient with suspected or known malignancy, either US or CT of the upper abdomen can demonstrate hepatic metastases or dilated biliary radicles, the hallmark of extrahepatic obstruction. Either study may also reveal a mass in the head of the pancreas. Percutaneous needle biopsy usually follows demonstration of liver metastases or a mass in the pancreatic head.

If extrahepatic biliary obstruction without a pancreatic mass is demonstrated, percutaneous transhepatic cholangiography (PTC) or endoscopic retrograde cholangiopancreatography (ERCP) should follow. These techniques may locate the exact site of obstruction and in some cases indicate the probable cause. The choice between PTC and ERCP depends on physician preference, endoscopic and radiologic expertise, and patient tolerance. Both studies can guide fine needle biopsies of any mass visualized.

In recent years, interventional radiologists have developed sophisticated techniques for both internal and external biliary drainage via the percutaneous route. Their purpose is palliation of obstructive jaundice, particularly in patients who are not surgical candidates. Percutaneous drainage is the procedure of choice for relief of obstructive jaundice due to Klatskin tumors—biliary duct cancers located at the junction of the hepatic ducts, so high in the porta hepatis that surgical bypass is impossible.

RETROPERITONEAL AND PELVIC LYMPH NODES

Lymphomas and cancers arising in the pelvic organs and gastrointestinal tract commonly spread to retroperitoneal and pelvic lymph nodes. Accurate staging of these diseases requires identification of involvement of these nodes. Lymphomas characteristically cause massive nodal replacement and bulky adenopathy, whereas the solid tumors often produce only partial involvement of nodes and therefore, in many cases, no lymph node enlargement.

US, CT, and bipedal lymphography can each image these lymph node areas. CT may detect enlarged nodes but requires a 1- to 2-cm size threshold for visualization. MRI offers no advantage compared to CT. Ultrasonography and lymphography allow visualization of normal-sized nodes. Visualization of homogeneously hypoechoic lymph nodes by US is suggestive of malignant disease independent of size. Lymphography can detect architectural abnormalities within nodes of normal or increased size. Lymphography, however, cannot image mesenteric and porta hepatis nodes and often fails to opacify the upper para-aortic nodes.

Computed tomography in many centers has become the procedure of choice for demonstrating bulky retroperitoneal adenopathy as usually seen in lymphomas and testicular carcinomas. Ultrasonography is probably not sufficiently reliable for routine lymph node staging, but it offers a convenient and inexpensive method for serial evaluations of enlarged nodes. In children and thin adults with little intra-abdominal fat, the occasional suboptimal CT examination may be complemented by US, which performs well in this circumstance. Lymphography offers increased sensitivity, especially for nodes involved with metastases from pelvic solid tumors, and is often used following a negative CT or US examination in selected cases when an increased degree of certainty is desired. Percutaneous fine needle biopsy can be used with any of these modalities to confirm the presence of tumor in a suspicious lymph node.

PELVIC MASSES

Primary cancers of the genitourinary tract and lower gastrointestinal tract often present as pelvic masses, first suspected on physical examination or suggested by a radiologic study (barium enema, intravenous urogram). The pelvic organs may be studied by several methods, including physical examination (optimally under anesthesia), barium examination of the small and large intestines, CT, US, MRI, and direct visualization with several endoscopic procedures.

When lesions of the gastrointestinal tract are suspected, barium studies are clearly indicated. In staging primary cancers of the genitourinary system, however, barium examinations can only indicate secondary effects: displacement and compression due to mass lesions. In this setting, US and CT are definitely superior and can offer considerable information on the location, extent, and possible origin of the mass and the presence or absence of regional lymph node involvement and ascites. MRI has shown promise in staging uterine and cervical cancers.

Endoluminal (transrectal or transvaginal) ultrasound is becoming established as the most accurate method for early diagnosis and/or staging of pelvic malignancies, including prostate, ovary, and rectal cancers. Furthermore, precise needle biopsy is possible when guided by these special ultrasound probes.

BRAIN METASTASES

MRI and CT have almost completely obviated the need for radionuclide scans, pneumoencephalography, and angiography in the evaluation of the patient with suspected brain metastases. The characteristic appearance of multiple enhancing lesions is virtually diagnostic of brain metastases in a patient with a known malignancy. MRI with contrast is particularly useful for brain lesions. The next most useful examinations arranged in order of descending sensitivities are MRI without contrast, high-dose contrast CT with delayed imaging, and contrast CT. Greater availability of MRI has improved diagnostic accuracy in the evaluation of intracranial masses, especially in the posterior fossa.

Difficulty arises when only a solitary lesion is present, particularly in a patient without previous malignancy. The differential diagnosis of a solitary brain lesion includes abscess, intracranial hemorrhage, benign tumor, primary malignancy, metastatic tumor from an occult primary site, and certain degenerative conditions. Unless the appearance is that of a vascular lesion, tissue diagnosis is required. Newly developed techniques for needle biopsy of brain with stereotactic localization are available but are probably underutilized and should make brain biopsy a much more acceptable procedure for many patients.

SKELETAL METASTASES

Bone is a frequent metastatic site for numerous primary cancers, including breast, lung, prostate, gastrointestinal tract, renal, and others. In a patient with bone pain at a particular location, a plain x-ray of the area is the most efficient examination. However, in screening asymptomatic patients or in the patient with numerous aches and pains, the radionuclide bone scan is far superior to the metastatic bone survey. The bone scan will detect many metastases that have not yet destroyed enough bone to make them visible on plain radiography. The scan abnormality may precede the plain film finding by as much as 6 months.

Skeletal uptake of the radionuclide (a technetium 99m—labeled phosphate compound) depends on new bone formation, usually evoked by the presence of metastatic tumor. Rare cases of falsely negative bone scans occur, however, even in the presence of widespread skeletal metastases. In a cancer patient with persistent bone pain, a negative bone scan does not completely exclude the possibility of metastatic disease, and plain films of the painful areas should be obtained. In addition, purely lytic lesions, such as seen in multiple myeloma, for example, may not stimulate sufficient bone metabolism to produce uptake on the scan. MRI is the most sensitive imaging modality for diagnosis of bone metastases, espccially involving the marrow, and should be used when clinical suspicion is high despite normal radiographs and NM bone scans. CT is favored for purely cortical bone lesions.

The interpretation of the NM scan is further complicated by its lack of specificity for metastatic disease; arthritis, trauma, metabolic bone disease, and osteomyelitis all can produce a positive bone scan. Correlation of the scan with the clinical situation and plain film views of the positive areas is essential to avoid falsely positive interpretation in cases of nonmalignant disease. The combination of negative films with a positive scan should be taken as evidence of early metastatic involvement.

Serial bone scans are useful in detecting disease progression by indicating the appearance of new lesions. The bone scan is not helpful in following response to therapy, however, since increased uptake may persist or even worsen as healing progresses.

SPINAL CORD

Patients with known malignancies may present with clinical manifestations suggesting spinal cord compression secondary to metastases. Emergent imaging of a tumor causing cord compression is required prior to radiation therapy, which should be administered promptly to prevent paralysis. Cord compression is ideally diagnosed by MRI, but if MRI is not available, contrast myelography with or without CT may be considered.

REFERENCES

American Cancer Society: Advances in cancer imaging. Cancer 67(suppl):1119–1284, 1991.
Ferrucci JT: Liver tumor imaging: Current concepts. AJR 155:473–484, 1990.
Gold RI, Seeger LL, Bassett LW, et al: An integrated approach to the evaluation of metastatic bone disease. Radiol Clin North Am 28:471–483, 1990.
Heitzman ER: The solitary pulmonary nodule. Contemp Diag Radiol 8(19):1–5, 1985.
Kline TS, Kannan V, Kline IK: Lymphadenopathy and aspiration biopsy cytology. Cancer 54:1076–1081, 1984.
Kopans DB, Meyer JE, Sadowsky N: Breast imaging. N Engl J Med 310:960–967, 1982.
Richter JM, Silverstein MD, Schapiro R: Suspected obstructive jaundice: A decision analysis of diagnostic strategies. Ann Intern Med 99:46–51, 1983.
Steckel RJ (ed): Diagnostic imaging. Semin Oncol 18:63–173, 1991.
Sze G, Milano E, Johnson C, et al: Detection of brain metastases: Comparison of contrast-enhanced MR with unenhanced MR and enhanced CT. AJNR 11:785–791, 1990.
Zeman RK (ed): Symposium on new imaging technology: Pitfalls and controversies. Radiol Clin North Am 23:379–583, 1985.

4
PRINCIPLES OF RADIATION ONCOLOGY

Duncan E. Savage

The clinical use of therapeutic radiation dates back almost to the discovery of x-rays in 1895, but the widespread application of modern radiotherapeutic techniques is only several decades old. Recent developments in radiation physics, computer technology, and radiobiology have contributed to major improvements in this field. The radiation oncologist possesses the tools to cure many malignancies and to palliate many more with minimal risk of serious side effects.

PHYSICS OF RADIATION

Without some understanding of radiation physics, little sense can be made of radiation therapy techniques or dosages. All forms of radiation in clinical use produce ionization in the target tissue. This ionization can lead to direct damage to cellular deoxyribonucleic acid (DNA) or form chemically reactive free radicals that in turn cause injury to DNA. The mechanism by which these reactions produce the clinically observed effects—tumor shrinkage, radiation damage to various tissues and organs, genetic changes, and induction of secondary malignancies—is incompletely understood.

Types of radiation in clinical use include high-energy x-rays, gamma rays, and certain particle beams (electrons, protons, and neutrons). The radiation may originate from natural sources such as naturally occurring radioactive elements (radium) and from man-made sources (e.g., x-rays, electron beams, gamma rays from cobalt-60). X-rays and gamma rays differ only in their sources of origin. X-rays are produced by acceleration of electrons striking nuclei in target atoms. Gamma rays are formed as by-products from decay of radioactive nuclei.

Three different radiation techniques are in general use today:

- Teletherapy—the use of beams of x-rays, gamma rays, or particles generated at a distance from the patient
- Brachytherapy—the use of encapsulated sources of ionizing radiation implanted directly into tissues or placed in natural body cavities; also called "interstitial" and "intracavitary" therapy
- Systemic therapy—the use of radioactive materials introduced systemically, relying on physiologic processes for localization (e.g., I–131 for differentiated thyroid cancer)

PHYSICAL PRINCIPLES

Regardless of the source of the radiation or the type of therapy, the same laws of radiation physics must be obeyed.

Energy

Both x-rays and gamma rays are part of the electromagnetic spectrum and are propagated at the speed of light. The energy of x-rays and gamma rays determines their ability to penetrate tissues and to produce effects in those tissues by transfering their energy. Higher-energy x-rays will retain a larger amount of their original dose at a given depth than lower-energy x-rays. Energy of x-rays is defined in terms of electron volts. A beam whose energy is less than 1 million eV (1 MeV) is called an orthovoltage beam, whereas beams with energies greater than 1 MeV are referred to as megavoltage beams.

The effects produced by x-ray beams are not energy specific. That is, no relationship exists between radiation energy and tumor curability. The biologic effects of ionizing radiation depend on the dose, which is a measure of energy absorbed, and is independent of the energy of the incident beam. The advantages of megavoltage radiation are due to its dose distribution characteristics rather than its energy level.

Inverse Square Law

All radiation from a point source falls off in intensity inversely as the square of the distance from that source. For example, consider a source of radiation 10 cm from a surface. The intensity at a point 10 cm below the surface would be one-fourth of that on the surface, ignoring absorption and scatter for the moment. The point 10 cm below the surface is twice as far from the source as a point on the surface; therefore, the intensity is 25% ($10^2/20^2 = 100/400 = 25\%$) as great. If the source-to-surface distance is now 100 cm, the intensity at a point 10 cm below the surface is 83% ($100^2/110^2 = 83\%$).

Lengthening the source-to-surface distance increases the depth dose. This simple principle is exploited in the design of x-ray therapy equipment. High-energy equipment today is usually designed with a source-to-skin distance (SSD) of 80 to 100 cm. Reduction in the SSD will produce a rapid fall-off in intensity beneath the skin. Equipment with an SSD in the range of 2 to 30 cm is available for the treatment of superficial lesions either on the skin or in body cavities. The inverse square law also explains both the strengths and weaknesses of brachytherapy. The very small SSD employed with this technique makes very high dosages possible, and the rapid fall-off in dose protects adjacent tissues. At the same time, however, this rapid fall-off limits these techniques to effective treatment volumes within 1 to 2 cm of the source.

Absorption and Scattering of X-rays

X-rays do not pass directly through tissue but are absorbed and scattered in the irradiated tissue. Absorption of radiation in tissues is dependent upon the energy of the incident radiation and the atomic structure of the irradiated material. Scattered x-rays also get absorbed and contribute to dosage. At energy levels below 600 keV, scattered radiation makes a major contribution to dosage. At megavoltage levels, scatter occurs almost completely in a forward direction and represents a much less important contribution to dosage. High-energy radiation, and the concomitant reduction in the contribution of scatter to dosage, makes possible the use of irregularly shaped portals without total disorganization of the underlying dose distributions. The mantle field used to treat Hodgkin's disease (Fig. 4–1), for example, would not be possible without megavoltage radiation units. The marked reduction in lateral scatter also permits sharper delineation of the beam edge in megavoltage radiation.

Electron Beam Therapy

Many linear accelerators in clinical use can produce beams of electrons for treatment of superficial lesions. Electron beams have the advantage of limiting the dose delivered to deeper critical structures. While x-ray beams contain a distribution of energies within a beam, electron beams contain a single initial energy. Electron beam therapy has found wide applicability in many clinical settings, especially in the treatment of breast and head and neck neoplasms.

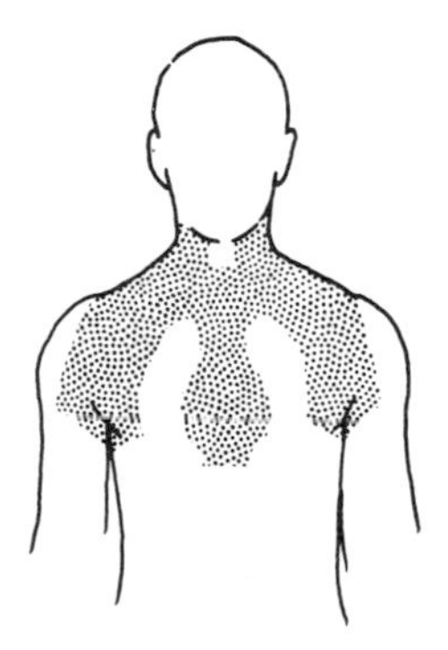

Figure 4–1. Mantle radiation field for the treatment of Hodgkin's disease. (*From* Haskell CM, Parker RG: Hodgkin's disease. *In* Haskell CM (ed): Cancer Treatment, 2nd ed. Philadelphia, WB Saunders, 1985, p. 772.)

ISODOSE CURVES

To utilize x-rays and gamma rays properly, details of the distribution of dosage within tissues must be available. Graphic representations of such distributions are known as isodose curves. These curves are dependent on energy, SSD, and area irradiated. They are expressed as percentages with reference to the maximum or peak tissue dose. Isodose curves operate on the assumption that tissues are homogeneous, which of course they are not, but this assumption is sufficiently accurate for clinical purposes.

Usually isodose curves are symmetric (Fig. 4–2), but with the use of wedge-shaped asymmetric filters placed in the beam, asymmetric isodose curves can be produced (Fig. 4–3). Isodose curves can also be drawn as lines of equal dosage surrounding implantable radioactive substances. These curves also assume tissue homogeneity. Such curves take

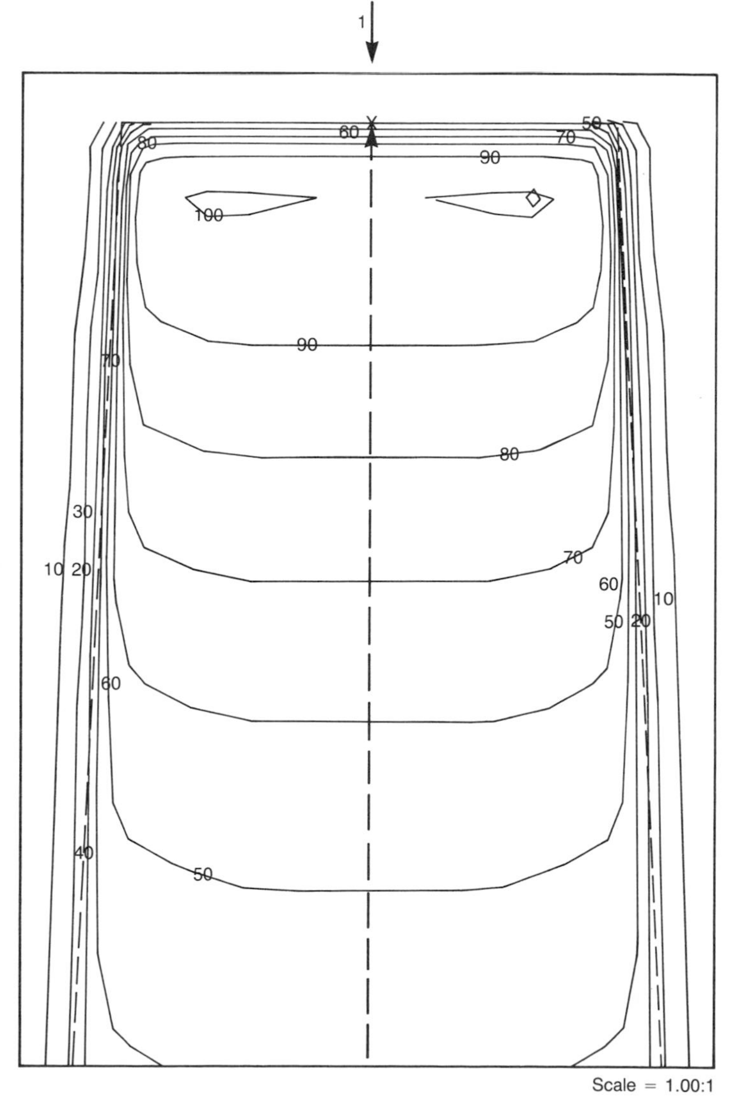

Figure 4–2. Example of an isodose curve for a 6-MeV linear accelerator, 100-cm source to skin distance and 10 × 10 cm field size.

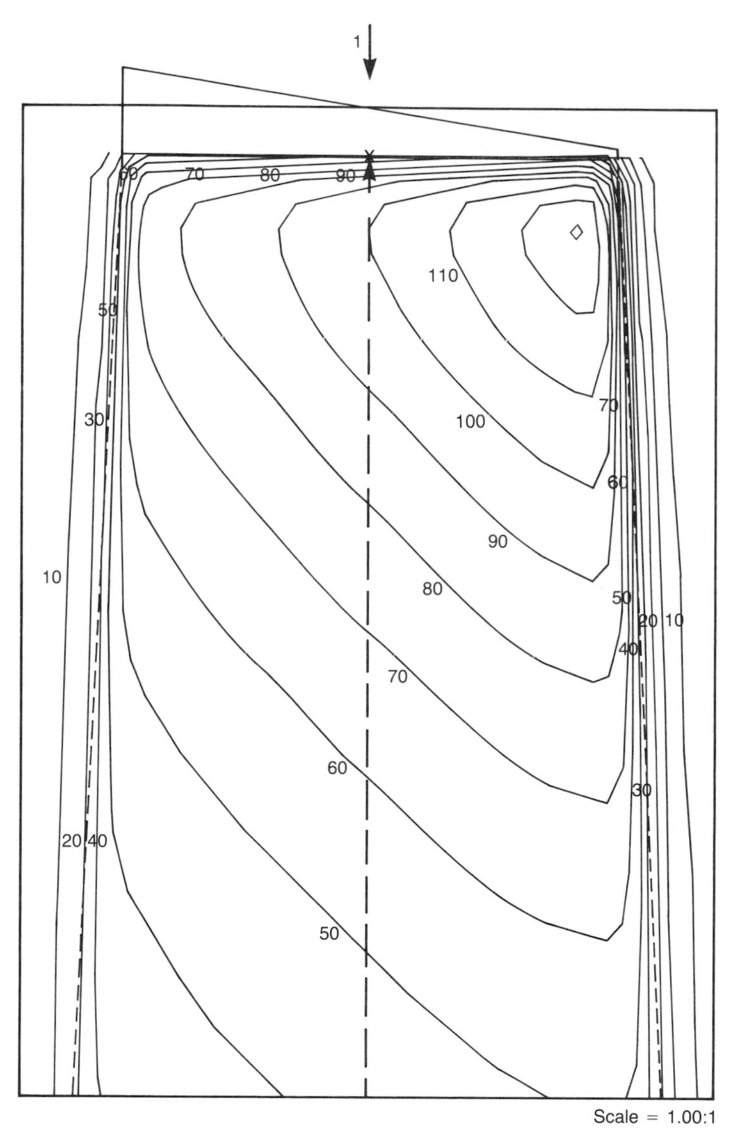

Figure 4–3. Asymmetrical (wedge) isodose curve for a 6-MeV linear accelerator, 100-cm source to skin distance and 10 × 10 cm field size. The position of the wedge filter across the beam is represented as if it were on the skin, although in practice it is attached to a tray on the machine head.

the form of concentric circles around a point source of radiation; in three dimensions these curves would consist of spherical shells surrounding the source. Linear sources produce more complex isodose lines, and such sources may be loaded (with isotope) nonuniformly to produce asymmetric dosage volumes.

TREATMENT PLANNING

Appropriate treatment of any deep-seated tumor requires precise anatomic knowledge of the tumor extent and appreciation of the radiation tolerance of adjacent normal tissues.

All available methods—clinical, radiologic, and surgical—are employed to delineate a treatment volume for the tumor under consideration. Ideally, the treatment volume includes all gross tumor, adjacent sites of suspected microscopic disease, and a margin of safety to allow for patient motion and divergence of the radiation beam. Given the isodose curves discussed above and a knowledge of the position and radiation sensitivity of adjacent structures, the radiation therapist selects and combines radiation fields to optimize the dose distribution within the treatment volume and minimize the dose to adjacent normal tissues.

This process of planning is made immeasurably easier by the use of a treatment planning computer that can store, move, and sum isodose curves from several treatment fields to calculate the spatial distribution of dose for an optimal plan. The computer can also accept data on tumor location and patient contours directly from a CT scanner. The final result consists of a computer-generated treatment plan (Fig. 4–4), often superimposed on a CT scan of the area in question. Although the computer generates the treatment plan, the radiation therapist selects and positions the radiation fields. The computer simply makes the necessary calculations very rapidly, allowing alternatives to be considered prior to the final decision. Interstitial and intracavitary radiation can be planned in the same manner. Historically, radium was the original radioactive material used for these purposes; however, the energy level of radium's gamma rays is unnecessarily high for clinical uses, and its first breakdown product is the radioactive gas radon. Both of these factors result in undue hazard for radiation personnel and other individuals in close contact with patients under treatment. Cesium 137 has replaced radium for intracavitary uses (uterus, vagina), and iridium 192 has become the principal material for interstitial work (oral cavity, neck, breast, perineum, anorectum).

Regardless of the expense of the computer and the sophistication of its treatment plan, the therapy will not succeed unless several more mundane, but equally important, requirements are met: the clinical information must be accurate and sufficient; the radiation technicians must be properly trained and meticulously careful to apply the treatment plan accurately and repeatedly to the patient; and the radiation physicists must ensure that the equipment is consistently delivering the prescribed doses at the prescribed energies.

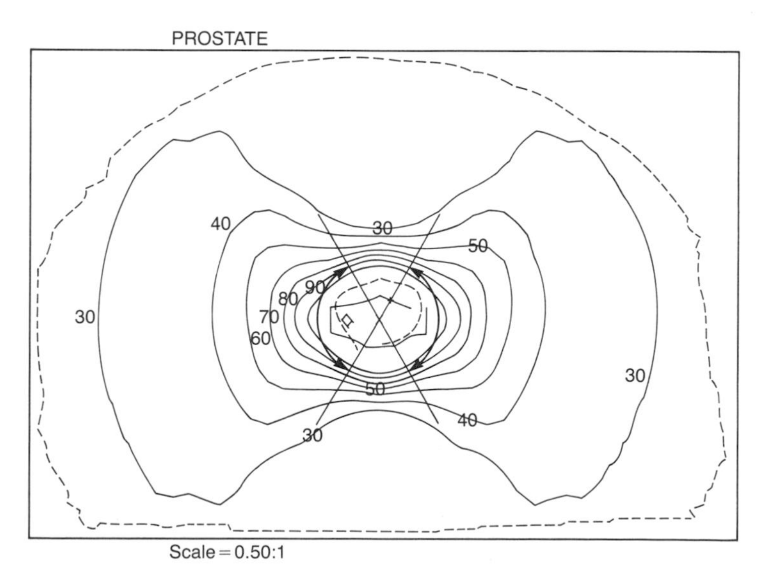

Figure 4–4. Computer-generated treatment plan. The patient outline and target volume, in this case the prostate, have been drawn by the computer directly from the CT scan. The size, position, and limits of the two laterally opposed beams have been selected manually, and the resulting combined curves, with relative dosage values, have been calculated and drawn automatically. On the computer screen (but not evident in this figure) all the detail of the CT scan is displayed.

DOSAGE AND FRACTIONATION

The unit of dose common to all clinical applications is the gray (Gy), which is defined as 1 joule of absorbed energy per kilogram of tissue. The gray has supplanted the rad, which is 0.01 Gy. The rad had been used for years, and many radiation oncologists and physicists use the centigray (cGy), which is equivalent to the rad.

The gray is a unique unit of dosage in medicine in that it is a unit of absorbed dose. In more familiar terms, it is as if penicillin were prescribed in terms of the amount actually affecting the bacterial cell wall rather than as the amount taken by the patient. Dose can be measured directly in the patient by small volume receptors (thermoluminescent capsules). Alternatively, dose can be calculated through the use of data obtained by radiating phantoms constructed to resemble human tissue.

The biologic effect of a given dose of radiation varies with the amount of time taken to deliver that dose and with the number of fractions into which that dose is divided. For example, 4500 cGy delivered to the pelvis in a single dose would produce major bowel complications and probably result in death, whereas the same total dose delivered over 5 weeks in 25 fractions is well within the acceptable range.

Most radiation therapy is delivered in five daily treatments per week, with the usual dose per treatment in the 180- to 200-cGy range. Clinical trials have examined other treatment schedules. The split course method consists of daily treatments until half the total dose is reached, followed by an interruption lasting 2 to 3 weeks before resuming treatment. Patients tolerate a split course better than continuous treatment, but the results are not as good. Multiple fractionation (also called hyperfractionation), treating patients twice daily and increasing the total number of fractions, has also been tried, and some evidence suggests that hyperfractionation produces superior local control, most notably in head and neck tumors. Trials using smaller numbers of fractions (i.e., three per week) appear to produce inferior results compared with conventional fractionation, and the complication and morbidity rate is greater. Under certain circumstances such as palliation of ulcerating masses, relatively large single doses at weekly or even greater intervals may be useful.

Clearly a statement of radiation dosage must contain more than a single number. Duration of treatment and number of fractions are more than technical issues; they are important determinants of biological effect.

BIOLOGICAL EFFECTS OF RADIATION

RADIOBIOLOGY

Radiobiologic principles provide a scientific foundation for the use of radiotherapy, despite the fact that the clinical practice of radiation oncology has developed empirically. Radiosensitivity of tumor cells in tissue culture can be determined by exposing the cells to increasing radiation dosages and measuring survival. The resulting cell survival curve (Fig. 4–5) can be used to define a D_0 for each cell population equal to the dose of radiation required to reduce the surviving fraction of cells to 37%. D_0 values for different tumors vary, but most adenocarcinomas and squamous cell carcinomas have D_0 values in the same range as most normal cells. The effectiveness of radiation in treating the majority of cancers therefore depends on factors other than inherent radiosensitivity.

The initial "shoulder" of the cell survival curve (Fig. 4–5) corresponds to a dose range in which cellular repair of sublethal radiation damage occurs. The use of fractionation schedules with small doses given repeatedly allows repair of sublethal damage between fractions. In other words, each fraction causes a "shoulder" effect in cell survival similar to the first portion of the cell survival curve. Since malignant cells possess inferior repair mechanisms, the treatment will have a differential effect on normal and neoplastic tissue. Fractionation and different time-dose relations can maximize the antitumor effects of radiation and minimize radiation complications in normal tissue.

Tumor shrinkage following radiation therapy depends not only on the effectiveness of the treatment but also on the growth fraction of the tumor, the cell cycle time, and the proportion of nonmalignant cells present. Rapid shrinkage may be gratifying to both patient and physician but may have no relationship to ultimate prognosis. Slow response is perfectly consistent with complete sterilization of malignant cells in a tumor with a low growth fraction, long cell cycle, and large proportion of fibrous and supporting tissues.

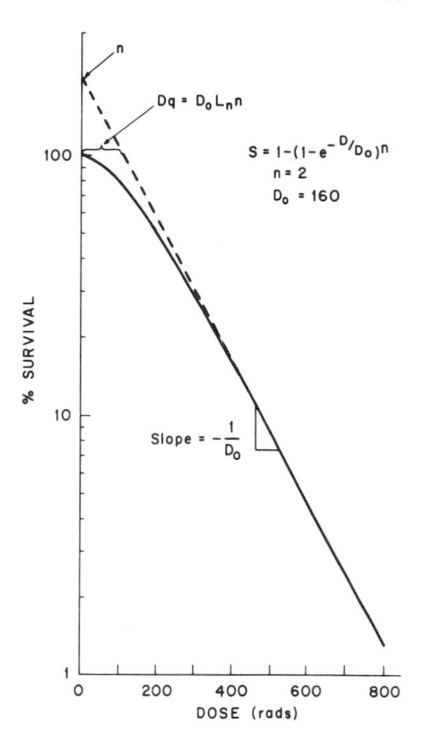

Figure 4–5. Theoretical cell-survival curve for mammalian cells exposed to a single dose of radiation. (*From* Prosnitz LR, Kapp DS, Weissberg JB: Radiotherapy. Reprinted by permission of the New England Journal of Medicine 309:771–777 and 834–840, 1983.)

The ability of normal tissues to recover from therapeutic doses of radiation may result from their low growth fractions and long cell cycle durations, which allow unirradiated cells time to move in and damaged cells opportunity to recover. However, the same cell kinetic features also explain the late damaging effects of radiation on normal tissues, which are thought to result from endothelial damage and progressive tissue ischemia.

SYSTEMIC EFFECTS

The acute adverse effects of both radiation therapy and chemotherapy have been exaggerated by the public media. Not all symptoms occurring during treatment are complications of therapy. Vomiting may signal peptic ulcer disease, small bowel obstruction, or hypercalcemia; changes in mental status may indicate central nervous system metastases, narcotic overdose, or metabolic abnormality. The recognition of treatment-related side effects should be left to a skilled oncologist, who will consider alternative diagnoses before labeling a symptom as a side effect of treatment.

General

Variable degrees of anorexia, lassitude, nausea, and vomiting may accompany radiation therapy. The intensity of these effects varies with several factors:

- Radiation energy—megavoltage therapy produces less severe side effects than orthovoltage.
- Volume irradiated—small treatment volumes produce fewer side effects.
- Fraction size—reduction in the dose per fraction by as little as 10% (i.e., from 200 to 180 cGy) reduces side effects.
- Site of irradiation—treatment of the upper abdomen, with or without inclusion of the liver, produces more severe systemic effects. Treatment of the brain and the extremities causes little if any distress, and treatment of the thorax and chest wall produces an intermediate level of symptoms.

- Individual variation—with the same treatment conditions, one patient will suffer severe side effects whereas another will remain asymptomatic.

Treatment of these symptoms consists primarily of reassurance by the radiation staff. In severe cases, temporary modification in the treatment course may be necessary.

Hematologic

Reduction in blood counts, especially the white blood count and platelet count, occurs commonly during and immediately following radiation therapy. The blood counts return to normal levels 3 to 6 months after treatment. The radiation dose and the amount of bone marrow included in the radiation field affect the degree of blood count suppression. Prior or concurrent myelosuppressive therapy, advanced age, and involvement of the marrow with tumor should prompt particular concern for the development of serious myelotoxicity. In most cases, if the white blood count falls below 2000 or the platelet count falls below 50,000, treatment should be suspended temporarily to allow for hematologic recovery.

EARLY LOCAL EFFECTS

Skin

The severe skin reactions that limited deep therapy with orthovoltage are no longer seen today in the era of megavoltage radiation. However, if the skin itself is the target and doses in excess of 4000 cGy are used, severe skin changes will occur. These reactions are dependent not only on dose, but also on the area and site irradiated. Small skin areas will tolerate higher doses than large areas. Warm, moist areas subject to trauma will develop more marked skin reactions at a lower dose and will take longer to heal than drier areas less subject to trauma. For example, the inframammary fold of an irradiated pendulous breast usually develops moist desquamation, whereas the rest of the breast receiving the same dose develops mild erythema only.

Temporary epilation of the scalp consistently follows single radiation doses greater than 300 cGy. Epilation occurring as a result of the treatment of brain tumors to currently accepted doses can be permanent.

Oropharynx and Esophagus

A mucositis characterized by erythema and progressing to a diphtheria-like membrane overlying the treated area invariably accompanies radiation of squamous cell cancers in this region. Swallowing and speech become painful, and the problem is aggravated by the associated mucosal dryness. Candidal overgrowth commonly occurs and is treated with topical or systemic antifungal agents.

Although this reaction produces discomfort, it can usually be tolerated except by elderly or malnourished patients. Management includes prescription of a soft diet, analgesics, ample oral fluids, and local anesthetic mouthwashes. Cessation of smoking is essential to minimize the degree of mucositis. The mucositis resolves approximately 14 days after completion of treatment.

Bowel

Irradiation of any abdominal site results in irradiation of the bowel. At almost any dose, diarrhea occurs. In most cases, diarrhea can be controlled with antidiarrheal agents and dietary modifications. Less than 2% of patients fail to respond to these measures and develop dehydration and occasionally bloody stools. In these cases therapy must be interrupted until the symptoms resolve. Symptoms may recur on resumption of treatment, making delivery of the planned course of treatment impossible.

Rectal reactions from external therapy are usually mild and consist of tenesmus and discomfort. Avoiding either constipation or diarrhea helps most patients.

Stomach

Radiation treatment of the stomach usually produces constitutional effects as described above. Doses of 1000 cGy in 1 week will cause hypochlorhydria, which explains the role of gastric irradiation in the treatment of peptic ulcer disease in the past. (With the advent of improved pharmacologic agents to reduce acid production, this practice has become obsolete.) At current dosages, no acute clinical problems follow gastric irradiation.

Bladder

Urinary frequency and dysuria often follow pelvic irradiation to doses above 3000 cGy. Urine cultures should be obtained in all such cases, since urinary tract infection, common in patients with pelvic malignancies, produces identical symptoms. Antibiotic therapy should be given to patients with positive cultures, but eradication of infection may not occur if a large tumor causes partial obstruction to urinary flow. Control of the tumor will usually permit successful treatment of the infection.

In cases with negative cultures, the symptoms of radiation cystitis may respond to pyridium, but frequently relief of symptoms must await completion of treatment.

Lung

Radiation pneumonitis may develop 1 to 3 months after completion of therapy. The symptoms include harsh, dry cough and mild exertional dyspnea. Fever and constitutional symptoms occur in severe cases. The chest x-ray reveals an infiltrate exactly corresponding to the treatment field. Sharp borders and failure to follow normal anatomic distribution distinguish this process radiologically from infectious pneumonia or progressive tumor. Treatment consists of observation unless symptoms are severe, in which case high doses of oral corticosteroids should be given. Once symptomatic relief has occurred, steroid doses should be tapered gradually to avoid resurgence of symptoms.

LATE LOCAL EFFECTS

Most late effects of radiation are irreversible and impose definite limits on dosage. The likelihood of these late effects usually precludes retreatment of areas previously treated to full doses, even when the tissues have apparently returned to normal. In other words, previously irradiated tissue "remembers" the radiation given in the past. Late effects of radiation may occur in organs and tissues that manifested no clinical evidence of acute effects.

Skin

Skin that has received 5000 cGy or more will be smoother than normal and lack the usual appendages. There may be some atrophy of the subcutaneous tissue as well. Irradiated skin responds poorly to trauma and in rare cases may form a nonhealing painful ulcer that requires plastic surgical efforts to correct. Lesser changes in the skin occur in response to changes in the endothelium of cutaneous blood vessels, giving rise to small vessel proliferation (telangiectasia). With the use of megavoltage equipment, serious skin complications are rare.

Oropharynx and Larynx

The late effects seen in skin may similarly occur in mucous membranes. In the oropharynx and larynx, ulceration is intensely painful and may require surgical correction for relief of symptoms.

Loss and distortions of taste occur during treatment of the mouth. The most severe changes follow treatment to the whole mouth with doses required to cure squamous cell cancers. Recovery of taste occurs gradually but may never be complete.

Dry mouth invariably accompanies radiation to the mouth and is worsened when the major salivary glands are included in the treatment volume as well. In addition to the discomfort it causes, xerostomia leads to extensive dental decay. Dental evaluation is necessary prior to the start of radiation to the oral cavity to identify existing caries and institute fluoride treatments to reduce the incidence of radiation-induced caries. Artificial salivary solutions are available and may help some patients. Recovery from dry mouth occurs over time but, like taste, may never be complete.

The late effects of radiation on the laryngeal cartilages cause pain and local sepsis. These effects occur more often when the cartilage itself is involved by tumor; many regard such involvement as a contraindication to radiation. Laryngectomy may be necessary for resolution of this problem.

Esophagus

Stenosis and stricture of the esophagus may follow radiation to this organ. Strictures resulting from radiation must be distinguished from recurrent tumor. This distinction usually requires endoscopy and biopsy or brushing. Treatment consists of bouginage or bypass procedures in severe cases. Perforation of the esophagus is almost invariably due to tumor rather than treatment.

Bowel

Ulceration of the bowel occurs following the treatment of uterine malignancies with intracavitary sources. Steroid enemas provide symptomatic relief; many cases require surgical diversion before healing can take place.

Chronic radiation damage to the small intestine occurs when the small bowel is immobile owing to adhesions. Abdominal radiation under this circumstance may result in the clinical syndrome of intermittent colic, obstipation, vomiting, diarrhea, and wasting. Barium examination reveals stenosed, ulcerated, dilated, and kinked loops of small bowel resembling a variety of benign diseases—sprue, regional enteritis, intestinal lymphoma, and other conditions.

Kidney

Early effects of radiation on the kidney are clinically silent, but late effects may totally destroy renal function. If a minimum of one-third of the kidney is shielded, some useful function can be preserved. The risk of renal damage imposes limits on treatment to the upper abdomen. Clinical features of chronic radiation nephritis include proteinuria, hypertension, and uremia. A syndrome of late malignant hypertension occurring 2 to 11 years following radiation to the kidney has also been recognized.

Central Nervous System

Late effects on the central nervous system are attributed to the effects on small vessels and therefore tend not to occur before 12 to 18 months following completion of therapy. Detectable late effects occur above doses of 6000 cGy given at 200 cGy daily.

Clinical syndromes arising from radiation effects on the brain depend on the anatomic site involved. Mental status, motor function, sensation, and vegetative functions may each be involved. Neurosurgical intervention with removal of foci of necrotic irradiated brain can result in symptomatic improvement.

Radiation fields for the treatment of cervical lymph nodes, thoracic tumors, para-aortic lymph nodes, and other sites include portions of the spinal cord. Doses lower than 4500 cGy in 4 weeks are considered safe, but given the extent of individual variation and the severe consequences of spinal cord injury, every effort is made to keep the dose to the cord below this level, if possible. The manifestations of cord damage depend on the location and the length of cord irradiated. The extent of damage may be mild (Lhermitte's sign) or severe (Brown-Séquard syndrome, transverse myelopathy).

Peripheral nerves, including the cauda equina, tolerate radiation doses well above the usual therapeutic range. Radiation damage to certain peripheral nerves (e.g., brachial plexus) occurs rarely.

Gonads

Radiation to the ovaries in doses above 1000 cGy produces cessation of menses and sterility. Recovery depends on total dose and patient age. Doses greater than 600 cGy to the testes produce sterility, but secondary sexual characteristics are not affected. Prior to the treatment of Hodgkin's disease with pelvic radiation in premenopausal women wishing to preserve fertility, the ovaries should be surgically relocated outside the planned radiation fields.

Liver

Hepatic failure develops in a significant fraction of patients who receive 2500 cGy or more to the entire liver. Consequently, radiation dose is severely limited in the treatment of malignant liver disease, and this limitation imposes problems for the delivery of adequate doses to the right lower thorax and right upper quadrant of the abdomen.

Lung

As little as 2000 cGy to an entire lung at 200 cGy daily will produce an alveolar exudate and subsequent irreversible fibrosis and volume loss. Careful examination of the chest x-rays of patients who have received chest wall irradiation (especially when axilla and supraclavicular triangle have been included) reveals evidence of pulmonary fibrosis and volume loss in almost every case. In the majority, these findings produce no symptoms. Radiation for carcinoma of the lung always causes the same late changes in the treatment volume. Meticulous treatment planning and delivery will minimize the amount of normal lung affected.

Heart

Inclusion of the heart in the treatment volume is unavoidable in the treatment of mediastinal Hodgkin's disease and most other intrathoracic malignancies. Radiation damage involves the pericardium most often and leads to pericardial effusion and chronic constrictive pericarditis. Patients receiving 4000 cGy or more to greater than 50% of the pericardium are at risk for these complications. A majority of patients demonstrate pericardial damage at autopsy examination.

Severe premature coronary artery disease has been described in young persons who received cardiac irradiation in the course of treatment of Hodgkin's disease. Interstitial myocardial fibrosis is also recognized in these patients, but the clinical significance of these findings is not clear.

Second Malignancies

Overwhelming evidence demonstrates that ionizing radiation is carcinogenic. Natural radiation, diagnostic x-rays, atomic weapons, and therapeutic radiation all are known to produce malignancies in laboratory animals and in humans. The exact frequency of second malignancies following therapeutic radiation is difficult to assess. Patients cured of one malignancy have an increased incidence of second tumors regardless of treatment. Also, cases of radiation-induced tumors are reported anecdotally; it is difficult to know the number of similarly treated patients surviving the same length of time who did not develop second tumors.

Nevertheless, therapeutic radiation definitely induces second tumors in some patients. Patients with Hodgkin's disease have been most extensively studied. Radiation has been reported to cause thyroid cancer, non-Hodgkin's lymphoma, various sarcomas, lung cancer, and various adenocarcinomas in Hodgkin's patients. However, the incidence of radiation-induced second malignancies is low: following radiation therapy alone for Hodgkin's disease, fewer than 1% of patients will develop acute leukemia; the rate of developing a secondary solid tumor is higher. Therapeutic radiation for other conditions has been associated with a wide variety of second malignancies.

RADIATION SENSITIZERS

Oxygen must be present in irradiated tissue for maximal cell kill. Hypoxic cells are about three times less sensitive to the effects of radiation. A prolonged course of radiation may gradually reduce the number of hypoxic cells as reduction in tumor size permits reoxygenation of the remaining mass. Treatment in the presence of hyperbaric oxygen seems to have an advantage, but technical difficulties and suspicion of an increased complication rate prevent widespread use of hyperbaric chambers.

Hypoxic cell sensitizers are agents capable of reproducing the effects of oxygen by sensitizing hypoxic cells to the effects of radiation. These drugs enhance the radiation sensitivity of tumor cells in vitro, but to date no clinical benefit from their use has been demonstrated. Research in this area continues. Radioprotective agents, designed to reduce the sensitivity of normal tissues to radiation effects, are also under study.

CONCLUSIONS

Enormous variation exists among individual patients in their tolerance of radiation. Some patients have received massive doses without adverse consequences, whereas others have sustained catastrophic results from small doses. As with any other therapeutic agent, no entirely risk-free dose exists. On the other hand, it is possible to reduce the complication rate of radiation therapy substantially by systematically underdosing. However, the cure of most tumors involves the use of dosages close to normal tissue tolerance. Limitation of complications can therefore occur only at the price of reduced chance of cure (Fig. 4–6). Clearly, this is too high a price to pay, and a certain incidence of radiation complications must be tolerated. Meticulous attention to the details of treatment planning and delivery can reduce this incidence to an acceptable minimum.

It is important to determine prior to treatment whether the object of therapy is cure or palliation. If the goal is cure, doses should be maximal and a substantial rate of complications should be anticipated. On the other hand, if the goal of treatment is palliation, then the dose delivered should be the smallest consistent with achieving symptomatic response. Complications should be avoided; if they occur, modifications in the treatment plan should be made to produce improved patient comfort.

FUTURE PROSPECTS

HYPERTHERMIA

Hyperthermia involves the heating of tumor tissue to 42°C for periods of 1 hour using microwave or ultrasound power sources. It preferentially kills oxygen-depleted cells, which

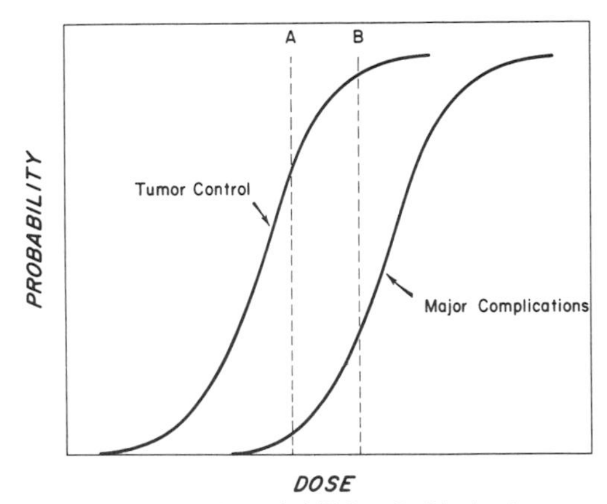

Figure 4–6. Theoretical curves describing the probabilities of achieving tumor control and development of major complications as a function of the radiation dose. A and B represent two different treatment programs. Treatment B offers a higher probability of tumor control, but at the cost of a greater likelihood of major complications. The choice between treatments A and B depends on whether the intent is palliative (A) or curative (B), whether salvage therapy is available in case of treatment failure, and whether the anticipated complications are life threatening or irreversible on the one hand or manageable and reversible on the other. (*From* Bloomer WD, Hellman S: Normal tissue responses to radiation therapy. Reprinted by permission of the New England Journal of Medicine 293:80–83, 1975.)

are less responsive to radiation. Patients with small superficial tumors have benefitted from this technique; however its use is limited by difficulties in directing heat to deep-seated tumors and reliable monitoring of the heat-delivery system.

HIGH DOSE RATE BRACHYTHERAPY

While conventional radioactive implants deliver 60 to 100 cGy/hr to a tumor, high-dose rate units have been developed to give radiation much more rapidly. These procedures are carried out in a sealed room, and the radioactive source can be advanced and retracted mechanically. This reduces the radiation exposure to personnel and can eliminate the need for inpatient hospitalization. High-dose rate brachytherapy has been used in curative settings (cervix and endometrial cancer) and also to palliate lumenal obstructions from lung and esophageal cancer.

INTRAOPERATIVE RADIATION THERAPY

Intraoperative radiation is currently used in some centers to treat locally advanced cancers. This technique delivers a single dose of 1500 to 2000 cGy by electron beam under direct vision at the time of surgery. It offers the theoretical advantage of directing radiation to sites where the risk of local recurrence is the greatest (e.g., residual microscopic or gross tumor). Intraoperative radiation has been used for carcinomas of the stomach and pancreas and extensive retroperitoneal sarcomas. The ultimate role of intraoperative radiation remains to be determined.

PARTICLE BEAM THERAPY

Neutrons have been the most widely studied type of particle therapy. Compelling evidence indicates that neutron irradiation offers superior results in the treatment of malignant salivary gland neoplasms. Current studies are exploring its use in the treatment of soft tissue sarcomas and prostate cancer. Proton beam therapy has been used to successfully treat chordomas and uveal melanomas. The advantage of protons is their unique dose distribution characteristics, allowing delivery of radiation at a specified depth within a structure, sparing adjacent critical structures in close proximity to the tumor.

REFERENCES

Fowler JF: The linear quadratic formula and progress in fractionated radiotherapy. Br J Radiol 62:679–694, 1989.

Hall EJ: Radiobiology for the Radiologist. Philadelphia, JB Lippincott, 1988.

Kahn FM: The Physics of Radiation Therapy. Baltimore, Williams & Wilkins, 1984.

Kohn HI, Fry RJM: Radiation carcinogenesis. N Engl J Med 310:504–510, 1984.

Perez CA, Brady LW: Principles and Practice of Radiation Oncology. Philadelphia, JB Lippincott, 1991.

Prosnitz LR, Kapp DS, Weissberg JB: Radiotherapy. N Engl J Med 309:771–777, 834–840, 1983.

Tucker MA, Coleman CN, Cox RS, et al: Risk of second cancers after treatment for Hodgkin's disease. N Engl J Med 318:76–81, 1988.

5
CLINICAL PHARMACOLOGY OF ANTINEOPLASTIC AGENTS

Timothy J. Woodlock
John E. Loughner

PRINCIPLES OF TREATMENT

Cancer chemotherapy is systemic treatment for malignancies that are incurable by surgery or radiation. Most anticancer medicines are nonspecific, injuring both malignant and normal cells. The primary goal of chemotherapy is to destroy the cancer and spare the host. Since the differences between normal and malignant cells are largely quantitative rather than qualitative, a very fine line separates therapeutic success from unacceptable toxicity.

Pharmacologic and biochemical factors determine cellular sensitivity and resistance to chemotherapy. The amounts of certain enzymes, the speed of certain metabolic reactions, and the presence of cell membrane receptors and of active transport mechanisms for particular antineoplastic drugs account for a tumor's innate sensitivity or resistance to chemotherapy. The ability of cells to repair chemical injury and to metabolize chemotherapeutic agents permits recovery from drug-induced tissue damage. Successful therapy requires that the repair mechanisms of the tumor cells be inadequate and those of the normal cells be sufficient for survival.

On a tissue basis, the efficacy of chemotherapy depends on the number of cells undergoing active cell division. A tumor consists of a mixed population of cancer cells; the actively dividing cells are most sensitive to chemotherapy. The nondividing cells remain relatively resistant, unless treatment continues until they enter the actively dividing population.

Although tumors may grow exponentially in vitro, tumor doubling time in vivo increases as the tumor mass enlarges. This slowing of cell division with increased tumor volume is probably related to tumor vascularity, hypoxia, and necrosis. By the time a cancer is clinically evident, most of its doublings are completed; more than 10^8 tumor cells exist, and the risk of metastasis is high (Fig. 5–1).

The log kill hypothesis of chemotherapy efficacy states that with each chemotherapy treatment some constant fraction of tumor cells die. If the tumor burden is between 10^8 and 10^{12} cells and the cell kill is between 2 and 5 logs, the need for repeated doses is apparent. According to this theory, chemotherapy will never completely eradicate a cancer, but experience shows that eradication is possible. Therefore, host defenses must eliminate the minimal residual after maximal log kill.

MECHANISMS OF ACTION

Deoxyribonucleic acid (DNA) synthesis is the primary target for most antineoplastic medications; additional chemotherapy targets include ribonucleic acid (RNA) transcription and microtubular binding (Fig. 5–2). Antimetabolites, which interfere with DNA synthesis, must be within the cell during S (synthesis) phase to be effective; they are cell-cycle specific. Chemotherapy that damages DNA, such as alkylating agents, does not require administration during S phase, because the affected cells die attempting replication with defective DNA. These agents are cell-cycle nonspecific. The distinction between cell-cycle specific and nonspecific is a relative rather than an absolute one. The specific agents are generally most effective against rapidly proliferating, highly active cancers. The nonspecific agents, because of their cycle independence, retain activity against slowly proliferating tumors.

THE RATIONALE FOR MULTIDRUG CHEMOTHERAPY

Gestational trophoblastic neoplasms and Burkitt's lymphomas are curable with single-agent methotrexate and cyclophosphamide, respectively. These tumors are rare and

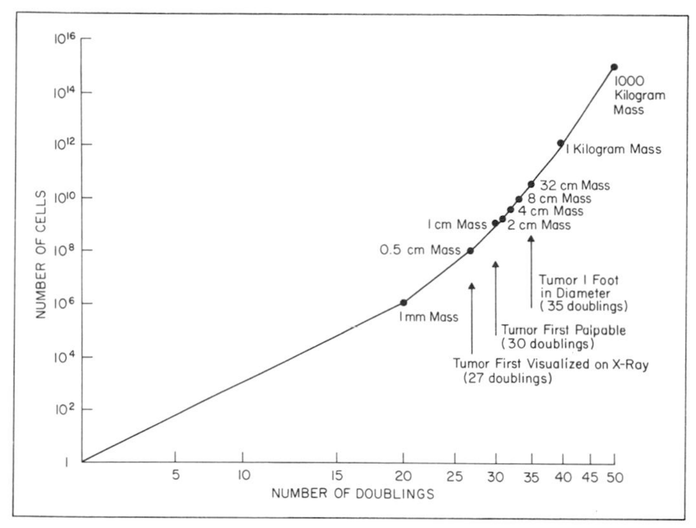

Figure 5–1. Theoretical tumor growth curve. (*From* Silver RT, Young RC, Holland JF: Some new aspects of cancer chemotherapy. Am J Med 63:772–787, 1977.)

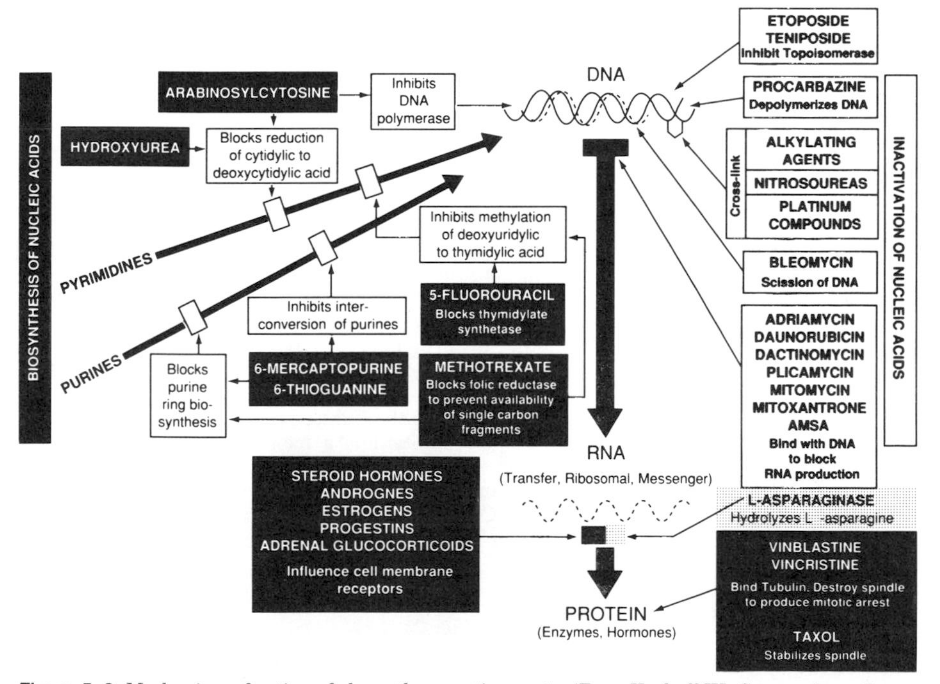

Figure 5–2. Mechanism of action of chemotherapeutic agents. (*From* Krakoff IH: Cancer chemotherapeutic and biologic agents. CA 41:264–278, 1991.)

exceptional; effective therapy for most tumors requires the greater efficacy of combinations of drugs. Initial empiric combinations included drugs with (1) antitumor activity, (2) different mechanisms, and (3) nonoverlapping drug toxicities. Drug combinations increase cell kill and decrease the development of drug resistance. The principal drawback of combination chemotherapy is superimposed toxicities requiring dose reductions of the individual agents to improve tolerance of the bone marrow, gastrointestinal tract, and the patient as a whole. Curative drug combinations for Hodgkin's disease and testicular cancer are successful because of the dissimilar toxicities and different mechanisms of action of the individually active agents.

ADJUVANT CHEMOTHERAPY

Adjuvant chemotherapy, the early or prophylactic use of cytotoxic drugs following surgery or radiation therapy, evolved from the systemic treatment of advanced disease. For patients with a high risk of developing metastases, active drugs for advanced disease are given early in an attempt to prevent or delay this occurrence. Numerous animal tumor models demonstrate the superior curative potential of early chemotherapy when existing tumor burdens are low.

Curative local therapy often fails because of initially occult systemic metastases, frequently established before the primary tumor becomes clinically detectable. Several factors allow the eradication of clinically occult metastatic disease, even in those cancers in which overt metastatic disease is incurable. As tumors enlarge, the proportion of actively proliferating cells (the growth fraction) decreases. Since most drugs act selectively on dividing cells, increased cytotoxicity occurs in smaller tumors with higher growth fractions. Tumor resistance becomes more likely with increasing cell burden. The purpose of treating subclinical disease is to eliminate the cancer before a resistant population of cells emerges. Finally, asymptomatic patients with good performance status tolerate chemotherapy better and respond more frequently than extremely ill patients. In patients with low tumor burdens, host defense mechanisms are better able to eliminate small numbers of residual cells.

CHEMOTHERAPY RESISTANCE

Chemotherapy is curative for many patients with gestational trophoblastic tumors, testicular cancer, acute leukemia, Hodgkin's disease, and non-Hodgkin's lymphoma. Adjuvant chemotherapy also improves the curability of Wilms' tumor, osteogenic sarcoma, rhabdomyosarcoma, and some breast cancers. Other cancers respond to systemic chemotherapy initially but then develop resistance or are constitutionally resistant. For those cancers that are intrinsically resistant to chemotherapy, many mechanisms of resistance exist, and research efforts focus on new or different treatments to circumvent these difficult cellular defenses. Exposure to a chemotherapy drug may also induce resistance to multiple other seemingly unrelated compounds. The term *multidrug resistance,* or MDR, describes this phenomenon, which involves antibiotic, vinca alkaloid, epipodophyllotoxin, and even some synthetic antineoplastic drugs. MDR is due to the induced and augmented expression of P-glycoprotein (P for permeability). P-glycoprotein is a membrane transport protein that actively pumps out the chemotherapy drugs before cell damage can occur. Efforts to circumvent MDR include the use of calcium channel blockers such as verapamil to bind to P-glycoprotein and inhibit its function. Current efforts have resulted in limited success with such "chemosensitizers" because drug resistance is a multifactorial problem.

THE ANTINEOPLASTIC AGENTS

ALKYLATING AGENTS

In 1942, the alkylating agent nitrogen mustard caused a transient but dramatic remission in a patient with advanced lymphosarcoma. This marked the beginning of the modern era of cancer chemotherapy. Alkylating agents (Table 5–1) possess highly reactive electrophilic alkyl groups that readily form covalent bonds with nucleophilic moieties of

Table 5–1. **ALKYLATING AGENTS**

DRUG	ADMINISTRATION PROCEDURE	SITES OF METABOLISM AND EXCRETION	TOXICITY
Mechlorethamine (Mustargen)	IV push	Systemic metabolism	Vesicant, GI, bone marrow
Cyclophosphamide (Cytoxan)	IV bolus Oral: 25-mg, 50-mg tablets	Hepatic metabolism, renal excretion	Bone marrow, GI, alopecia, hemorrhagic cystitis
Ifosfamide (Ifex)	IV infusion	Hepatic metabolism, renal excretion	Hemorrhagic cystitis, bone marrow, GI, alopecia, CNS
Chlorambucil (Leukeran)	Oral: 2-mg tablets	Systemic metabolism	Bone marrow
Melphalan (Alkeran)	Oral: 2-mg tablets IV: investigational	Systemic metabolism	Bone marrow
Carmustine (BiCNU)	Slow IV infusion	Hepatic metabolism, renal excretion	Delayed bone marrow, GI, renal, pulmonary, hepatic
Lomustine (CeeNU)	Oral: 10-mg, 40-mg, 100-mg capsules	Hepatic metabolism, renal excretion	Delayed bone marrow, GI, pulmonary, hepatic, renal
Streptozocin (Zanosar)	Direct IV injection	Hepatic metabolism, renal excretion	GI, hyperglycemia, renal, hepatic
Dacarbazine (DTIC)	Slow IV infusion	Hepatic metabolism, renal excretion	GI, vesicant, bone marrow, alopecia
Busulfan (Myleran)	Oral: 2-mg tablets	Hepatic metabolism, renal excretion	Bone marrow, adrenal insufficiency, pulmonary fibrosis
Thiotepa	IV, IM intravesical, IT	Hepatic metabolism, renal excretion	Bone marrow

cellular constituents, including structural proteins, enzymes, lipids, and nucleic acids. Alkylation of DNA accounts not only for the antitumor effects but also for the mutagenicity, carcinogenicity, and teratogenicity of these compounds. The alkylating agents are cell-cycle phase nonspecific. Although they may damage nonproliferating cells, the greatest cytotoxicity occurs in rapidly proliferating cells. Proliferating cells may be less able to repair damaged DNA before cell division leads to irreversible changes and eventual cell death.

Nitrogen Mustard (Mechlorethamine, Mustargen)

The prototype of all alkylating agents is nitrogen mustard. Nitrogen mustard causes both intrastrand and interstrand DNA cross links. Resistance to nitrogen mustard is due to decreased drug uptake and increased capacity for DNA repair. Nitrogen mustard undergoes systemic metabolism, so neither hepatic nor renal dysfunction necessitates dose adjustments.

Nitrogen mustard is a potent vesicant; contact with the skin or eyes may cause serious injury. Extravasation of the drug results in severe tissue necrosis. Severe nausea and vomiting are common and occur 1 to 4 hours after drug administration. Bone marrow suppression, with leukopenia more prominent than thrombocytopenia, is maximal at 7 to 10 days and usually recovers by the third or fourth week. Other toxicities include alopecia, menstrual irregularities, sterility, and skin rashes.

Mechlorethamine (Mustargen) is dispensed in a 10-mg vial. Indications for mechlorethamine include treatment of advanced Hodgkin's disease and topical therapy for mycosis fungoides.

Cyclophosphamide (Cytoxan)

Cyclophosphamide requires activation by microsomal enzymes in the liver. The urinary excretion of these metabolites causes the bladder complication associated with this drug.

As much as 60% of a dose appears in the urine within 24 hours. Cyclophosphamide is active orally or intravenously and is not a local irritant or vesicant. Absorption from the gastrointestinal tract is variable and incomplete.

Bone marrow suppression, particularly granulocytopenia 7 to 14 days after drug administration, is dose limiting. Reversible alopecia is common following high-dose intravenous therapy. Cyclophosphamide occasionally produces a sterile hemorrhagic cystitis secondary to the renal excretion of toxic metabolites. Cystitis may occur within the first few days following high-dose intravenous administration or after months of treatment with small oral doses. Increased fluid intake dilutes the concentration of metabolites within the bladder and decreases the risk of cystitis. Possible long-term complications include bladder fibrosis and bladder cancer. Sterility and skin hyperpigmentation may occur. There are rare cases of irreversible pulmonary fibrosis. Following extremely large intravenous doses, congestive heart failure and hyponatremia may develop.

Cyclophosphamide is an extremely versatile antineoplastic drug. It is available in 25- and 50-mg tablets as well as 100-, 200-, and 500-mg vials for injection. The oral dose is 1 to 3 mg/kg/day. The intravenous dose is 1.0 to 1.5 g/m^2 every 3 to 4 weeks. Cyclophosphamide is a valuable agent in combination chemotherapy regimens for Hodgkin's and non-Hodgkin's lymphomas, multiple myeloma, macroglobulinemia, and chronic lymphocytic leukemia. It is also effective in carcinomas of the breast, ovary, and lung. It is an important part of many bone marrow transplant regimens.

Ifosfamide (Ifex)

A structural analogue of cyclophosphamide, ifosfamide also requires hepatic activation. The activated metabolites function as cell-cycle nonspecific alkylators with a different range of activity from cyclophosphamide. Ifosfamide metabolism differs from that of cyclophosphamide: hydrolysis in the liver and kidneys produces 100 times more chloroacetaldehyde, possibly accounting for the neurotoxicity of ifosfamide. In addition, hemorrhagic cystitis is far more common with ifosfamide because its metabolism generates larger amounts of 4-hydroxy-ifosfamide and acrolein than cyclophosphamide. Mesna infusion concurrent with ifosfamide administration inactivates these metabolites in the bladder and significantly decreases the incidence of hemorrhagic cystitis.

The neurotoxicity of ifosfamide—altered mental status, cerebellar and cranial nerve dysfunction, weakness, and seizures—is usually reversible. Other toxicities include nausea, vomiting, myelosuppression, alopecia, and hepatotoxicity. Nephrotoxicity also occurs and is more common after prior cisplatin therapy.

The long half-life of ifosfamide together with its need for hepatic activation make infusional or multiple fractionated treatments optimal. Dosages range from 1.0 to 1.5 g/m^2/day for 5 days, usually in combination with other chemotherapeutic agents. Ifosfamide is an important part of curative salvage therapy for testicular cancer. Current studies will better define the promising role of ifosfamide in the treatment of soft tissue sarcomas, small cell and non–small cell lung cancers, cervical and other gynecologic cancers, hematologic malignancies, and pediatric cancers.

Chlorambucil (Leukeran)

Chlorambucil is an aromatic derivative of nitrogen mustard. In comparison with nitrogen mustard, its antitumor effects and toxicity are delayed and cumulative over time. Chlorambucil is an oral medication, available as 2-mg tablets. Although toxicity is generally mild and predictable, prolonged continuous administration may lead to profound bone marrow suppression and rarely damage to the liver and skin. Daily doses should not exceed 2 to 4 mg, and periodic complete blood counts are advisable. An alternative regimen consists of a single dose of 0.4 to 0.8 mg/kg every 2 weeks.

Chronic lymphocytic leukemia, Waldenström's macroglobulinemia, and other indolent lymphoproliferative disorders are sensitive to chlorambucil. Chlorambucil is also active against carcinomas of the breast and ovary, although cyclophosphamide is more commonly used and more suitable for combination therapy.

Melphalan (L-Phenylalanine Mustard, L-Pam, Alkeran)

Melphalan is a well-tolerated, oral phenylalanine derivative of nitrogen mustard. The usual treatment course consists of 0.7 to 1.0 mg/kg administered over 4 to 7 days, repeated every 4 to 6 weeks. It is commercially available as a 2-mg tablet. Bone marrow suppression (especially thrombocytopenia) is common and usually mild, although it is occasionally severe and prolonged. Less common side effects include sterility, pulmonary fibrosis, and secondary malignancies.

Melphalan is effective treatment for multiple myeloma and carcinomas of the breast and ovary. Melphalan may be useful for short-term perfusion treatment of malignant melanoma involving the extremities and in bone marrow transplant regimens.

BCNU (Carmustine, BiCNU) and CCNU (Lomustine, CeeNU)

The nitrosoureas are a subclass of alkylating agents with marked lipid solubility, lack of cross-resistance with conventional alkylating agents, and delayed and cumulative bone marrow toxicity. Initial studies with BCNU suggested that it acts as a cell-cycle phase nonspecific agent. Subsequent studies found that nonproliferating cells are more sensitive, indicating that BCNU affects both resting and proliferating cells. The lipid solubility of the nitrosoureas facilitates their penetration into the central nervous system, with corresponding activity in the treatment of primary brain tumors.

Administered intravenously, BCNU may produce severe burning pain along the vein. A 30- to 60-minute infusion minimizes discomfort. Intense flushing and conjunctival reddening may also occur during drug administration. In many patients, nausea and vomiting occur 2 to 6 hours after treatment. The major dose-limiting toxicity is bone marrow suppression, often delayed until 4 to 6 weeks after treatment and lasting 1 to 2 weeks before recovery. Thrombocytopenia predominates and occurs earlier than leukopenia. Bone marrow suppression is dose related and cumulative over a period of several months. Dose-related pulmonary fibrosis is another potentially serious nitrosourea complication.

BCNU is commercially available for injection in 100-mg vials. The usual dose is 200 to 240 mg/m^2 given intravenously over 1 to 3 days, repeated every 6 to 8 weeks. CCNU is commercially available in 10-, 40-, and 100-mg capsules. The usual dose is 100 to 130 mg/m^2 given as a single oral dose and repeated every 6 to 8 weeks. Patients with bone marrow suppression or compromised renal function require dose modification to avoid serious hematologic toxicity. These agents have significant activity in both Hodgkin's and non-Hodgkin's lymphomas. They are also useful in the management of primary brain tumors, small cell anaplastic lung cancer, multiple myeloma, and some gastrointestinal cancers and in bone marrow transplantation.

Streptozocin (Zanosar)

Streptozocin (formerly called streptozotocin) is a methyl nitrosourea antibiotic. Although cytotoxicity is probably due to alkylation of DNA, there are distinct differences from the other nitrosoureas. Streptozocin is a cell-cycle phase–specific inhibitor of DNA synthesis. In addition, this drug inhibits pyrimidine nucleotide synthesis and interferes with enzymes involved in gluconeogenesis. These biochemical effects result in damage to pancreatic islet cells, causing selective antitumor activity against islet cell carcinomas. Streptozocin is not cross-resistant with other nitrosoureas.

The metabolism and excretion of streptozocin resemble those of other nitrosoureas. Renal excretion accounts for removal of the majority of the drug and its metabolites. The limiting toxicity is a dose-independent renal dysfunction, manifested by reversible proteinuria and azotemia. Renal tubular acidosis may occur. Nausea and vomiting develop in most patients. Mild hepatic dysfunction limited to transient elevations of transaminase enzymes is possible. Unlike other nitrosoureas, single-agent streptozocin does not cause dose-limiting hematologic depression, although severe bone marrow toxicity occasionally develops. Effects on glucose metabolism are usually not clinically significant, and if glycosuria occurs, it is most often due to renal tubular toxicity.

Streptozocin (Zanosar) is available in 1-g vials. The usual dose is 1.0 to 1.5 g/m^2 weekly or a 5-day schedule of 0.5 g/m^2/day repeated every 2 to 4 weeks. Streptozocin has a unique role in the treatment of pancreatic islet cell tumors, with a reported response rate of 60%. Carcinoid tumors also respond to streptozocin.

Dacarbazine (DTIC)

Dacarbazine is an imidazole carboxamide derivative with cytotoxic activity due to alkylation and to inhibition of purine metabolism. Dacarbazine undergoes activation in the liver. The renal tubules secrete the drug, with approximately half of an administered dose detectable in the urine. Impaired renal function necessitates a dose reduction.

Most patients experience moderate to severe nausea and vomiting shortly after drug administration. Symptoms usually subside by the second to third day despite continued treatment. Mild to moderate bone marrow suppression generally occurs between days 10 and 15 but may be delayed. Less common toxicities include a flulike syndrome, alopecia, facial flushing, and hepatic, renal, and cerebral dysfunction.

Dacarbazine is available in 100- and 200-mg vials, which require protection from light. The administration of dacarbazine requires meticulous care because subcutaneous extravasation produces potentially severe tissue damage. The usual dose is a 5-day intravenous infusion of 150 to 250 mg/m^2/day. An alternative schedule is 450 to 650 mg/m^2 repeated every 3 to 4 weeks. Dacarbazine is active in the treatment of malignant melanoma with response rates of 20% as a single agent and 50% in combination with cisplatin, nitrosourea, and tamoxifen. Intra-arterial dacarbazine is an experimental treatment for regional melanoma. Intravenous dacarbazine is also active against Hodgkin's disease, and it may have activity against other lymphomas and some sarcomas.

Busulfan (Myleran)

Busulfan is a bifunctional alkylating agent with good oral absorption. It is available in 2-mg tablets. The drug undergoes extensive systemic metabolism followed by urinary excretion. Granulocytes are exceptionally sensitive to busulfan. For this reason, busulfan is useful in the treatment of myeloproliferative disorders, particularly chronic granulocytic leukemia. The treatment consists of a loading dose of 4 to 6 mg/m^2/day, followed by low-dose continuous administration to maintain the leukocyte count at or below 15,000/mm^3. Intermittent therapy as required by the leukocyte count is an alternative. Although generally well tolerated, chronic administration may lead to widespread cytologic abnormalities, irreversible pulmonary fibrosis, hyperpigmentation resembling Addison's disease, amenorrhea, sterility, gynecomastia, cataracts, and secondary malignancies.

Thiotepa (Triethylenethiophosphoramide)

Thiotepa is an alkylating agent administered by parenteral and intracavitary routes; 85% of the drug is excreted in the urine. Generally well tolerated, the major toxicity of thiotepa is bone marrow suppression. Most current combination chemotherapy regimens requiring an alkylating agent include cyclophosphamide rather than thiotepa. Since thiotepa does not require metabolic activation and lacks vesicant properties, it is useful in the treatment of pleural, pericardial, and peritoneal effusions. Thiotepa is also active in treating superficial bladder cancers by direct instillation. Thiotepa is available in 15-mg vials. Doses and schedules vary according to the type of cancer and route of administration.

ANTIMETABOLITES

The antimetabolites are a group of drugs that inhibit important enzymes and act as pseudosubstrates, interfering with the synthesis of macromolecules essential for cellular integrity and function. Table 5–2 summarizes the mechanisms of action and resistance of these agents.

Methotrexate

With activity against childhood leukemia demonstrated in 1947, the folic acid antagonists were the second group of clinically active antineoplastic agents. At present, only methotrexate is commercially available. Methotrexate, a derivative of folic acid, is a potent inhibitor of the enzyme dihydrofolate reductase. Inhibition of this enzyme results in depletion of intracellular tetrahydrofolate coenzymes required for the de novo synthesis of purines, thymidylate, and methionine. Therefore, methotrexate interferes with DNA, RNA, and protein synthesis and is cell-cycle phase specific for S phase. In most cases, resistance is due to increased cellular levels of the target enzyme dihydrofolate reductase.

Table 5–2. **ANTIMETABOLITES**

DRUG	ADMINISTRATION PROCEDURE	SITES OF METABOLISM AND EXCRETION	TOXICITY
Methotrexate	IV push, IM, IT Oral: 2.5-mg tablets	Hepatic metabolism, renal excretion	Bone marrow, mucositis, GI, hepatic fibrosis
5-Fluorouracil (5-FU)	IV push, IV infusion	Renal and hepatic excretion	Bone marrow, GI, CNS, rash
Cytarabine, ARA-C (Cytosar)	SQ, IT, IM, IV push, IV infusion	Systemic metabolism, renal excretion	Bone marrow, GI, pulmonary, ocular, neurologic
Mercaptopurine (Purinethol)	Oral: 50-mg tablets	Hepatic metabolism, renal excretion	Bone marrow, cholestatic jaundice, GI
Thioguanine	Oral: 40-mg tablets	Hepatic metabolism, renal excretion	Bone marrow, hepatic
Fludarabine (Fludara)	IV bolus	Systemic metabolism, renal and hepatic excretion	Bone marrow, CNS, GI, fatigue
Deoxycoformycin (Pentostatin)	IV bolus	Renal excretion	Renal, CNS, ocular, GI, altered T-cell immunity

Decreased drug transport into cells and alterations in the target enzyme may also cause resistance.

Readily absorbed from the gastrointestinal tract, methotrexate distributes widely throughout the body, except for the central nervous system. Since the toxicity of methotrexate depends on duration of exposure as well as concentration, factors that prolong plasma levels may dramatically increase systemic toxicity. Pleural effusions and ascites act as third-space reservoirs for the drug, leading to prolonged plasma methotrexate levels and increased toxicity. Methotrexate is excreted primarily by the kidney, and impaired renal function necessitates a dose reduction.

Dose-limiting toxicities are bone marrow suppression and gastrointestinal mucositis. The buccal mucosa is particularly sensitive, and painful shallow ulcers are common. More severe toxicity includes diarrhea and gastrointestinal bleeding. These toxic effects develop within 3 to 10 days following treatment and usually disappear after 7 days. Effects on granulocytes and platelets are equal in frequency and severity. Uncommon side effects include hepatic fibrosis and cirrhosis, which occur in 3 to 5% of patients taking methotrexate for prolonged periods. A rare syndrome of pulmonary infiltrates accompanied by fever and peripheral blood eosinophilia may occur. Skin rash, usually maculopapular and involving the upper trunk and neck, occurs in 10 to 20% of patients.

Intrathecal administration of methotrexate may produce nausea, vomiting, arachnoiditis, dementia, peripheral neuropathy, seizures, coma, mucositis, and bone marrow suppression. Major complications occur most commonly in adults and usually appear after 1 to 2 weeks of treatment. The maximum dose should be 12 mg, regardless of the patient's body surface area. Intrathecal administration requires preservative-free methotrexate combined with preservative-free 0.9% sodium chloride solution at a concentration of 1 to 2 mg/ml. Twenty-four to forty-eight hours of leucovorin (folinic acid) administration after intrathecal methotrexate may diminish systemic toxicity.

Methotrexate is commercially available in 2.5-mg tablets and as injectable solution in 5- and 50-mg vials. A 20-mg vial of preservative-free methotrexate is available for intrathecal treatment. Conventional doses of methotrexate in combination chemotherapy regimens range from 40 to 60 mg/m^2 intravenously twice monthly. High-dose methotrexate regimens may contain doses as high as 12 g/m^2 intravenously weekly, with leucovorin rescue and scrupulous monitoring of renal function to prevent systemic toxicity.

Methotrexate is an integral part of the highly successful treatment of acute lymphocytic leukemia of childhood and gestational choriocarcinoma. It is also active against head and neck cancers and in combination with other agents in the treatment of breast and lung cancers, non-Hodgkin's lymphoma, and osteogenic sarcoma. Intrathecal methotrexate is most effective in prophylaxis for meningeal acute lymphocytic leukemia, but it is also used in the treatment of established carcinomatous meningitis of all types.

High-Dose Methotrexate with Leucovorin Rescue. In 1953, Goldin and colleagues introduced the use of potentially lethal doses of methotrexate followed by the antidote leucovorin (citrovorum factor, folinic acid). Leucovorin replenishes the depleted tetrahydrofolate pool caused by methotrexate inhibition of dihydrofolate reductase. The efficacy of this therapy is due to differences in the ability of leucovorin to reverse the effects of methotrexate in susceptible normal tissue and in tumor.

The major route of excretion of methotrexate is renal; high-dose methotrexate may precipitate in the renal tubules, lowering the rate of drug excretion and leading to unexpected toxicity and renal damage. Administration of large volumes of intravenous fluids and alkalinization of the urine decrease the risk of renal toxicity. Serum creatinine and plasma methotrexate levels 24 to 48 hours after drug administration determine whether delayed clearance is occurring and whether increased doses of leucovorin will be necessary. Leucovorin administration begins 24 hours after methotrexate and continues until the plasma methotrexate level falls below 5×10^{-8} M.

High-dose methotrexate may produce striking but transient elevations in hepatic enzymes. As long as these return to pretreatment levels, no dose modification is necessary. Other toxicities resemble those with conventional methotrexate therapy.

High-dose methotrexate with leucovorin rescue is an accepted part of adjuvant treatment for osteogenic sarcoma. Several combination regimens for the treatment of aggressive non-Hodgkin's lymphomas include high-dose methotrexate. However, randomized trials comparing conventional-dose methotrexate with high-dose methotrexate for these lymphomas are lacking. Randomized trials have shown no advantage for high-dose methotrexate therapy for head and neck cancer and small cell lung cancer. The National Cancer Institute estimates a 6% mortality rate with high-dose methotrexate regimens, and methotrexate with leucovorin rescue is very expensive. High-dose methotrexate remains investigational; safe administration and monitoring require specialized techniques and expertise.

5-Fluorouracil (5-FU)

Following conversion to nucleotides, fluorouracil has two important effects on cellular metabolism: (1) inhibition of thymidylate synthetase, a key enzyme in the production of thymine nucleotides, and (2) incorporation into RNA, which impairs ribosomal RNA synthesis. 5-FU requires activation within cells. Since this activation depends on a series of enzymatic reactions, alterations in any of these enzymes may result in drug resistance. Approximately 20% of the parent drug is excreted unchanged in the urine. The liver metabolizes the remaining 80%.

The major toxicities of 5-FU resemble those of methotrexate. Oral mucositis and diarrhea provide the earliest indication of toxicity. Nausea and vomiting are usually mild but vary with the intensity of treatment. Bone marrow toxicity is schedule dependent but is usually mild to moderate, with the blood count nadir between days 7 and 10 and recovery within the subsequent 7 to 10 days. Less common side effects include skin rash, mild alopecia, hyperpigmentation, and conjunctivitis. A reversible cerebellar syndrome occurs in 2% of patients.

5-FU is available in 500-mg ampules. Although a number of different schedules and routes of administration exist, some evidence indicates that optimal therapeutic results occur with doses sufficient to produce at least mild toxicity. Many centers favor a well-tolerated regimen of 12 mg/kg/day (450 mg/m^2/day) for 5 days by intravenous bolus. A well-tolerated alternative schedule is 15 mg/kg/week. As a single agent, 5-FU is active in the treatment of advanced gastrointestinal cancer, particularly of colorectal origin. In combination with other agents, 5-FU is effective treatment for carcinomas of the breast, prostate, and endometrium. Responses also occur occasionally in hepatomas, carcinoids, and islet cell tumors of the pancreas.

Hepatic artery infusion of 5-FU or its derivative, FUdR, remains controversial; some patients respond to hepatic artery infusion even after progression with intravenous 5-FU. The patients who derive maximal benefit are those with metastatic disease confined to the liver. There are no controlled studies that demonstrate survival benefit for this expensive and invasive approach to 5-FU delivery.

Biochemical modulators of 5-FU activity such as thymidine, uridine, PALA, and most commonly leucovorin attempt to overcome resistance and improve the efficacy of 5-FU.

Leucovorin increases the intracellular concentration of reduced folates, which results in prolonged inhibition of thymidylate synthetase and prolonged inhibition of DNA synthesis. Clinically this results in increased response rates, particularly in colorectal cancer where 5-FU plus leucovorin is now the standard treatment for advanced disease and a potentially important part of the adjuvant treatment of colon cancer. Levamisole, an antihelminthic agent, improves the effectiveness of 5-FU in the adjuvant treatment of colon cancer. It is unclear whether this occurs by immunomodulatory effect or by biomodulation of 5-FU.

Cytarabine (Cytosar, Ara-C, Cytosine Arabinoside)

Cytarabine is an analogue of the naturally occurring nucleosides cytidine and deoxycytidine. It is a competitive inhibitor of DNA polymerase, inhibiting DNA synthesis while exerting only minor effects on RNA and protein synthesis. In view of its effect on DNA synthesis, cytarabine is cell-cycle phase specific for S phase. Alterations in drug activation and catabolism cause drug resistance.

The major dose-limiting toxicity is bone marrow suppression, with granulocytopenia occurring 12 to 18 days after therapy followed by recovery within 3 to 4 weeks. Reversible megaloblastic changes are common. Nausea and vomiting occur in the majority of patients, but continuous infusion of the drug improves tolerance; mucositis occurs in some patients. Transient elevations of hepatic enzymes occur but are not usually clinically significant. Since the liver is the major site of drug inactivation, severe hepatic dysfunction necessitates dose modifications to avoid serious toxicity.

Cytarabine is available in 100- and 500-mg vials. Cytarabine is active in the treatment of acute myelogenous leukemia in combination with thioguanine or daunorubicin or both. Repeated injections or continuous infusions maximize the advantages of the S phase specificity and short plasma half-life of cytarabine. The bolus dose of cytarabine is 100 mg/m^2 twice daily by the intravenous or subcutaneous route for a period of 7 days. The cytarabine infusion dose is 100 mg/m^2 for 7 days. Cytarabine is also active against acute lymphocytic leukemia and non-Hodgkin's lymphomas.

Because cytarabine disappears slowly from the cerebrospinal fluid, intrathecal cytarabine is an alternative to methotrexate in the treatment of meningeal leukemia. The dose for intrathecal use is 10 to 70 mg/m^2 every 3 to 7 days.

Treatment of refractory acute leukemia with high-dose cytarabine results in complete remission rates of 20 to 50%. The cytarabine dose is 3 g/m^2 over 1 hour, repeated every 12 hours for 3 to 6 days. Additional toxicity—neurotoxicity (cerebellar ataxia), corneal toxicity, diarrhea, pancreatitis, and skin rashes—occurs with these regimens. Steroid eye drops during treatment decrease corneal toxicity.

Azacitidine

Azacitidine is a cytidine analogue that interferes with protein synthesis and ribosomal RNA processing, competitively inhibits enzymes involved in pyrimidine synthesis, and is incorporated into nucleic acids. Azacitidine is cell-cycle phase specific for S phase. From 80 to 90% of the drug appears in the urine within 24 hours.

Nausea and vomiting occur in the majority of patients beginning within 1 to 3 hours after treatment. Intravenous infusion or subcutaneous injection improves gastrointestinal tolerance. Diarrhea, fever, and hypotension also occur. The major dose-limiting toxicity is bone marrow suppression. Azacitidine is hepatotoxic, and the risk of severe hepatic damage is greatest in patients with preexisting hepatic dysfunction. Azacitidine is an investigational agent useful in treating refractory acute myelogenous leukemia. It is available from the National Cancer Institute in 100-mg vials.

6-Mercaptopurine (Mercaptopurine, Purinethol)

Mercaptopurine, an analogue of hypoxanthine, inhibits de novo purine nucleotide formation. Mercaptopurine is also incorporated into both DNA and RNA. Decreased or absent levels of the mercaptopurine-activating enzyme result in resistance. The drug is cell-cycle phase specific for S phase. Oral mercaptopurine has variable absorption from the gastrointestinal tract. The liver extensively metabolizes mercaptopurine to inactive compounds ultimately excreted in the urine. Xanthine oxidase plays an important role in mercaptopurine metabolism. Coadministration of allopurinol (a xanthine oxidase inhibitor) potentiates mercaptopurine toxicity. Therefore, with concomitant allopurinol the dose of mercaptopurine is one-third the usual dose.

The dose-limiting toxicity is bone marrow suppression. A second major toxicity is cholestatic jaundice, which develops in about one-third of patients. Jaundice usually clears promptly with drug discontinuation. Minor toxicities include anorexia, nausea, vomiting, mouth ulcers, and rarely dermatitis and drug fever.

The usual oral dose of mercaptopurine is 50 to 90 mg/m^2 daily. The drug is given as a single daily dose continuously, with dose adjustment according to blood counts and tumor response. The most common use for mercaptopurine is in maintenance therapy of acute lymphoblastic leukemia.

Thioguanine

Once activated, thioguanine integrates into DNA, which largely accounts for its cytotoxicity. The drug also integrates into RNA and inhibits purine synthesis. Thioguanine is cell-cycle phase specific for S phase. In most cases, resistance to thioguanine is due to deficiency of the activating enzyme. Oral administration of thioguanine results in slow and incomplete absorption from the gastrointestinal tract, and approximately 40% of the dose appears in the urine.

The major toxicity is bone marrow suppression, which may be delayed and profound. Recovery usually occurs within 7 days after drug discontinuation. Other side effects resemble those of mercaptopurine, although thioguanine may be slightly less toxic. Thioguanine is commercially available in 40-mg tablets and the dose is 2 mg/kg/day. The most common use for thioguanine is in multiple drug combination therapy for myelogenous leukemias.

Fludarabine

An analogue of ara-C and ara-A, fludarabine interferes with DNA synthesis by inhibiting ribonucleotide reductase and DNA polymerase alpha. Fludarabine is currently available in 50-mg vials for intravenous injection and is excreted primarily by the kidneys. It is generally well tolerated, and its most common side effects include myelosuppression, nausea and vomiting, diarrhea, fatigue, and abnormalities of liver and renal function. Fludarabine is particularly useful for refractory chronic lymphocytic leukemia, with an aggregate response rate of 56%. Studies also reveal activity against low-grade non-Hodgkin's lymphomas, Hodgkin's disease, and mycosis fungoides.

Deoxycoformycin (Pentostatin)

Deoxycoformycin irreversibly inhibits adenosine deaminase, an enzyme found at highest levels in lymphoid tissues, especially T cells. Inhibition of adenosine deaminase impairs DNA and RNA synthesis, damages DNA integrity, and interferes with ATP-dependent cell functions. It is excreted primarily by the kidneys, and its principal side effects include myelosuppression, renal failure, lethargy, and seizures. Immunosuppression due to lymphoid damage increases the risk of secondary infections, especially disseminated herpes zoster. Deoxycoformycin produces a 90% response rate in hairy cell leukemia and is also active in chronic lymphocytic leukemia, mycosis fungoides, prolymphocytic leukemia, acute T-cell leukemia, and T-cell lymphomas. The usual dose is 4 mg/m^2 every one or two weeks. The treatment of acute leukemias requires higher doses, which also result in substantially increased severe toxicity.

ANTITUMOR ANTIBIOTICS

The antitumor antibiotics are microbial products with a wide range of effects on cellular processes. Among these drugs are some of the most active agents used in current chemotherapeutic regimens. Antibiotic research is one of the most promising areas for future drug discoveries, both for new drugs and for derivatives of current drugs with less toxicity (Table 5–3).

Table 5–3. **ANTIBIOTICS**

DRUG	ADMINISTRATION PROCEDURE	SITES OF METABOLISM AND EXCRETION	TOXICITY
Bleomycin (Blenoxane)	IV, SQ, IM, intracavity	Renal excretion	Fever, mucositis, skin, pulmonary fibrosis
Dactinomycin (Cosmegen)	IV bolus	Renal excretion	Vesicant, bone marrow, GI, alopecia
Daunorubicin (Cerubidine)	IV bolus	Hepatic metabolism and excretion	Vesicant, bone marrow, GI, alopecia, cardiac
Doxorubicin (Adriamycin)	IV bolus, infusion	Hepatic metabolism and excretion	Vesicant, bone marrow, GI, alopecia, cardiac
Mitoxantrone (Novantrone)	IV bolus	Hepatic metabolism and excretion	Bone marrow, cardiac, GI, alopecia
Mitomycin (Mutamycin)	IV bolus, intravesical	Hepatic metabolism	Vesicant, bone marrow, hemolytic/uremic syndrome, pulmonary fibrosis
Plicamycin (Mithracin)	IV bolus, infusion	Renal excretion	Bone marrow, hepatic, GI, hypocalcemia

Doxorubicin (Adriamycin) and Daunorubicin (Cerubidine)

Despite similar chemical structures and pharmacologic behaviors, the anthracycline antibiotics doxorubicin and daunorubicin differ in antitumor activity. Both drugs bind tightly to DNA by intercalation. This produces inhibition of DNA synthesis, but effects on RNA and protein synthesis also occur. Interaction with DNA also leads to breaks in the DNA strand and chromosomal damage. Resistance to these agents is related to impaired transport across cell membranes and decreased drug retention. Cytotoxicity occurs in both proliferating and nonproliferating cells; however, cycling cells in S phase appear to be most sensitive. The metabolism of these drugs is quite similar; rapid and extensive metabolism occurs in the liver. Approximately 40 to 50% of an administered dose appears in the bile and 10% in the urine.

Adriamycin and daunorubicin produce similar toxicity. Nausea and vomiting occur frequently. Stomatitis is common and usually dose related. Generalized alopecia occurs in virtually all patients and is reversible after therapy. During intravenous administration a "flare" reaction may occur with an urticarialike eruption over the injection site or proximally. This is generally not painful or serious and responds to an antihistamine. Extravasation causes a very different, painful redness at the injection site. Tissue necrosis will occur; the tissue damage is proportional to the amount of drug extravasated. Other side effects include fever, chills, flushing, and hypersensitivity. Drug excretion causes a red-tinged urine. Bone marrow suppression, primarily leukopenia, is dose limiting, with the nadir occurring at 10 to 14 days and recovery usually by day 21.

Cardiac toxicity is a distinctive problem with Adriamycin and daunorubicin treatment. Acute changes in the electrocardiogram and arrhythmias may occur in the first few days following drug administration; these changes are generally reversible and rarely necessitate treatment cessation. In contrast, a severe and progressive cardiomyopathy develops in approximately 3% of patients receiving more than a cumulative dose of 400 mg/m^2 of Adriamycin. A similar cardiomyopathy occurs when the total dose of daunorubicin exceeds 600 mg/m^2. This complication is fatal in approximately 50% of patients. Increased risk factors for cardiac toxicity are age greater than 70 years, hypertension, preexisting cardiac disease, concomitant administration of cyclophosphamide, and prior cardiac radiation. To minimize cardiac toxicity in patients with significant risk factors, cumulative doses less than 400 to 450 mg/m^2 are advisable. Patients with severe underlying cardiac disease will not tolerate even minimal Adriamycin or daunorubicin doses.

Serial radionuclide angiography (MUGA or ERNA scan) is the most successful noninvasive method for detection of early anthracycline cardiac damage. New doxorubicin-like compounds such as mitoxantrone and 4-epirubicin diminish the risk of cardiac toxicity while retaining much of the antineoplastic activity. Current research efforts include the development of drugs that protect the heart from toxicity without compromising the antineoplastic activity of the anthracycline.

Adriamycin is one of the most frequently used anticancer agents because of its activity against a wide variety of neoplastic disorders. In combination with other agents, Adriamycin is extremely effective in treating Hodgkin's and non-Hodgkin's lymphomas, acute leukemias, breast cancer, sarcomas, and pediatric malignancies. Adriamycin also has activity in the treatment of multiple myeloma and carcinomas of the lung, ovary, thyroid, bladder, prostate, and stomach. The dose of Adriamycin ranges from 60 to 90 mg/m^2 given over 1 to 3 days and repeated every 3 to 4 weeks. An alternative schedule is 20 mg/m^2 per week; nausea, vomiting, and possibly cardiac toxicity may decrease with the weekly regimen, but activity may also decrease. Because of extensive hepatic metabolism of the anthracyclines, hepatic dysfunction or biliary obstruction necessitates significant dose modification.

In contrast to Adriamycin, daunorubicin has a limited spectrum of activity and is used primarily to treat acute lymphocytic and myelogenous leukemias. Daunorubicin is particularly useful for induction of remission, and doses range from 30 to 60 mg/m^2/day for 2 to 3 consecutive days.

Mitoxantrone (Novantrone)

Structurally related to Adriamycin, mitoxantrone is an anthracenedione that binds to DNA, causing strand breaks and inhibiting DNA synthesis. It is cell-cycle phase nonspecific. Its primary route of elimination is via the biliary system, and dose adjustments are necessary when hyperbilirubinemia exists. Bone marrow suppression is its dose-limiting toxicity. Mitoxantrone is less cardiotoxic than adriamycin, and it is not a vesicant. It may cause alopecia, mucositis, nausea, and vomiting. It is active in combination chemotherapy for refractory acute nonlymphocytic leukemia (dose: 10 to 12 mg/m^2 for 5 days) and breast cancer and non-Hodgkin's lymphoma (dose: 10 to 14 mg/m^2).

Actinomycin D (Dactinomycin, Cosmegen)

Actinomycin D inhibits DNA-directed RNA synthesis by intercalating with DNA bases. At higher concentrations, inhibition of DNA synthesis occurs. Actinomycin D is cell-cycle phase nonspecific. Impaired cellular penetration of the drug results in drug resistance. Significant metabolism does not occur, and excretion of the drug by fecal and urinary routes is prolonged.

Common side effects include nausea, vomiting, mucositis, diarrhea, alopecia, and acneiform skin eruptions. Dose-limiting toxicity is bone marrow suppression, with the nadir occurring at 7 to 15 days and recovery within the next 7 days. Tissue necrosis may result from local extravasation. Actinomycin D is available in 500-μg vials. The usual dose in children is 15 μg/kg/day for 5 consecutive days, repeated every 3 to 4 weeks. In adults, the dose is 2 mg/m^2 every 3 to 4 weeks.

Actinomycin D is most useful for treating pediatric malignancies, particularly Wilms' tumor. Actinomycin D also has activity against gestational trophoblastic neoplasms and against sarcomas.

Bleomycin (Blenoxane)

Bleomycin binds to DNA and produces both single-strand and double-strand breaks, thereby inhibiting DNA synthesis. Both cycling and noncycling cells are sensitive, but proliferating cells demonstrate enhanced sensitivity. Resistance to bleomycin results from enzymatic drug inactivation. Approximately 50 to 60% of an administered dose appears unchanged in the urine within 24 hours. Severe renal dysfunction prolongs the half-life, and a dose reduction of 50% is necessary.

Unlike the toxicities of the majority of chemotherapeutic agents, the acute toxicities of bleomycin are minimal, but its chronic toxicities may be severe and life threatening. Bleomycin rarely causes bone marrow suppression and is therefore a useful agent in multidrug regimens. Mucositis is common and dose related. Reversible skin toxicities include hyperpigmentation, erythema, hyperkeratosis, and nail changes. Partial alopecia occurs in 10 to 20% of patients. The most severe acute toxicity consists of fever, myalgia, and shaking chills in about 25% of patients. This usually occurs 4 to 6 hours after drug administration. In about 1% of patients, a severe reaction consisting of fever, chills, hypotension, wheezing, and confusion occurs and may be fatal. Virtually all of these reactions arise in patients with lymphoma. Gastrointestinal side effects are infrequent.

The most severe bleomycin toxicity occurs in the lungs. Pulmonary toxicity affects 5 to 10% of patients and may be fatal in 1%. Risk factors include age greater than 70 years, total dose over 400 U, prior radiotherapy to the lungs, and a history of underlying pulmonary disease. Clinical findings consist of dyspnea, tachypnea, nonproductive cough, and fever. Fine, dry rales at the bases and a diffuse interstitial or patchy basilar infiltrate on chest x-ray may be early, although nonspecific, findings. Pathologic examination of the lungs reveals interstitial edema, intra-alveolar hyaline membrane formation, alveolar squamous metaplasia, and, in later stages, fibrosis. Although generally dose related, pulmonary toxicity may rarely occur after the first few doses. Pulmonary function studies usually show restrictive disease and abnormal carbon monoxide diffusion capacity, but these tests are poorly predictive of incipient clinical pulmonary toxicity. Therapy for the clinical syndrome is supportive and requires discontinuation of bleomycin. The role of corticosteroids in this disorder is unclear, but beneficial effects may occur. Patients surviving the acute pulmonary decompensation may recover significant pulmonary function.

Whether high inspired oxygen concentrations precipitate bleomycin pulmonary toxicity remains controversial. Minimizing oxygen concentrations for patients receiving both bleomycin and supplemental oxygen is prudent. An increased risk of bleomycin pulmonary toxicity also occurs in patients receiving both bleomycin and methotrexate, particularly high-dose methotrexate—e.g., in the M-BACOD regimen for non-Hodgkin's lymphoma (Chap. 10).

Bleomycin is usually given intravenously or subcutaneously. It is also effective intracavitary treatment for malignant pleural effusions, pericardial effusions, and ascites. The dose of bleomycin is a weekly or twice weekly injection of 5 to 20 U/m^2. In combination with other agents, it produces high response rates and durable remissions in Hodgkin's disease, non-Hodgkin's lymphomas, and testicular cancers. Squamous cell carcinomas, particularly of the head and neck, also occasionally respond transiently. Bleomycin is available in 15-U vials.

Mitomycin C (Mutamycin)

Mitomycin C is an alkylating agent that produces interstrand cross links, single-strand cleavage of DNA, and chromosomal breaks. It inhibits DNA synthesis and is cell-cycle phase nonspecific. Mitomycin C may be active against tumors resistant to conventional alkylating agents. The liver is the primary site of mitomycin C metabolism; less than 10% of the parent drug is detectable in the urine.

Delayed, cumulative, and frequently serious bone marrow suppression (particularly thrombocytopenia) greatly reduces the clinical utility of mitomycin C. The blood count nadir occurs at 3 to 4 weeks, and recovery may not occur for another 1 to 3 weeks. Other toxicities such as nausea, vomiting, alopecia, and stomatitis are usually mild and occur in a minority of patients. Extravasation of the drug may cause severe tissue necrosis.

Two other less common but potentially fatal toxicities of mitomycin C are a hemolytic-uremic syndrome and pulmonary fibrosis. The hemolytic-uremic syndrome is not dose-related and is frequently fatal. It presents with proteinuria, hematuria, thrombocytopenia, and microangiopathic hemolytic anemia. Most patients die of renal failure within a few months. The pulmonary fibrosis appears to be a hypersensitivity reaction and generally occurs after cumulative doses greater than 50 mg.

Mitomycin C is available in 5- and 20-mg vials. The dose is 10 to 20 mg/m^2 intravenously every 6 to 8 weeks. Mitomycin C has activity against breast cancer, non–small cell lung cancer, and some gastrointestinal cancers. As intravesical therapy for superficial bladder cancer, 20 to 40 mg of mitomycin C is instilled weekly for 8 weeks.

Plicamycin (Mithracin)

Plicamycin (formerly called mithramycin) binds reversibly to DNA and inhibits RNA synthesis; it also inhibits osteoclasts, preventing resorption of bone, making it a valuable treatment for hypercalcemia. Little information is available about the pharmacology of plicamycin.

Plicamycin possesses a variety of unusual and serious toxicities. The most important is a hemorrhagic diathesis. Thrombocytopenia, altered platelet function, vascular damage, depression of clotting factors, and increased fibrinolytic activity contribute to this toxicity. Elevation of liver enzymes, particularly transaminases and LDH, is universal and may be marked. Other toxicities include anorexia, nausea, vomiting, a flulike syndrome, changes in mental status, impaired renal function, and various electrolyte abnormalities, including hypocalcemia. Stomatitis and leukopenia are uncommon.

The above-mentioned toxicities were common in the past when high-dose plicamycin was used in the treatment of testicular cancer. Currently, plicamycin is employed almost exclusively to control malignant hypercalcemia and at much lower doses (15 to 25 μg/kg). This dose results in minimal toxicity except for transient elevations of liver enzymes. Optimal administration is by intravenous bolus injection with appropriate care to avoid extravasation and consequent tissue necrosis. Serum calcium levels usually decrease within 24 to 48 hours; additional doses may be needed every 4 to 7 days if the serum calcium remains abnormal. Plicamycin is available in a 2500-μg vial.

VINCA ALKALOIDS

Derived from the periwinkle plant, the vinca alkaloids are mitotic inhibitors that disrupt the mitotic spindle assembly, interrupting cell division in metaphase. These drugs are cell-cycle phase specific for M (mitosis) phase (Table 5–4). Despite their minimal structural difference, vinblastine and vincristine are non–cross-resistant in clinical practice.

Vinblastine (Velban)

Vinblastine is excreted primarily in the bile. Compromised hepatic function requires dose modification. The dose-limiting toxicity is bone marrow suppression, occurring within 5 to 9 days with subsequent recovery within 14 to 21 days. Effects on the granulocytic series predominate. At conventional doses, other side effects are generally mild and well tolerated; however, larger doses may cause severe toxicities. These include transient nausea, vomiting, mucositis, abdominal pain, constipation, malaise, myalgias, alopecia, peripheral neuropathy, and painful extravasation.

Dispensed in a 10-mg vial, vinblastine is an extremely effective agent in the treatment of advanced Hodgkin's disease as part of the ABVD regimen (Chap. 9). It also is part of combination regimens for testicular cancer, breast cancer, and non–small cell lung cancer.

Table 5–4. **MISCELLANEOUS ANTINEOPLASTIC DRUGS**

DRUG	ADMINISTRATION PROCEDURE	SITES OF METABOLISM AND EXCRETION	TOXICITY
Vincristine (Oncovin)	IV push, infusion	Hepatic metabolism and excretion	Vesicant, neuropathy, alopecia
Vinblastine (Velban)	IV push, infusion	Hepatic metabolism and excretion	Vesicant, neuropathy, bone marrow, alopecia
Etoposide (VePesid)	Slow IV infusion Oral: 50-mg capsules	Hepatic metabolism, renal and hepatic excretion	Bone marrow, GI, alopecia, hypotension
Cisplatin (Platinol)	IV infusion	Renal excretion	Renal, GI, ototoxic, neuropathy
Carboplatin (Paraplatin)	IV bolus	Renal excretion	Bone marrow, GI, ototoxic, neuropathy
Procarbazine (Matulane)	Oral: 50-mg capsules	Hepatic metabolism, renal excretion	Bone marrow, CNS, neuropathy, skin
Hydroxyurea (Hydrea)	Oral: 500-mg capsules	Hepatic metabolism, renal excretion	Bone marrow
Asparaginase (Elspar)–*E. coli*	IM, IV infusion	Systemic metabolism	Anaphylaxis, hepatic, GI, CNS, metabolic
Altretamine (Hexalen)	Oral: 50-mg capsules	Hepatic metabolism, renal excretion	GI, neuropathy, bone marrow, CNS

In combination with other myelosuppressive drugs, the dose is 6 mg/m^2. As a single agent, the dose may approach 15 mg/m^2 (0.3 to 0.4 mg/kg) every 3 to 4 weeks.

Vincristine (Oncovin)

In contrast to vinblastine, the dose-limiting toxicity of vincristine is a mixed motor-sensory and autonomic neuropathy. Vincristine binds to tubulin (which forms the neurotubules), resulting in axonal degeneration and clinical neurotoxicity. The earliest clinical sign is depression of the Achilles tendon reflex, and the earliest symptom is paresthesia of the fingers and toes. Although nerve function may normalize following the cessation of therapy, continuation of the drug may lead to severe and disabling paresthesias, areflexia, and weakness. Other side effects include myalgias, especially in the jaw and neck area, cramping abdominal pain, and constipation. Less frequent side effects include orthostatic hypotension, difficulty in micturition, inappropriate secretion of antidiuretic hormone, and cranial neuropathy. Mild and reversible alopecia is common. Vincristine has minimal effects on the bone marrow and is useful in combination with myelosuppressive drugs, particularly in patients with compromised bone marrow function.

Vincristine is available for intravenous injection only. It is a vesicant. The usual dose is 1.4 mg/m^2, repeated at weekly intervals depending on individual tolerance. Some recommend a maximum dose of 2 mg. Vincristine is important in combination chemotherapy for acute leukemia, Hodgkin's disease, non-Hodgkin's lymphoma, small cell lung cancer, and others.

EPIPODOPHYLLOTOXINS

The epipodophyllotoxins are semisynthetic podophyllotoxin derivatives that prevent cells from entering into mitosis. These drugs also inhibit nucleoside transport and incorporation into RNA and DNA. The two drugs in this category include commercially available etoposide (VP-16, VePesid) and VM-26 (teniposide), an investigational drug (see Table 5–4).

Etoposide (VePesid, VP-16)

Etoposide is active when given orally and by intravenous infusion. Approximately 45% of the drug appears in the urine and 15% in the feces. The dose-limiting toxicity is bone marrow suppression. Leukopenia and thrombocytopenia occur, with a nadir by day 14 and recovery usually by day 20 to 22. Gastrointestinal toxicity is usually mild, and alopecia occurs in nearly all patients.

Etoposide is available in 100-mg vials and as 50-mg capsules. Intravenous infusion requires 30 to 60 minutes; faster infusion rates may cause hypotension and headaches. There are many dosage schedules: (1) a 3-day schedule of 125 mg/m^2 intravenously; (2) twice the intravenous dosage orally; (3) daily doses of 50 to 100 mg/m^2 orally for prolonged periods; and others. Etoposide is active against small cell and non–small cell lung cancers and testicular cancer. It is also effective in non-Hodgkin's lymphomas and other hematologic malignancies, as well as Kaposi's sarcoma and some childhood cancers.

VM-26 (Teniposide)

VM-26 is an investigational epipodophyllotoxin administered by intravenous infusion. The major dose-limiting toxicity is bone marrow suppression, with a leukopenic nadir around day 14 and recovery by day 20 to 22 after treatment. There is mild gastrointestinal toxicity and mild alopecia. Hypersensitivity reactions are more common than with etoposide. Teniposide infusions require 30 to 60 minutes to prevent hypotension. For investigational use it is available in 50-mg vials, with a usual dose of 100 mg/m^2/week, or 50 mg/m^2 twice a week for 4 to 6 weeks. Research protocols use VM-26 primarily for hematologic malignancies.

MISCELLANEOUS AGENTS

The agents discussed below do not fit into any of the previously described classes of anticancer drugs because their mechanisms of action are either unknown or unique (see (Table 5–4).

Cisplatin (Platinol) and Carboplatin (Paraplatin)

Of the many platinum derivatives with antitumor activity, only *cis*-diamminedichloroplatinum (cisplatin) and CBDCA (carboplatin) are currently available for clinical use. These drugs share the same mechanism of action–they bind to DNA and form both intra- and interstrand DNA cross links. This results in inhibition of DNA synthesis with lesser effects on RNA and protein synthesis. Cisplatin and carboplatin kill cells in all stages of the cell cycle. Clinically they are not cross-resistant with conventional alkylating agents or with each other. The major route of excretion is renal.

The dose-limiting toxicity of cisplatin is renal damage. Pathologic changes in the renal tubules and collecting ducts resemble mercurial damage. Vigorous hydration and diuresis minimize the dose-related cisplatin renal toxicity. Avoidance of concomitant nephrotoxic drugs, such as aminoglycosides, is also advisable. Ototoxicity—usually tinnitus and hearing loss at high frequencies—may ultimately result in irreversible deafness. Nausea and vomiting are often severe and protracted. Asymptomatic hypomagnesemia occurs frequently and is due to renal tubular damage. Anaphylactic reactions, hemolytic anemia, and peripheral neuropathies also occur. Cisplatin is particularly useful in combination with other agents because of its minimal bone marrow toxicity.

Carboplatin is less nephrotoxic, ototoxic, and neurotoxic. It is easier to administer than cisplatin because hydration and diuresis are unnecessary. The dose-limiting toxicity of carboplatin is bone marrow suppression with a nadir count at 21 days and recovery at 28 days after treatment. Anemia also occurs and is dose related. Nausea and vomiting are significantly less common and less severe than with cisplatin. Hypersensitivity reactions, similar to those with cisplatin, occur in 2% of patients.

Cisplatin doses range from 20 mg/m^2 to 120 mg/m^2 by intravenous infusion repeated every 3 to 4 weeks. Pretreatment consists of intravenous hydration and antiemetics; diuretics are optional with lower doses (20 to 40 mg/m^2). Antiemetic support should continue for more than 24 to 48 hours after treatment. High doses of cisplatin (greater than 100 mg/m^2) can be administered in high concentrations of sodium chloride (3%) with minimal renal toxicity. With dose escalation, however, ototoxicity, neuropathy, and gastrointestinal toxicity become evident and dose limiting. Other methods to avoid cisplatin toxicity include the investigational use of "chemo-protectors" such as DDTC and the substitution of other platinum derivatives such as carboplatin and CHIP.

Carboplatin doses range from 300 mg/m^2 to 400 mg/m^2 by a 15-minute intravenous infusion, without hydration or forced diuresis, repeated every 4 weeks. Patients with impaired renal function require significant dose reductions.

Cisplatin is an essential part of curative chemotherapy regimens for testicular cancer and extragonadal germ cell tumors. It also plays an important role in the treatment of ovarian cancer and small cell lung cancer. Cisplatin results in palliative benefit for bladder, esophageal, head and neck, and non–small cell lung cancers. Carboplatin is equally effective in the curative treatment of ovarian cancer and is also effective salvage therapy for ovarian cancer patients who progress after initial cisplatin. Carboplatin is also active against testicular cancer, particularly seminoma; currently, carboplatin is an important part of high-dose chemotherapy with autologous bone marrow transplants for refractory testicular cancer. Studies to define the role of carboplatin in initial therapy for testicular cancer, lung cancer, head and neck cancer, and other primary sites are in progress.

Procarbazine (Matulane)

The precise mechanism of action of procarbazine is unclear. It inhibits DNA and RNA synthesis and produces phase-nonspecific effects on the cell cycle. Procarbazine is not cross-resistant with alkylating agents or other antitumor drugs. Completely absorbed from the gastrointestinal tract, procarbazine also readily penetrates into the central nervous system. The primary route of excretion is via the kidneys.

The dose-limiting toxicity of procarbazine is bone marrow suppression. Potential neurologic toxicity includes altered mental status and peripheral neuropathy. Reversible ataxia and myalgias may also occur. Procarbazine is a weak inhibitor of monoamine oxidase; concomitant exposure to sympathomimetic agents, tricyclic antidepressants, or tyramine-containing foods may result in hypertensive episodes. Procarbazine also potentiates the sedative effects of phenothiazines, barbiturates, and narcotics. Following alcohol ingestion, procarbazine may cause a disulfiram-like reaction characterized by facial flushing, headache, and sweating. Nausea and vomiting are common after treatment. Hypersensitivity reactions, including severe skin rashes, are possible with procarbazine.

Procarbazine is commercially available in 50-mg capsules. The daily dose is 100 to 200 mg daily in three or four doses. Bone marrow toxicity usually limits procarbazine treatment to intermittent 14- to 21-day courses. Dose reductions are required for patients with renal or hepatic dysfunction. The most common use for procarbazine is as part of multiple drug therapy for Hodgkin's disease. Procarbazine also has limited activity against non-Hodgkin's lymphomas, lung cancer, and malignant brain tumors.

Hydroxyurea (Hydrea)

Hydroxyurea inhibits DNA synthesis by inhibition of ribonucleotide reductase. It is cell-cycle phase specific for S phase and is well absorbed from the gastrointestinal tract. After metabolism in the liver, the primary route of drug excretion is renal. Although no firm guidelines exist, patients with severely compromised renal function require dose reductions. The major dose-limiting toxicity is bone marrow suppression, manifested by leukopenia and megaloblastosis. Reversal of cytopenias usually occurs rapidly. Other side effects are infrequent and generally mild, and consist of nausea, vomiting, mucosal ulcerations, and dermatologic reactions.

Hydroxyurea is available commercially as 500-mg capsules. The most common indication is in chronic granulocytic leukemia as an alternative to busulfan. The rapid onset of action of hydroxyurea makes it very useful treatment for life-threatening leukocytosis associated with either acute leukemia or blast crisis. In such cases, the dose is 80 mg/kg/day for one or two doses. The usual dose is 20 to 30 mg/kg/day or 80 mg/kg every 3 days, adjusted for blood counts.

L-Asparaginase (Elspar)

L-Asparaginase, the only enzyme currently used in treating cancer, hydrolyzes asparagine to aspartic acid and ammonia. The antitumor activity of this agent depends on the requirement of some tumors for an exogenous source of the essential amino acid L-asparagine due to an impaired capacity for de novo synthesis. Asparagine deficiency primarily interferes with protein synthesis, but it may subsequently inhibit DNA and RNA synthesis as well. The factors that determine plasma disappearance are not well defined. The most serious toxicity of L-asparaginase is anaphylaxis, which occurs in approximately 10% of patients, more frequently with intravenous than with intramuscular administration, and more likely after repeated doses. A 10-U intradermal skin test may detect hypersensitivity prior to systemic therapy. Patients who develop hypersensitivity from a preparation derived from one source may tolerate a preparation from another source. L-Asparaginase may produce liver and central nervous system dysfunction, pancreatitis, hyperglycemia, hypoalbuminemia, and depression of clotting factors, particularly fibrinogen. Nausea and vomiting occur commonly.

L-Asparaginase is commercially available in 10,000-U vials. Its primary use is in the induction phase of treatment for acute lymphocytic leukemia and lymphoblastic lymphoma. One schedule of administration is 6000 IU/m^2 intramuscularly three times a week for a total of nine doses. Another regimen is 1000 IU/kg intravenously by short infusion for a period of 10 days.

Mitotane (o,p′-DDD, Lysodren)

Mitotane has a direct effect on normal and neoplastic adrenocortical tissue, manifested by reductions in adrenocorticosteroid levels and degeneration of the adrenal cortex. Gastrointestinal absorption is incomplete. About 25% appears in the urine as a water-soluble metabolite. Common side effects include gastrointestinal intolerance, central nervous system reactions, and dermatitis. In most cases, these effects are dose related. Rarely, visual disturbances, retinopathy, proteinuria, and hematuria also occur. Severe physiologic stress may result in adrenal insufficiency after mitotane treatment.

Mitotane is commercially available as 500-mg tablets, administered in a total daily amount of 8 to 10 g in divided doses. Dose escalations depend on patient tolerance. The only indication for mitotane is the treatment of locally advanced and metastatic adrenocortical carcinoma.

Amsacrine (m-AMSA)

Amsacrine is an acridine that intercalates into DNA, causing strand breakage and inhibition of DNA synthesis. Usually given intravenously, it also has good gastrointestinal absorption. Amsacrine undergoes liver metabolism and biliary excretion, so hepatic dysfunction or biliary obstruction necessitates dose reductions. Most common amsacrine toxicities include myelosuppression, nausea, vomiting, and phlebitis. At higher antileukemic doses, neurotoxicity, cardiac toxicity, hypersensitivity, and hepatic toxicity also occur.

As a single agent, amsacrine produces a 15 to 30% complete remission rate in acute myelogenous leukemia. Currently, amsacrine and cytarabine are part of intensive consolidation therapy for patients with acute myelogenous leukemia in complete remission. Doses range from 50 to 150 mg/m^2 daily for 5 days.

Hexamethylmelamine (Altretamine, Hexalen)

The mechanism of action of hexamethylmelamine is unknown. Following oral administration and gastrointestinal absorption, hexamethylmelamine undergoes extensive demethylation in the liver followed by urinary excretion. Gastrointestinal intolerance is dose limiting. Most patients develop moderate bone marrow depression. Some patients experience a dose-related cumulative neurologic toxicity manifested by paresthesias, muscle weakness, and ataxia resembling Parkinson's disease. Alterations in mental status and mood also occur. Although the mechanism of this neurotoxicity is unknown, pyridoxine in a dose of 100 mg three times daily is a possibly effective countermeasure. A dose reduction may also decrease these adverse reactions. Pruritus and skin rashes also occur rarely.

Hexamethylmelamine is available as 50-mg capsules. The drug is active against ovarian cancer, both as a frequent part of initial combination therapy and also in the treatment of refractory disease. It has some activity reported against lymphomas, lung cancer, head and neck cancer, and carcinomas of the bladder, cervix, and breast. As a single agent, hexamethylmelamine is used at 260 mg/m^2/day for 14 to 21 days, repeated every 28 days. Divided doses, four times a day, minimize gastrointestinal toxicity.

Suramin

Suramin (also known as Antrypol, Moranyl, and Naganol) was initially employed for the treatment of oncocerciasis, trypanosomiasis, and African sleeping sickness. A glycosaminoglycan agonist-antagonist, suramin inhibits a broad spectrum of growth-regulatory enzymes. Suramin inhibits cell growth by binding to heparin-binding growth factors (i.e., platelet-derived growth factor [PDGF]) and interfering with the binding of these growth factors with their appropriate receptors. It also impairs cell growth by inhibiting DNA polymerase, reverse transcription (RNA to DNA), protein kinase C, transferrin binding, and other growth factors. Early clinical trials of suramin for prostate cancer show promising pain responses and objective responses in tumor size and prostate-specific antigen levels. Indolent lymphomas may also be responsive to suramin. Confirmatory studies and investigation of suramin activity in other cancers are underway. Suramin toxicity results from accumulation of glycosaminoglycans, producing an "acquired mucopolysaccharidosis syndrome." Clinical suramin toxicity includes impaired cell-mediated immunity and myelosuppression, reversible adrenal insufficiency, and neurotoxicity ranging from transient paresthesias to a severe polyradiculoneuropathy. Additional toxicities include rashes, keratopathy, elevated liver enzymes, coagulopathy, and renal toxicity.

Taxol

Taxol is derived from the bark of the western yew *(Taxus brevifolia)*; currently one tree provides enough bark for only two or three antitumor doses. Intensive efforts to synthesize taxol or a closely related product are underway. Unlike the vinca alkaloids that inhibit polymerization of tubulin, taxol uniquely stabilizes the microtubules, promotes their formation, and resists their disassembly. Cells appear to enter into mitosis prematurely with inappropriate preparation, and cell death follows. Initial clinical studies favored continuous infusion dosing to decrease the bronchospasm and hypotension (attributed to the taxol diluent) common with bolus dosing. Premedication with steroids and antihistamines is still necessary to prevent or decrease hypersensitivity reactions. Bone marrow toxicity is dose limiting. Other potential toxicities include peripheral neuropathies, mucositis, total alopecia, bradycardia, myalgias, lethargy, and weakness. Taxol produces a 30% response rate for relapsed or resistant ovarian cancer. In breast cancer studies, 48% of resistant patients responded to taxol; many had received previous Adriamycin. Early studies also reveal activity against acute myelogenous leukemia and malignant melanoma.

HORMONAL AGENTS

Hormones influence the growth and function of many normal tissues; some tumors retain this responsiveness to hormonal therapy. Normal hormone action depends on binding to a specific cytoplasmic protein receptor. Once binding between hormone and receptor occurs, the hormone-receptor complex undergoes a conformational change that facilitates binding to nuclear chromatin. This causes the synthesis of specific messenger RNAs, which in turn direct the synthesis of new proteins. The antitumor activity of some hormonal agents depends on the same sequence of events. Other agents, such as the antiestrogens, derive their antitumor effect by interfering with these processes.

Estrogens

The most commonly used estrogen is the nonsteroidal synthetic hormone diethylstilbestrol (DES), which is effective in treating prostate cancer. DES is available in tablets or capsules ranging from 0.1 mg to 25 mg. It is inexpensive and has excellent gastrointestinal absorption. Acute toxicity is dose related and includes nausea, vomiting, fluid retention, rare liver dysfunction, and thromboembolism, as well as exacerbated hypertension and congestive heart failure. In males, it causes impotence and gynecomastia. In females, it causes increased migraines, breast tenderness, vaginal bleeding, and can exacerbate endometriosis. Long-term estrogen therapy increases the risk of endometrial cancer, possibly breast cancer, and vaginal neoplasms in the daughters of estrogen-treated pregnant mothers.

In men, DES appears to inhibit prostate cancer growth by feedback inhibition of the hypothalamic-pituitary axis. Production of both luteinizing hormone (LH) and testosterone decreases, frequently to castrate levels. Deprived of testosterone stimulus, prostate cancer regresses rapidly, resulting in significant symptomatic relief in 70 to 80% of previously untreated patients. The usual DES dose is 1 mg daily. If no response occurs and if serum testosterone is not at castrate levels with a 1-mg dose, some investigators advise a dose escalation to 3 mg daily. A 5-mg daily dose results in excessive cardiac and vascular morbidity.

Tamoxifen (Nolvadex)

The only clinically available antiestrogen in the United States is tamoxifen (Nolvadex). In the breast cancer cell, tamoxifen competitively binds to cytoplasmic estrogen receptors and deprives the cells of proliferative estrogen stimulation. Additionally, after the antiestrogen-receptor complex translocates to the cancer cell nucleus, direct cell injury may occur. Cell death and breast cancer regression follow.

Tamoxifen is extremely well tolerated; only 3% of patients discontinue treatment because of toxicity. It is available in 10-mg tablets; the recommended dosage is 10 mg twice daily. Pharmacologic clearance is very slow and independent of liver and renal function. The only common side effects are hot flashes and minimal nausea. Rare side effects include vomiting, rash, vaginal discharge, and lowered blood counts (thrombocytopenia). One potentially dangerous side effect that occurs in 2 to 5% of patients with bone metastases is called tamoxifen flare. In this flare, bone pain increases and hypercalcemia occurs 1 or 2 weeks after beginning tamoxifen (also rarely with other hormonal agents). Provided analgesics and calcium-lowering therapy, patients may continue tamoxifen, and most experience a significant response.

Tamoxifen is effective treatment for breast cancer, both in females and in males. It is also used with varying results for some patients with endometrial and ovarian cancers and in combination with chemotherapy for malignant melanoma.

Progestins (Megace, Provera)

The most commonly used progestational agents in cancer treatment are megestrol acetate (Megace) and medroxyprogesterone acetate (Provera). These compounds have minimal androgenic and fluid-retaining effects. Their precise mechanism of action is poorly understood, although they are known to interfere with the actions of estrogens, androgens, and gonadotropins.

Megace is available in 20- and 40-mg tablets. Provera is primarily used as an intramuscular preparation. Both are metabolized by the liver and excreted by the kidneys. Side effects are minimal and include only fluid retention, weight gain, and mild nausea. For hormonally responsive breast cancer, Megace is frequently the second or third hormone treatment following success with oophorectomy or tamoxifen, or both. The usual dose is 40 mg four times a day. Progestins can also induce a 30 to 35% response rate in metastatic uterine cancer. This efficacy and low toxicity make progestins the preferred treatment for uterine cancer that is no longer amenable to radiation or surgery. The dosage is 160 to 320 mg/day for Megace and 500 to 1500 mg/day for Provera. Megace has limited effect against prostate cancer that is no longer sensitive to estrogen treatment. Renal cancer may sporadically respond to progestins. The weight gain and appetite stimulation of Megace is sometimes helpful in treating tumor cachexia.

Androgens (Halotestin)

Androgens are useful treatment for women with hormone-responsive breast cancer after progression on earlier hormonal therapy. These agents also have useful anabolic properties for cachectic and debilitated patients and to stimulate bone marrow function. The daily dosage of fluoxymesterone (Halotestin) is 10 mg twice daily. Fluoxymesterone and certain other androgens may cause cholestatic jaundice. The major side effect is virilization.

LHRH Agonists (Leuprolide, Goserelin)

Leuprolide (Lupron) and goserelin (Zoladex) are synthetic analogues of luteinizing hormone (LH)–releasing hormone (LHRH). Continued use significantly decreases LH levels and gonadal testosterone secretion. As primary treatment for metastatic prostate cancer, LHRH agonists are as effective as DES or orchiectomy.

During the first several weeks of LHRH agonist treatment, symptoms may increase owing to acute increases in testosterone levels before suppression occurs. This "flare" is preventable by 2 weeks of low-dose (1 mg/day) DES or the coadministration of flutamide (an antiandrogen). Other toxicities include hot flashes, nausea, peripheral edema, decreased libido, and impotence. LHRH agonists lack the cardiovascular toxicity of DES. The principal drawbacks of LHRH agonists are the requirement for daily injections or monthly depot injections and expense—over $100 for a 2-week supply.

Flutamide (Eulexin)

Flutamide is an antiandrogen that interferes with the binding and intracellular translocation of dihydrotestosterone. Because flutamide's major site of action is at the level of the cancer cell as opposed to the pituitary-gonadal axis, serum testosterone levels do not decrease and may actually increase. Thus, potency may be preserved with flutamide. Side effects include flushing, diarrhea, and gynecomastia. Flutamide is available as 125-mg capsules; the usual dose is 250 mg three times a day. Flutamide is expensive and may cost more than $200 per month.

Aminoglutethimide (Cytadren)

Aminoglutethimide treatment produces a "medical adrenalectomy." It has two sites of action: within the adrenal gland, it inhibits the enzymatic conversion of cholesterol to pregnenolone, and peripherally it blocks the aromatization of androgenic precursors to estrogens. Aminoglutethimide thereby blocks adrenal steroidogenesis and prevents non-adrenal estrogen production. Concomitant glucocorticoids prevent compensatory increases in ACTH secretion that could overcome the aminoglutethimide blockade. In the treatment of breast cancer, aminoglutethimide produces results comparable to surgical adrenalectomy and has the advantages of rapid reversibility and avoidance of major surgery.

Aminoglutethimide toxicity may be considerable. Lethargy and fatigue are nearly universal but improve with time. Generalized rashes are also common. Central nervous system reactions, including nystagmus, ataxia, and somnolence, may also occur.

Aminoglutethimide is available in 250-mg tablets; the drug is well absorbed by the oral route and is excreted by the kidney. The usual dose is 250 mg orally four times a day together with 40 mg of hydrocortisone daily. An alternative regimen is 250 mg twice a day, which does not require the addition of hydrocortisone. As treatment for metastatic breast cancer, aminoglutethimide is comparable to other second- or third-line hormonal manipulations. It also has some activity against prostate cancer that is no longer responsive to DES.

Corticosteroids

The corticosteroids affect cellular metabolism and produce widespread alterations in many organ systems. Cytotoxicity for malignant lymphoid cells is dependent on the presence of specific glucocorticoid receptors. Prednisone is available in 1-, 2.5-, 5-, 10-, 20-, and 50-mg tablets. The usual doses range from 40 to 100 mg/m^2 over 1 to 2 weeks in combination with cytotoxic drugs. Prednisone is an important part of the treatment of acute lymphocytic leukemia, chronic lymphocytic leukemia, lymphomas, and multiple myeloma, and has activity against breast cancer. Steroids may help control hypercalcemia associated with breast cancer, myeloma, and lymphoid malignancies and may temporarily alleviate symptoms from lymphangitic pulmonary metastases.

Dexamethasone (Decadron) is a more potent and longer-acting steroid, commonly used to treat cerebral edema and as an antiemetic. Available for both oral (0.25-, 0.5-, 1.5-, and 4-mg tablets) and parenteral administration (4 mg/ml in 5- and 25-ml vials), therapy for cerebral edema begins with a 10-mg loading dose followed by 4 mg four times daily. A larger dose may provide additional benefit when the clinical situation remains unsatisfactory. Side effects are dependent on the dose and duration of therapy. Fluid retention, hypokalemic alkalosis, subcutaneous tissue atrophy, centripetal obesity, myopathy, osteoporosis, cataracts, and suppression of the hypothalamic-pituitary-adrenal axis occur regularly. Steroids may complicate the management of hypertension and diabetes. Opportunistic organisms may infect patients with steroid-suppressed immune responses.

CHEMOTHERAPY TOXICITY

The antiproliferative action of chemotherapy causes injury to normal tissues as well as to neoplastic tissue. Thus, the common side effects of alopecia, mucositis, and bone marrow suppression are an understandable consequence of the nonspecific nature of cancer chemotherapy. Other less obvious injuries can occur, particularly with prolonged therapy. Serious toxicities to the bone marrow, lung, heart, liver, and kidney may resemble cancer progression or worsening comorbid disease states. The distinction between cancer progression and treatment toxicity is critical to the decision to continue or modify the chemotherapy regimen. Table 5–5 summarizes organ-specific chemotherapy toxicities.

HEMATOLOGIC TOXICITY

The most common side effect of cancer chemotherapy is myelosuppression. With the exception of hormonal therapy, all drugs can cause some bone marrow injury. Bleomycin,

Table 5–5. **CHEMOTHERAPY TOXICITY: MEDICATIONS MOST LIKELY TO CAUSE TOXICITY**

PULMONARY	CARDIAC	HEPATIC	RENAL
Bleomycin	Doxorubicin (Adriamycin)	Methotrexate	Cisplatin
Mitomycin	Daunorubicin	Mercaptopurine	Streptozocin
Carmustine (BCNU)	Mitoxantrone	L-Asparaginase	Methotrexate
Busulfan	Cyclophosphamide (high-dose)	Carmustine (BCNU)	Ifosfamide
		Cyclophosphamide (high-dose)	Mitomycin
		Streptozocin	
		Cytarabine	

vincristine, cisplatin, and L-asparaginase are usually marrow sparing, unless their metabolism is impaired or extremely high doses are used.

Leukopenia generally occurs first because of the short half-life of circulating granulocytes (6 hours). Thrombocytopenia follows because of the 5- to 7-day half-life of platelets. Occasionally, thrombocytopenia will be more severe and more persistent, particularly after administration of a nitrosourea. Because most marrows recover within 21 to 28 days, the interval between chemotherapy treatments is usually 3 to 4 weeks. Notable exceptions are the nitrosoureas and mitomycin C, which usually require intervals of 4 to 6 weeks.

Anemia is a frequent consequence of both cancer (by marrow invasion or as a chronic disease) and cancer treatment. Peripheral macrocytosis and marrow megaloblastoid changes characteristically occur with marrow injury and recovery after chemotherapy, especially with the antimetabolites. Mitomycin C occasionally causes an unpredictable and frequently fatal microangiopathic hemolytic anemia, renal failure, and thrombocytopenia.

Chemotherapy, by itself, rarely causes severe anemia that necessitates transfusion. Age, previous therapy, bone marrow involvement, and blood loss may contribute to lowered marrow reserves in cancer patients receiving chemotherapy.

PULMONARY TOXICITY

Lung injury from chemotherapy is relatively uncommon but potentially fatal. It occurs sporadically after therapy with busulfan, cyclophosphamide, chlorambucil, melphalan, methotrexate, cytosine arabinoside, and procarbazine. Bleomycin, mitomycin C, and the nitrosoureas, however, are the most likely drugs to cause clinically significant pulmonary toxicity. Nitrosourea lung injury appears to be dose related; incidence increases after a total dose of BCNU of 1000 mg/m^2, so that by a dose of 1500 mg/m^2, 50% of patients will have detectable pulmonary impairment. Bleomycin and mitomycin C pulmonary toxicity can occur after very small total doses but are also more likely at higher doses. They can cause an unpredictable, rapidly progressing, severe pulmonary fibrosis that is possibly exacerbated by oxygen therapy.

CARDIAC TOXICITY

Adriamycin, daunorubicin, and to a lesser degree mitoxantrone are the chemotherapeutic agents most commonly associated with cardiac injury. The antitumor antibiotic section of this chapter discusses this more completely. Cyclophosphamide and nitrogen mustard, in the higher doses used for bone marrow transplantation, cause an uncommon, frequently fatal, acute congestive heart failure due to myocardial necrosis. Diethylstilbestrol clearly increases cardiovascular deaths; the risk is lower with daily doses of 1 mg rather than 5 mg. Amsacrine also uncommonly causes acute ventricular arrhythmias and chronic, cumulative, dose-related heart failure. Bleomycin, mitomycin C, actinomycin D, VP-16, and VM-26 cause rare cases of possible cardiac toxicity.

HEPATIC TOXICITY

Some chemotherapeutic agents cause hepatic toxicity (see Table 5–5). Methotrexate in daily oral doses is well known to cause hepatic fibrosis and cirrhosis. This is much less

Table 5–6. **DOSE MODIFICATION WITH HEPATIC DYSFUNCTION (% OF USUAL DOSE)**

DRUG	BILIRUBIN <2 MG/DL	BILIRUBIN 2.0–3.0 MG/DL	BILIRUBIN 3.1–5.0 MG/DL	BILIRUBIN >5 MG/DL
Doxorubicin (Adriamycin)	100	50	25	0
Daunorubicin	100	50	25	0
Mitoxantrone	100	50	25	0
Vincristine	100	50	25	0
Vinblastine	100	50	25	0
Cyclophosphamide	100	100	100	100
Etoposide	100	100	50	0
Fluorouracil	100	100	100	100
Methotrexate	100	100	100	100
Taxol (Investigational)	100	0	0	0

common with intermittent parenteral doses; however, acute hepatocellular injury can occur with high-dose methotrexate. Cholestasis and hepatocellular injury can occur with mercaptopurine, and the development of liver function abnormalities on routine blood tests necessitates treatment discontinuation. Cytosine arabinoside and the nitrosoureas can cause transient increases in hepatic enzymes that rarely limit their usefulness. L-Asparaginase can cause diffuse fatty metamorphosis with significant hepatic dysfunction in 42 to 82% of patients. Plicamycin (mithramycin) in small doses for the treatment of hypercalcemia may cause transient elevations of the liver transaminases, but significant hepatic toxicity is unlikely. Other chemotherapeutic agents result in increased systemic toxicity in the presence of hepatic dysfunction, and Table 5–6 outlines suggested dose modifications.

RENAL TOXICITY

Some chemotherapeutic agents (see Table 5–5) cause acute and irreversible renal toxicity. Cisplatin nephrotoxicity is dose limiting and potentially severe, ranging from mild reversible azotemia to tubular necrosis and irreversible renal failure. For a more complete discussion refer to the cisplatin section of this chapter. Up to 65% of patients who receive streptozocin develop renal dysfunction, and the toxicity is lethal in 11%. The cause is acute tubular injury, resulting in massive proteinuria, hypokalemia, proximal renal tubular acidosis, and the Fanconi syndrome. Nitrosoureas can cause delayed glomerular damage, resulting in insidious progressive renal dysfunction, most commonly occurring at total doses greater than 1500 mg/m^2. The prognosis is unpredictable and may be fatal. Methotrexate causes renal damage by precipitation within the renal tubules; brisk diuresis and urinary alkalinization minimize the risk of renal toxicity. Methotrexate renal failure is usually reversible, but significant systemic methotrexate toxicity usually occurs as a result of decreased methotrexate renal clearance. High-dose cyclophosphamide

Table 5–7. **DOSE MODIFICATION WITH RENAL DYSFUNCTION (% OF USUAL DOSE)**

DRUG	CREATININE <1.5 MG/DL	CREATININE 1.5–2.0 MG/DL	CREATININE 2.1–3.5 MG/DL
Cisplatin	100	100	25–50
Ifosfamide	100	100	75
Bleomycin	100	100	0
Fluorouracil	100	100	100
Cyclophosphamide	100	100	100
Methotrexate	50–100	25–50	0
Streptozocin	100	50	0
Lomustine	100	65	50
Vincristine	100	100	100
Vinblastine	100	100	100

therapy (greater than 50 mg/kg) can cause water intoxication and hyponatremia due to renal tubular damage; this is uncommon with standard-dose therapy. Mitomycin C causes renal damage by a microangiopathic hemolytic uremic syndrome that is frequently fatal. Some data suggest 5-azacitidine may cause proximal renal tubular dysfunction. Table 5–7 indicates dose modifications for chemotherapy in the presence of renal functional impairment in order to prevent unacceptable toxicity.

REFERENCES

General Chemotherapy Reviews

Black DJ, Livingston RB: Antineoplastic drugs in 1990. A review (Part I and Part II). Drugs 39:489–501, 652–673, 1990.

Deuchars KL, Ling V: P-glycoprotein and multidrug resistance in cancer chemotherapy. Semin Oncol 16:156–165, 1989.

Epstein RJ: Drug-induced DNA damage and tumor chemosensitivity. J Clin Oncol 8:2062–2084, 1990.

Krakoff IH: Cancer chemotherapeutic and biologic agents. CA 41:264–278, 1991.

Selected Chemotherapy References

Canetta R, Bragman K, Smaldone L, Rozencweig M: Carboplatin: Current status and future prospects. Cancer Treat Rev 15(suppl B):17–32, 1988.

Chun HG, Leyland-Jones B, Cheson BD: Fludarabine phosphate: A synthetic purine antimetabolite with significant activity against lymphoid malignancies. J Clin Oncol 9:175–188, 1991.

Dorr RT: New findings in the pharmacokinetic, metabolic, and drug-resistance aspects of mitomycin C. Semin Oncol 15(suppl 4):32–41, 1988.

Gandara DR, Perez EA, Wiebe V, DeGregorio MW: Cisplatin chemoprotection and rescue: Pharmacologic modulation of toxicity. Semin Oncol 18(suppl 3):49–55, 1991.

Love RR: Tamoxifen therapy in primary breast cancer: Biology, efficacy, and side effects. J Clin Oncol 7:803–815, 1989.

McGuire WP, Rowinsky EK, Rosenshein NB, et al: Taxol: A unique antineoplastic agent with significant activity in advanced ovarian epithelial neoplasms. Ann Intern Med 111:273–279, 1989.

O'Dwyer PJ, Leyland-Jones B, Alonso MT, et al: Etoposide (VP–16–213): Current status of an active anticancer drug. N Engl J Med 312:692–700, 1985.

Pinedo HM, Peters GFJ: Fluorouracil: Biochemistry and pharmacology. J Clin Oncol 6:1653–1664, 1988.

Sarosy G: Ifosfamide: Pharmacologic overview. Semin Oncol 16(suppl 3):2–8, 1989.

Stein CA, LaRocca RV, Thomas R, et al: Suramin: An anticancer drug with a unique mechanism of action. J Clin Oncol 7:499–508, 1989.

Chemotherapy Toxicity Reviews

Averette HE, Boike GM, Jarrell MA: Effects of cancer chemotherapy on gonadal function and reproductive capacity. CA 40:199–209, 1990.

Boivin JF: Second cancers and other late side effects of cancer treatment. Cancer 65:770–775, 1990.

Doll DC, Ringenberg QS, Yarbro JW: Vascular toxicity associated with antineoplastic agents. J Clin Oncol 4:1405–1417, 1986.

Ehrke MJ, Mihich E, Berd D, Mastrangelo MJ: Effects of anticancer drugs on the immune system in humans. Semin Oncol 16:230–253, 1989.

Filastre JP, Viotte G, Morin JP, Moulin B: Nephrotoxicity of antitumoral agents. Adv Nephrol 17:175–218, 1988.

Lehne G, Lote K: Pulmonary toxicity of cytotoxic and immunosuppressive agents. Acta Oncol 29:13–124, 1990.

Rudolph R, Larson DL: Etiology and treatment of chemotherapeutic agent extravasation injuries: A review. J Clin Oncol 5:1116–1126, 1987.

Schwartz RG, McKenzie WB, Alexander J, et al: Congestive heart failure and left ventricular dysfunction complicating doxorubicin therapy. Am J Med 82:1109–1118, 1987.

6
BIOTHERAPY OF CANCER

Alex Yuang-Chi Chang

Biotherapy is a revolutionary new approach to cancer treatment. In marked contrast to other treatment modalities, biotherapy utilizes the living system. With the premise that neoplastic disease represents a failure of the immune system, investigators have endeavored to treat malignancy by attempts to restore immune competence.

Early studies utilized many nonspecific immune stimulants, such as bacille Calmette-Guérin (BCG) and levamisole, which produced tumor responses in animal models and in early clinical trials but were almost universally unsuccessful in larger controlled clinical studies. More specific activation of the immune system by promoting recognition of tumor antigens utilizing tumor vaccines plus nonspecific immune stimulants was attempted but proved to be only minimally effective.

Recently, significant advances in biotechnology have greatly improved the purity and availability of biologically active molecules and consequently our understanding of the immune system. Specific effector cells in the immune system, including subsets of lymphocytes and macrophages as well as cell products such as cytokines and monoclonal antibodies, have been isolated and show promising value not only in the detection and treatment of advanced disease, but also in the prevention of recurrence of malignancy.

Cytokines are polypeptide proteins produced by cells of the immune system that serve as messengers between cells. They are produced and function at a specific local site and are rarely detectable in the blood. They act by binding to specific surface membrane receptors and generating a second messenger to the nucleus, causing gene activation or suppression. Recombinant DNA and hybridoma techniques can produce large quantities of these cytokines and specific monoclonal antibodies for clinical trials, which will facilitate the wider application of biotherapy.

INTERFERON

Human interferon represents the prototype immunoregulatory protein used in cancer therapy. Initially discovered in 1957 as an antiviral agent, interferon also has antiproliferative and immunomodulatory functions. Interferon consists of three species: alpha, beta, and gamma, with alpha occurring as multiple subspecies. Natural interferons are produced from cell preparations and cultures: alpha interferon from leukocytes, beta interferon from fibroblasts, and gamma interferon (a lymphokine) from T lymphocytes. All three subtypes of interferon are currently produced by recombinant DNA technology. These products are purified and available in large quantities.

Interferons act by binding to cell-surface receptors. Alpha and beta interferons share one receptor, whereas gamma interferon binds to a different receptor. This binding induces secondary messages that alter proliferative activity by inhibiting protein and DNA synthesis. These secondary messages also modulate the immune response by increasing membrane antigen expression, augmenting humoral activity when the interferon is given after antigenic challenge, altering oncogene expression, and stimulating natural killer cells, monocytes, macrophages, and cytotoxic T cells. These responses vary with the type of interferon and the time course of application. Thus, interferons are potent agents that exert diverse effects on a wide range of target cells and organs.

Most cancer treatment programs have used alpha interferon. Responses occur in both heavily pretreated and previously untreated patients. The highest response rates (40 to 90%) have been seen in hairy cell leukemia, Kaposi's sarcoma, cutaneous T-cell lymphomas, and chronic myelogenous leukemia. Response rates of 90% have been reported in hairy cell leukemia; however, the complete response rate is low (see Chapter 8). Interferon also produces responses in renal cell carcinoma, multiple myeloma, melanoma, and non-Hodgkin's lymphoma, with response rates ranging from 20 to 40%. Lung, breast, and colon cancers are only minimally responsive to interferon.

Interferon is primarily cytostatic when in direct contact with tumor cells. Optimal dosages and durations of treatment are not yet well defined. Use of interferon(s) in combination with chemotherapy or radiation is currently being explored. There are now reports of improved response rates in colorectal cancer when alpha interferon is combined with 5-fluorouracil and in multiple myeloma when alpha interferon is used with cyclophosphamide, melphalan, BCNU, prednisone, and vincristine. The U.S. Food and Drug Administration has approved alpha interferon for the treatment of hairy cell leukemia, Kaposi's sarcoma associated with AIDS, and condyloma accumulata (genital warts). Gamma interferon is approved for the treatment of chronic granulomatous disease.

Interferon toxicity can be both acute and chronic. A flulike syndrome occurs acutely and is characterized by fever, chills, myalgia, headache, and malaise. This toxicity is greatest with initial doses, responds to antipyretics and anti-inflammatory agents, and decreases with subsequent doses. Additional subacute and chronic toxicities include mild myelosuppression, nausea, vomiting, anorexia, weight loss, increased liver transaminase levels, proteinuria, and fatigue, which is sometimes profound and dose limiting. Rare chronic effects include severe central nervous system toxicity, peripheral neuropathy, cardiac arrhythmias, congestive heart failure, hypocalcemia, and hyperkalemia.

MONOCLONAL ANTIBODIES

The use of monoclonal antibodies specific for tumor cell antigens represents an attractive approach to cancer detection and treatment. In theory, the ability to focus therapy specifically on tumor cells and avoid toxicity to normal tissues should circumvent the principal limitation of conventional chemotherapy.

Large quantities of pure monoclonal antibodies for clinical use have been produced by hybridomas. Hybridoma technology utilizes the antibody response of rodents that are inoculated with the patient's tumor cells. The animal's B lymphocytes are then collected and subsequently fused in vitro with a highly proliferative cell line, creating a cell culture that produces large quantities of tumor-specific antibodies. The monoclonal antibodies are infused into the patient and localize in tumor tissue. As effectors, monoclonal antibodies have been directed in vivo against specific T-cell antigens in acute lymphoblastic leukemia and cutaneous T-cell lymphomas. Decreases in circulating T cells and skin plaques were noted transiently. Clinical trials have also studied the effects of monoclonal antibodies in patients with melanoma or breast, colon, lung, and renal cell carcinomas with some responses in small numbers of patients. However, in these trials the antibody specificity for malignant cells was found to be relative and not absolute, resulting in cross-reactivity with normal tissue. Tumor cell antigenic heterogeneity and antigenic modulation further frustrate efforts to treat human malignancies with monoclonal antibodies.

Toxicity of monoclonal antibody therapy has been appreciable, with fevers, chills, dyspnea, wheezing, hypotension, nausea, vomiting, skin rashes, and anaphylactoid reactions. Because these first-generation monoclonal antibodies are of murine origin, patients may produce antibodies against them and develop serum sickness–like toxicity; thus, the use of these monoclonal antibodies may be limited. Second (chimeric) and third (humanized) generations of monoclonal antibodies are being developed to reduce side effects and increase specificity. For patients undergoing autologous bone marrow transplantation, monoclonal antibody treatment of the bone marrow in vitro to purge malignant cells avoids systemic toxicity.

As vectors, monoclonal antibodies have been conjugated with both radioisotopes and cytotoxic agents. Investigational efforts have used the antibody-radioisotope conjugates to detect subclinical cancer deposits. The local accumulation of monoclonal antibody-isotope conjugates has also been proposed as a "magic bullet" for specific delivery of radiation to tumor deposits. Conjugation of monoclonal antibodies with toxins (such as ricin A chain) and cytotoxic agents is also being investigated as a specific delivery system of the toxin or drug to the malignant cells, sparing the normal cells of the patient, or the bone marrow preparation when used in vitro.

Limitations of immune conjugates include varying degrees of (1) cross-reactivity with normal tissue as a result of less than absolute monoclonal antibody specificity, (2) uptake of conjugates by the liver and spleen, (3) loss of antibody specificity after conjugation, (4) heterogeneous tumor antigens and antigenic modulation, and (5) inadequate delivery of the conjugates to the tumor. In addition, monoclonal antibody conjugates cause the same toxicities as nonconjugated monoclonal antibodies. Monoclonal antibody techniques for clinical use are currently in their infancy. Potential exists for efficacy and toxicity. Extensive research efforts continue in this rapidly developing field.

INTERLEUKIN 2

Produced by helper T cells, interleukin 2 (IL-2) is a lymphokine that supports the growth of activated T cells that bear an IL-2 receptor. Both in vitro and in vivo, IL-2 induces proliferation of this T-cell subset and promotes differentiation of null cells into cytotoxic cells (lymphokine-activated killer cells, LAK). It can also induce lymphocytes to produce tumor necrosis factor (TNF), gamma interferon, and possibly other cytokines. Produced by recombinant DNA technology, IL-2 has been used alone and with LAK lymphocytes in the treatment of malignancies. IL-2 has also had some success in partially correcting the T-cell abnormalities of AIDS patients.

Recent clinical studies with IL-2 and LAK cell preparations have generated wide interest. In this program, the patient's lymphocytes are collected and then exposed to IL-2 in vitro. The null subset of the lymphocytes transforms into LAK cells; then the expanded population of LAK cells is reinfused into the patient with additional IL-2 to maintain LAK cell effectiveness. These circulating LAK cells then may destroy malignant cells in vivo, but they do not affect normal cells. High-dose IL-2 alone and IL-2/LAK produce similar results.

IL-2/LAK clinical trials have demonstrated responses in 20% of patients with refractory and metastatic renal cell carcinoma and melanoma. Lower response rates were seen in colon cancers. The principal toxicity encountered was significant fluid retention in the majority of patients, often resulting in pulmonary edema and occasionally requiring artifical ventilation. The interstitial fluid accumulation is caused by the effect of tumor necrosis factor on endothelial cells, which produces nitrous oxide and subsequent vasodilation and capillary leak. Treatment-related deaths have been reported. Interleukins other than IL-2 have been cloned and are being evaluated for cancer treatment.

MACROPHAGES

Macrophages are an important component of the immune surveillance system. When activated by a T-cell lymphokine, macrophage-activating factor (MAF), macrophages recognize and lyse many types of tumor cells but do not affect normal cells. The cytolytic process requires direct contact between the macrophage and the tumor cell. Tumor cell recognition by macrophages is independent of surface antigens; thus, malignant cell heterogeneity does not result in treatment resistance.

The most efficient method of macrophage activation uses activating agents packaged in liposomes. The infused liposomes are phagocytized and processed by macrophages, resulting in macrophage effectors that are capable of destroying tumor cells.

TUMOR-INFILTRATING LYMPHOCYTES

Tumor-infiltrating lymphocytes (TIL) are a unique subset of lymphocytes that invade and destroy autologous malignant tumors. They are present in essentially all tumors and have unique lytic specificity for each tumor. TIL represent beneficial host recognition and response to malignancy but are present in only small numbers. They are considered to be 50 to 100 times more potent than LAK cells. Investigators have been able to isolate TIL from tumors by labor-intensive, technically complex procedures. TIL are then greatly increased in number by exposing them to IL-2 in culture. Prior to reinfusion of TIL and IL-2, the patient is immunosuppressed with cyclophosphamide or total body irradiation. Preliminary clinical trials show a high response rate but short response duration. Clinical trials with TIL modified by gene transduction are ongoing.

TUMOR NECROSIS FACTOR

Produced by macrophages, tumor necrosis factor (TNF) is a cytokine that is selectively cytotoxic for a wide variety of tumor cells. The name for this cytokine is derived from the ability of TNF to induce hemorrhagic necrosis when directly injected into tumors or given in high intravenous doses in animal models. Utilization of recombinant TNF in treating malignancies is hindered by its additional actions, including regulation of the hematopoietic and immune systems and mediation of endotoxic shock, general inflammation, cachexia of chronic disease, and coagulation activation. Initial clinical trials demonstrated significant toxicity, including hypotension, fever, chills, fatigue, nausea, vomiting, and local irritation at the injection site. Tumor response has been minimal, most likely due to inadequate TNF levels. Recent research has focused on local delivery of TNF directly to tumor tissues either by liposomes or tumor-infiltrating lymphocytes.

TUMOR VACCINES

Vaccines against infectious diseases promote specific recognition and efficient destruction of the infectious agents. Similarly, tumor vaccines are an attempt to utilize the immune system to recognize and destroy malignant cells. This principle is predicated on the fact that tumor cells have uniquely identifiable membrane surface antigens that differ from those of normal cells. Because these tumor cells have propagated unopposed by the host's immune system, an immune stimulant together with tumor cell antigens is required to specifically sensitize the immune surveillance system.

Tumor vaccine preparation requires excising an adequate amount of tumor from the patient. Tumor cells are then rendered nonviable by mechanical and enzymatic disruption as well as by irradiation. To augment antigenicity, tumor cell lysates are mixed with immune adjuvants such as Freund's, bacille Calmette-Guérin (BCG), *Corynebacterium parvum*, and more recently Newcastle disease virus (NDV). The vaccine is given intradermally, and immune response is measured by the delayed-type hypersensitivity skin reaction.

Early clinical trials focused on melanoma and renal cell carcinoma. More recent studies have included colon and breast carcinoma. In a small percent of patients, responses are dramatic and prolonged. Patients most likely to respond have low tumor volume and minimal tumor surface antigen heterogenicity. Improved response rates occur when tumor vaccines are supplemented with systemic recombinant cytokines or lymphokines such as IL-1, IL-2, and interferon.

REFERENCES

Beutler B, Cerami A. Cachectin: More than a tumor necrosis factor. N Engl J Med 316:379–385, 1987.

Borden EC, Sondel PM: Lymphokines and cytokines: Immunotherapy realized. Cancer 65:800–814, 1990.

Dillman RO: Monoclonal antibodies for treating cancer. Ann Intern Med 111:592–603, 1989.

Fidler IJ: Critical factors in the biology of human cancer metastasis: Twenty-eight G.H.A. Clowes Memorial Award Lecture. Cancer Res 50:6130–6138, 1990.

Goldenberg DM, Blumenthal RD, Sharkey RM. Biological and clinical perspectives of cancer imaging and therapy with radiolabeled antibodies. Semin Cancer Biol 1:217–225, 1990.

Golomb HM: Interferons: Present and future use in cancer therapy. J Clin Oncol 4:123–125, 1986.

Mitchell MS, Harel W, Kempf RA, et al: Active specific immunotherapy for melanoma. J Clin Oncol 8:856–869, 1990.

Rosenberg SA, Lotze MT, Muul LM, et al: A progress report on the treatment of 157 patients with advanced cancer using lymphokine-activated killer cells and interleukin–2 or high dose interleukin-2 alone. N Engl J Med 316:859–897, 1987.

Rosenberg SA, Packard BS, Aebersold PM, et al: Use of tumor-infiltrating lymphocytes and interleukin-2 in the immunotherapy of patients with metastatic melanoma. N Engl J Med 319:1676–1680, 1988.

Rosenberg SA: Gene transfer into humans: Immunotherapy of patients with advanced melanoma, using tumor infiltrating lymphocytes modified by retroviral gene transduction. N Engl J Med 323:570–578, 1990.

7
ACUTE LEUKEMIAS

Jacob M. Rowe

The acute leukemias are diseases of the pluripotent stem cell, expressing themselves either as disorders of the hematopoietic system (acute myelogenous leukemia [AML]) or of the lymphoid system (acute lymphoblastic leukemia [ALL]). In spite of a high initial response rate following optimal therapy, the majority of adults with acute leukemia will die from the disease.

INCIDENCE AND EPIDEMIOLOGY

The incidence of acute leukemia in adults is 3.5 cases per 100,000 population per year. It is the leading cause of cancer deaths in adults less than 35 years of age. In adults the incidence of AML is much higher than ALL, the reverse of the incidence in childhood (Fig. 7–1).

Although the cause of acute leukemia remains unknown in the majority of patients, several risk factors related to an increased incidence have been identified. Leukemia following radiation exposure has been documented by the Atomic Bomb Casualty Com-

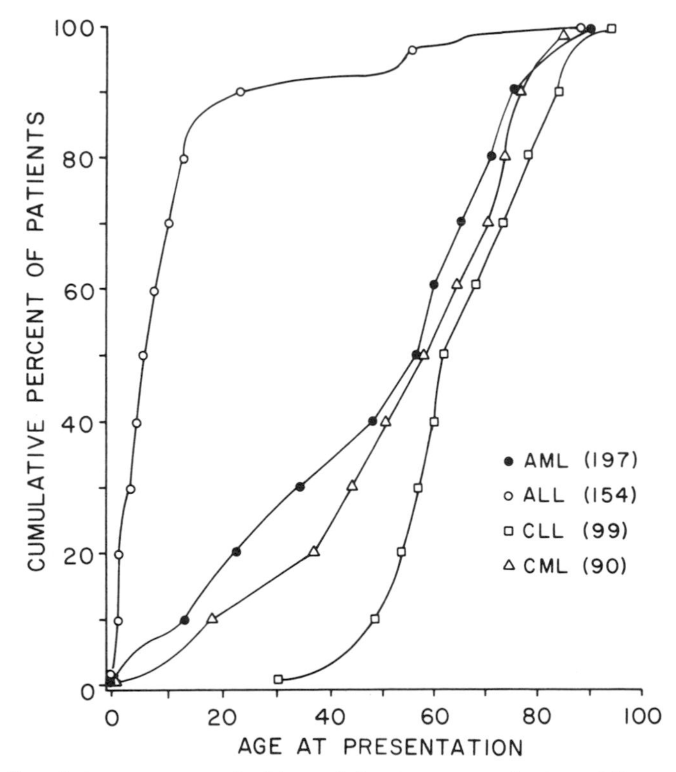

Figure 7–1. Cumulative percentage of subjects of the given age at the time of diagnosis with acute myeloid (AML), acute lymphocytic (ALL), chronic myeloid (CML), and chronic lymphocytic (CLL) leukemias. Number of patients with each type of leukemia shown in parentheses. (*From* Rowe JM: Clinical and laboratory features of the myeloid and lymphocytic leukemias. Am J Med Tech 49:103–109, 1983.)

mission in Hiroshima and Nagasaki. Benzene exposure has been closely associated with the subsequent development of leukemia, and chemical leukemogens have been identified in animal models. Cytotoxic therapy, especially alkylating agents, increases the risk for developing leukemia. These therapy-related leukemias, or secondary leukemias, have a poorer prognosis than de novo leukemias not associated with prior cytotoxic therapy. The combination of alkylating therapy and radiation therapy, as was frequently administered in the past to patients with Hodgkin's disease, confers the highest risk for subsequent development of acute leukemia—almost invariably AML.

ACUTE MYELOGENOUS LEUKEMIA

This is a disease of the myeloid or hematopoietic stem cell (Fig. 7–2). As a result, all cell lines are likely to be qualitatively defective, irrespective of the actual cell count.

CLINICAL AND LABORATORY FEATURES

Most patients with AML present with progressive fatigue and commonly have evidence for infection or a bleeding diathesis. The white blood count is usually elevated but may be normal or low. Anemia is present and is often profound. Thrombocytopenia is also common, and patients may present with petechiae, ecchymoses, hematuria, or gastrointestinal bleeding. Hemorrhage in the central nervous system is a rare but often fatal complication of acute leukemia. In the monocytic and myelomonocytic variants, there may be signs of extramedullary involvement, including gum hypertrophy, skin infiltration (leukemia cutis), or meningeal leukemia. Rarely, a solid tumor mass known as a chloroma or granulocytic sarcoma may be the only presenting sign in acute myeloid leukemia.

Examination of the peripheral blood smear may reveal dysplastic changes in the red

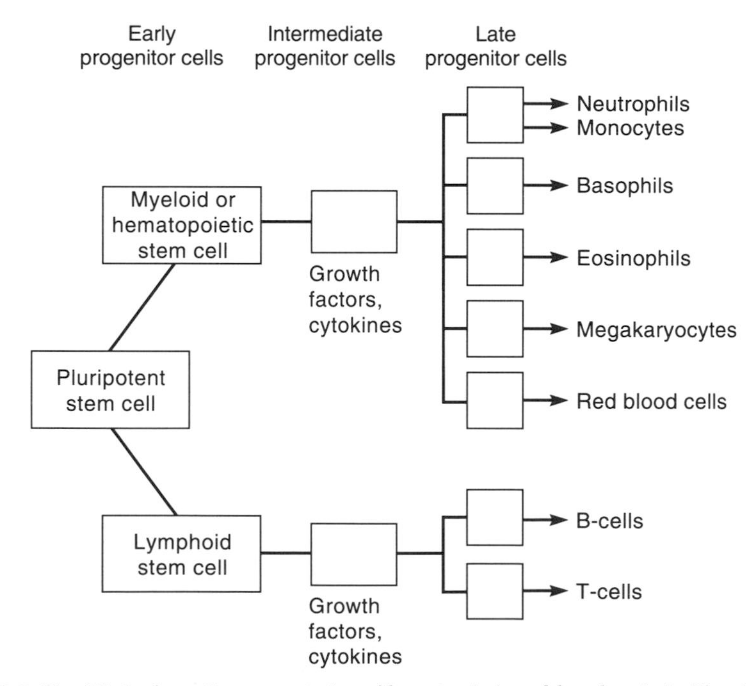

Figure 7–2. Simplified schematic representation of hematopoiesis and lymphopoiesis. The pluripotent stem cell differentiates into hematopoietic and lymphoid stem cells. Intermediate and late progenitors develop under the influence of growth factors and cytokines. Acute leukemias usually originate from clonal abnormalities at the stem cell level, explaining the various clinical expressions of these malignancies.

cells, granulocytes, and platelets. Myeloid immaturity is often present, and the diagnosis may be based on the presence of typical blast cells in the peripheral blood. The bone marrow is usually hypercellular and is often replaced with the leukemic blast cells. Uncommonly, the bone marrow may be hypocellular; in this case, the diagnosis may be somewhat more difficult to establish and will depend on a very precise morphologic delineation of the cells that are present.

The rapid turnover of leukemic blasts produces a hypermetabolic state with elevated lactate dehydrogenase (LDH) and uric acid levels. Electrolyte imbalances such as hypokalemia and hypophosphatemia are common features at presentation. Care must be taken to distinguish several laboratory abnormalities due to the ongoing metabolism or lysis of blast cells in the collected specimen prior to lab processing. Pseudohyperkalemia may be confirmed by checking an anticoagulated plasma specimen. Pseudohypoglycemia occurs as a result of glucose utilization by blast cells. Pseudohypoxemia due to rapid oxygen consumption by leukocytes, known as "leukocyte larceny," may make it impossible to determine the arterial blood oxygen accurately.

CLASSIFICATION

The traditional classification of AML is based on morphologic and histochemical characteristics of the peripheral blood and bone marrow cells. Recently, cytogenetic analysis and flow cytometric studies with immunophenotyping have provided invaluable additional information and may have special prognostic value in the classification of AML. Certain cell types may predict for particular clinical features such as the increased incidence of disseminated intravascular coagulation with the promyelocytic variant. However, all the subtypes of AML have overlapping clinical syndromes and are fundamentally the same disease and respond to identical therapy. One of the most widely used morphologic classifications (described by the French, American, British [FAB] group) relates the morphology of leukemic cells to their presumed hematopoietic counterparts. Several types of AML (M1–M7) have been described: M1 represents undifferentiated myeloblastic leukemia; the M2 variant, differentiated myeloblastic leukemia, has classic myeloblasts with Auer rods; M3 is promyelocytic leukemia; M4 is myelomonocytic leukemia; M5 is monocytic leukemia; M6 describes erythroleukemia; and M7 is megakaryoblastic leukemia, or what was formerly often referred to as acute myelofibrosis.

CYTOGENETICS

Clonal cytogenetic abnormalities, defined using banding techniques, are present in the majority of patients with newly diagnosed AML. Certain cytogenetic abnormalities may be found in both acute myeloid and acute lymphoblastic leukemias, but some are found exclusively in AML; these include t(8;21)(q22;q22) and 16q22. These abnormalities have been associated with a better overall prognosis, although it is very difficult to apply such information to the management of an individual patient. Other cytogenetic abnormalities often seen in AML are t(15;17), trisomy 8, and 11q23 (associated with classic monoblastic morphology). Abnormalities of chromosomes 5 and 7 (del 5q and del 7q) are commonly seen in therapy-related AML or in elderly patients with de novo AML. These variants are often associated with a more resistant form of the disease, with a somewhat lesser likelihood of attaining a complete remission.

TREATMENT

Induction Therapy

This most commonly consists of an anthracycline or its analogue—drugs such as daunorubicin, idarubicin, or mitoxantrone—together with cytosine arabinoside. A typical proven induction regimen for AML consists of daunorubicin 60 mg/m^2 on days 1 to 3 together with cytosine arabinoside 100 mg/m^2 by continuous infusion for 7 days. Results from cooperative group trials reveal that the overall remission rate using such a regimen is 65%, with a larger percent of patients under the age of 40 obtaining a complete remission. Typically, a day 14 bone marrow sample is examined and, if there is unequivocal residual leukemia, a second course of therapy, in identical doses, is administered at that time. As many as 25 to 40% of patients will require two courses of induction chemotherapy to attain a complete remission. There appears to be no prognostic significance for patients who require two initial courses of induction therapy to attain such a remission.

The length of hospitalization for induction chemotherapy is 4 to 6 weeks, during which time the patient will have a 2- to 4-week period of absolute pancytopenia. During this period the patient will be multiply transfused with red cells and platelets and will require multiple antibiotics and isolation for life-threatening infections.

Postremission Therapy

Once the patient has entered a complete remission, the only hope of long-term survival rests in some form of postremission therapy. In individuals less than 45 years of age who have a histocompatible sibling, most hematologists and oncologists recommend an allogeneic bone marrow transplant (see Chapter 31), which offers such patients a 50% chance of long-term disease-free survival. Actually, the relapse rate following transplantation is low, on the order of 15 to 20%, but the peritransplant mortality, primarily from graft-versus-host disease and interstitial pneumonitis, may be as high as 25 to 30%.

Conventional intensive consolidation therapy typically employs high doses of cytosine arabinoside with or without an anthracycline or other antileukemic agents. Regimens vary from one to approximately six complete cycles of high-dose chemotherapy. There is no clear evidence that one form of consolidation therapy is better than another.

A promising avenue for postremission therapy employs autologous bone marrow transplantation. The advantage of such a procedure is that all individuals have a donor; it can be offered to patients up to the age of 60 years (or to somewhat older patients if they are very fit); and the procedural mortality is lower than with allogeneic transplants. The overall mortality for AML patients in first remission is just under 10%. A disadvantage of this procedure, when compared with allogeneic transplantation, is the absence of the immunologic effect of graft versus leukemia, which is now recognized to have major antileukemic properties. Another disadvantage is the potential reinfusion of leukemic cells, although most evidence suggests that most patients relapse postautotransplantation because of residual leukemia due to failure to eradicate the disease rather than due to the reinfusion of contaminated leukemic bone marrow. Many methods of cleansing or purging bone marrow are employed, some using monoclonal antibodies or cytotoxic agents such as 4-hydroxyperoxycyclophosphamide (4-HC) or mafosphamide (this is more commonly used in Europe). There are no unequivocal data that demonstrate that purging is of value in the therapy of AML.

Autologous transplantation for postremission therapy in AML has the potential to achieve long-term disease-free survival in up to 40 to 50% of patients. Major clinical trials are in progress to evaluate prospectively the role of autologous bone marrow transplantation, comparing it to a more conventional established consolidation regimen using chemotherapy alone. Because of the absence of the major complications associated with allogeneic bone marrow transplantation, such as graft-versus-host disease or interstitial pneumonitis, it may be better to think of autologous bone marrow transplantation as the most intensive form of consolidation therapy. Clinical trials may simply demonstrate whether such therapy has added curative potential.

Refractory AML

Unfortunately, the majority of patients with AML will relapse. Once the patient has relapsed, the only therapy with curative potential is bone marrow transplantation. Once a patient has relapsed, the first step is reinduction into a second complete remission. If the patient has had a first remission of greater than 6 months, there is a 50 to 65% chance of obtaining a second complete remission using a standard regimen such as mitoxantrone, 12 mg/m^2 for 5 days, together with VP-16, 100 mg/m^2 for 5 days, or using high doses of cytosine arabinoside, 2 to 3 g/m^2 $\times$ 8 to 12 doses. Refractory AML patients who never attained a complete remission with standard therapy—primary treatment failures—or those who relapsed after a very short first remission, are best entered in experimental clinical trials to determine the efficacy of newer agents as well as combinations of established agents to evaluate the best regimen for such patients. Currently, it is possible to reinduce 20 to 30% of these refractory patients into complete remission. The role of cytokines such as interferons or interleukins (IL-2) in prolonging the duration of the second remission is being investigated. Cytosine arabinoside in low doses of 10 mg/m^2 every 12 hours for 21 days, given as maintenance therapy, may also significantly prolong the remission duration.

Supportive Care

Major improvements have taken place over the past 2 decades in the supportive care of the patient with acute leukemia, and these developments are responsible, in part, for the improved results in the therapy of AML.

Infections remain the main threat for the absolutely neutropenic patient. The management of the febrile neutropenic patient must be empiric, since infections in such patients are life threatening and delay to await results of cultures is unwise (see Chap. 28). When absolutely neutropenic patients become febrile, even without an obvious source, they must be placed on broad-spectrum antibiotics that will provide effective coverage against gram-negative organisms. Traditionally, two antibiotics are used: usually a semisynthetic penicillin with an aminoglycoside. In the future, it may be possible to use a single broad-spectrum antibiotic such as one of the newer beta-lactamase–resistant antibiotics (i.e., imipenem or ceftazidine). The empiric addition of specific antistaphylococcal antibiotics is recommended by some authorities because nearly all leukemic patients now have central venous catheters, and 50% of initial fevers are due to gram-positive infections. However, treatment delay awaiting positive blood cultures is much more likely to be fatal in the case of gram-positive infections than with gram-negative infections.

With the advent of superior broad-spectrum antibiotics, fewer patients are dying of bacterial sepsis, and the major cause of death, especially in young adults with acute leukemia, is fungal infection, either with *Candida* species or *Aspergillus*. *Mucor* sepsis is a less common fungal pathogen, but it is especially important in the diabetic patient. The therapy of fungal infections represents a unique challenge. If treatment is deferred until cultures demonstrate systemic fungal infection, the outcome is likely to be fatal. Therefore, if a patient remains febrile 24 to 48 hours after institution of broad-spectrum antibiotics, coverage with amphotericin B is initiated. Certain circumstances increase the likelihood of fungal infections, and in these instances prophylactic amphotericin B may be considered. Special high-risk groups include patients with prior therapy with high-dose corticosteroids, protracted granulocytopenia prior to admission to the hospital, and prior fungal sepsis during the preceding few months.

The use of white cell transfusion remains controversial. There is marked variability of the white cell product employed and the ability of the blood bank to deliver the product to the patient within a few hours of collection from the donor. White cell transfusion should be considered in life-threatening conditions such as documented gram-negative infections with hemodynamic compromise, resistance to standard antimicrobial therapy, or invasive aspergillosis. The use of growth factors such as granulocyte-macrophage colony-stimulating factor (GM-CSF) is now being evaluated in several prospective clinical trials to see if these recombinant cytokines may reduce the period of neutropenia and the mortality and morbidity related to infections. No unequivocal evidence supports the use of prophylactic antimicrobial therapy before a patient becomes febrile or the use of gut-sterilizing antibiotics or sterilized food products. The mainstay of prophylaxis rests with placing patients in reverse isolation with meticulous hand washing by all health care personnel.

Management of profoundly pancytopenic patients requires repeated red cell and platelet transfusions. With multiple platelet transfusions, patients develop alloimmunization and become progressively more refractory to subsequent platelet transfusion. Alloimmunization may be reduced by using special filters for both red cells and platelets, single-donor HLA-matched and family donors, or platelets from ABO-compatible donors. Because many patients will subsequently undergo bone marrow transplantation, it is critically important to administer blood products that are negative for cytomegalovirus (CMV) to those patients who are CMV negative at presentation. Such a precaution may decrease the incidence of fatal complications from CMV in the bone marrow transplant setting (Chap. 31).

Cell lysis from cytotoxic therapy produces a large amount of uric acid, which must be excreted by the kidneys and may cause acute renal failure. To prevent this complication, all patients with a high leukemia burden should be started on allopurinol and receive vigorous IV hydration prior to initiating cytotoxic therapy (Chap. 23).

Unusual Complications

Disseminated intravascular coagulopathy (DIC) may develop in any patient with acute leukemia but is more likely in promyelocytic leukemia. DIC, if not present initially, may develop during therapy when cells are lysed and release thrombogenic material. Optimal management of DIC in promyelocytic leukemia remains controversial, but a useful guideline is as follows: (1) frequent monitoring of coagulation parameters; (2) if there is no evidence of clinical bleeding and only mild coagulation abnormalities, close observation without the addition of prophylactic heparin; and (3) if the patient develops evidence of clinical bleeding or evidence of severe DIC, institute low doses of heparin, 300 to 500 units per hour by continuous infusion, together with twice daily platelets and cryoprecipitate or fresh frozen plasma. When the tumor burden has been significantly reduced, it will usually be possible to stop both the heparin and the replacement therapy.

Hyperleukocytic leukemias often require emergent therapy, especially if signs of leukostasis are present. Clinical features include dyspnea and central nervous system (CNS) signs and symptoms, as well as funduscopic findings of distended vessels, blurred disc margins, and hemorrhagic infiltrates. To relieve the signs of leukostasis and to avoid complications related to massive tumor lysis, leukapheresis should be employed. Patients are leukapheresed until the blast count is less than 50,000, at which point standard antileukemic therapy is given.

Meningeal leukemia most commonly occurs in the lymphoblastic leukemias and the monocytic variants of AML. Unless the patient has CNS signs or symptoms, cerebrospinal fluid should not be examined until the blasts have cleared from the peripheral blood because the cerebrospinal fluid may become contaminated with leukemic blasts from the peripheral blood, especially during a traumatic spinal tap. If meningeal leukemia is present, therapy, given by lumbar puncture or via an Omaya reservoir, consists of methotrexate, 12 to 15 mg, and/or cytosine arabinoside, 30 to 50 mg. Intrathecal therapy is given every 3 days until the cerebrospinal fluid is clear on at least two to three occasions. Although the cerebrospinal fluid can be successfully cleared and the patients may attain a complete peripheral remission, the CNS remains a site of potential relapse. The use of cranial irradiation in uncomplicated meningeal leukemia is not considered standard therapy in AML.

ACUTE LYMPHOBLASTIC LEUKEMIA

Unlike ALL of childhood, in which the majority of children can be cured, the long-term survival for adult patients with ALL remains dismal. Established poor prognostic factors include a high white count at presentation ($>$25,000 to 30,000/μL), the presence of the Philadelphia chromosome with the (9:22) translocation, bulky disease such as a mediastinal mass, pure B-cell ALL, and adult age. Clinical and laboratory features are similar to the presenting characteristics for AML.

CLASSIFICATION

Morphologic classification of ALL is less useful than it is for AML, and for practical purposes it is far better to base therapeutic decisions on the immunophenotypic and cytogenetic analyses. Eighty percent of adult ALL comprise non-T, non-B cells with surface markers that indicate B-cell precursors. Twenty percent of adult ALL are of T-cell origin and 1 to 2% are of B-cell type. Most of these leukemias demonstrate the common ALL antigen (CALLA) on the cell surface, as well as the presence of the intracellular enzymes such as terminal deoxynucleotidyl transferase (TdT).

CYTOGENETICS

The most common cytogenetic abnormality in adult ALL is also one that confers a poor prognosis. The Philadelphia chromosome (Ph^1), t(9;22)(q34;q11) can be found in approximately 25% of newly diagnosed patients with ALL. A very small fraction of these patients may be exhibiting the lymphoid blast crisis of chronic myelogenous leukemia without known antecedent abnormalities in the blood counts. The Ph^1 chromosome is found most commonly in non-T, non-B cell ALL and is never found in T-cell ALL. It tends to occur in older adults and always expresses early B-lineage–associated antigens in immunophenotypic analysis. This may be one of the reasons why T-cell ALL in adults does not appear to be an adverse prognostic factor as it is in childhood ALL. Other common cytogenetic abnormalities in ALL are t(4;11)(q21;q23), t(1;19)(q23;p13), and t(8;14)(q24;q32). The t(1;19)(q23;p13) is associated with the pre-B phenotype, whereas the t(8;14)(q24;q32) abnormality appears to be most specific for the rare B-cell ALL.

TREATMENT

Induction Therapy

Irrespective of the phenotype or cytogenetic abnormality, all patients with ALL receive identical induction regimens that usually contain prednisone, vincristine, and an anthracycline. A significant number of patients may go into remission using prednisone and vincristine alone, but other drugs have been added to increase the proportion of complete remitters. Induction therapy in ALL yields a 70 to 80% complete remission rate, which then must be followed by additional therapy.

Postremission Therapy

Following induction therapy, patients require prolonged maintenance therapy (from 9 to 24 months). This therapy utilizes alternating regimens of several effective drugs, including anthracyclines, cytosine arabinoside, cyclophosphamide, methotrexate, asparaginase, vincristine, and prednisone. The majority of such maintenance programs can be administered on an outpatient basis.

Central Nervous System Prophylaxis

CNS treatment is mandated even if no meningeal involvement was documented at presentation. It may not be critical to administer CNS prophylaxis at induction, but it is employed throughout most maintenance or intensification regimens. In adults, it is not critical whether one uses cranial irradiation, intrathecal prophylaxis, or systemic therapy with high-dose cytosine arabinoside—all appear to provide satisfactory CNS prophylaxis, preventing late CNS relapses.

Relapsed ALL

The majority of patients with ALL will relapse. The success of reinduction therapy depends on the duration of the first remission. Patients who have had a first remission of 18 months or more have an almost equal likelihood of achieving a second remission as they did at presentation. For such patients, it is not necessary to utilize a new non–cross-resistant regimen for reinduction. However, patients who relapse after a very brief first remission or while receiving maintenance chemotherapy, are likely to require the use of non–cross-resistant agents, and achieving a second remission is difficult. Irrespective of the duration of the first remission, once the patient has relapsed, the outcome is always fatal without bone marrow transplantation.

Bone Marrow Transplantation

Experience with bone marrow transplantation for ALL—both allogeneic and autologous—is much more limited than it is for AML. Results of allogeneic transplants in adults in first remission ALL have shown long-term disease-free survival rates on the order of 50 to 60%, much like those in AML. Patients who have relapsed with ALL who are under 50 years of age and have a histocompatible sibling should be referred for allogeneic transplantation after a second or subsequent remission has been attained. If no donor is available, they should be referred to centers employing trials using autologous bone marrow transplantation, with or without purging with monoclonal antibodies. As in AML, there is no evidence that purging is superior to autotransplants without purging.

Supportive Care

Supportive care for patients with ALL is similar to that used in AML and will not be repeated here. Additional risks for ALL patients include steroid exposure and the tumor lysis syndrome. Induction therapy includes high doses of corticosteroids, which increase the incidence of opportunistic infections such as *Pneumocystis carinii*. Furthermore, fevers may be masked for a time, and diagnosis of infections may be delayed. Additionally, fungal infections are probably more common in ALL patients receiving high doses of corticosteroids.

The tumor lysis syndrome may occur in ALL patients with high cell counts when treatment with corticosteroids is instituted. The most common abnormalities are hypocalcemia, hyperkalemia, hyperphosphatemia, hyperuricemia, elevated creatinine, blood urea nitrogen, and LDH (Chap. 23). In order to ameliorate or prevent this condition, leukapheresis is used to reduce high cell counts; patients are begun on allopurinol, 300 to 600 mg orally per day; and for those at significant risk for development of tumor lysis syndrome, vigorous hydration with urinary alkalinization is employed.

SUMMARY

Acute leukemias have been, and remain, among the most aggressive and lethal malignancies in adults. Improvements in the therapy and long-term outcome of this disease have been based on using better agents to achieve and prolong remission, improving supportive care measures, and using both autologous and allogeneic bone marrow transplantation. The role of cytokines and growth factors in the care of such patients should be defined in this decade.

REFERENCES

Bennett JM, Catovosky D, et al: Proposals for the classification of the acute leukemias. Br J Haematol 51:189–199, 1982.
Cassileth PA, Begg CB, Silber R, et al: Prolonged unmaintained remission after intensive consolidation therapy in adult acute non-lymphocytic leukemia. Cancer Treat Rep 71:137–140, 1987.
Champlin R, Gale RP: Acute myelogenous leukemia, recent advances in therapy. Blood 69:1551–1562, 1987.
Forman SJ, Blume KG: Allogeneic bone marrow transplantation for acute leukemia. Hematol/Oncol Clin of North Am 4:515–533, 1990.
Hoelzer D, Thiel E, Loeffler H, et al: Prognostic factors in a multicenter study for treatment of acute lymphoblastic leukemia. Blood 71:123–131, 1988.
Hussein KK, Dahlberg S, et al: Treatment for acute lymphoblastic leukemia in adults with intensive induction, consolidation and maintenance chemotherapy. Blood 73:578–563, 1989.
Mayer RJ: Allogeneic transplantation versus intensive chemotherapy in first remission acute leukemia: Is there a "best" choice? J Clin Oncol 6:1532–1534, 1988.
Thomas ED, Buchner CD, Banaji M, et al: One hundred patients with acute leukemia treated by chemotherapy, total body irradiation, allogeneic bone marrow transplantation. Blood 49:511–533, 1977.
Yeager AM, Kaizer H, Santos GW, et al: Autologous bone marrow transplantation in patients with acute non-lymphocytic leukemia using ex vivo marrow treatment with 4-hydroxyperoxycyclophosphamide. N Engl J Med 315:141–147, 1986.

8
THE CHRONIC LEUKEMIAS

John M. Bennett

In 1991, approximately 17,000 new cases of chronic leukemia were diagnosed in the United States. These leukemias include chronic granulocytic leukemia (CGL), atypical chronic myeloid leukemia (aCML), the chronic (mature) B and T lymphoid leukemias (CLL), and hairy cell leukemia. The term *chronic* refers to a cell type that is relatively well differentiated, in contrast to the immature blast cells of the acute leukemias. The implication that these diseases have chronic durations is misleading; the median survival of patients with these leukemias is in the range of 4 years.

CHRONIC GRANULOCYTIC LEUKEMIA

CGL is biphasic: the first phase is a chronic indolent disease that progresses over a period of months to years to an accelerated phase that moves rapidly to a fulminant neoplastic process indistinguishable from de novo acute leukemia. Peak incidence occurs between ages 30 and 60 years. Considerable data implicate ionizing radiation as a causative factor in the etiology of CGL. Other risk factors are unknown.

The diagnosis of CGL involves chromosomal analysis to demonstrate the Philadelphia (Ph^1) chromosome (present in 90% of cases). Patients present with splenomegaly and an elevated leukocyte count comprising neutrophils, bands, metamyelocytes, myelocytes, and a small percentage of promyelocytes and myeloblasts. Basophils and eosinophils are often present. The platelet count may be normal, increased, or slightly depressed. Anemia is usually mild. Leukocyte alkaline phosphatase is decreased. Bone marrow blasts do not exceed 5%.

The Ph^1 chromosome represents a reciprocal translocation from chromosome 22 to chromosome 9, written as t(9q+;22q−). The c-*abl* proto-oncogene is located on 9q, and the c-*sis* proto-oncogene is located on 22q. The role of these oncogenes in CGL is not clear. In approximately 10% of cases the Ph^1 chromosome will not be seen owing to masking by other complex chromosomal rearrangements. In these cases, as well as in the typical translocations, a specific DNA probe will localize a translocation of the c-*abl* oncogene to the breakpoint cluster region (bcr) of chromosome 22. This fusion gene *(bcr/abl)* transcribes a hybrid mRNA that is translated into a 210-kd protein. Recent studies have indicated that the fusion protein can produce myeloid leukemias in rats. The presence of the *bcr-abl* rearrangement has become the signature for CGL. Atypical CML resembles CGL clinically but lacks the fusion gene. This disease must also be distinguished from chronic myelomonocytic leukemia (CMML), which is characterized by monocytosis and morphologic dysplasia.

CHRONIC PHASE

The goal of therapy in the early phase of CGL is to reduce the greatly expanded granulocyte cell mass over a period of several weeks to months. Although therapy is not indicated solely for leukocyte counts up to 50,000, most patients have weight loss, decreased appetite, and abdominal discomfort from an enlarged spleen and therefore require treatment for symptomatic relief.

The majority of patients with early CGL respond to a variety of agents. The alkylating agents have been the most popular, with busulfan (Myleran) considered by most authorities to be the treatment of choice. The initial schedule involves oral administration of 8 to 10 mg daily, with weekly complete blood counts, and a downward adjustment of dosage by 50% for every 50% reduction in the leukocyte count. Once the white count reaches the normal range (8000 to 12,000), the hemoglobin usually returns to normal along with the platelet count. Either continuation of a small maintenance dose of 2 to 4 mg daily or intermittent therapy when the leukocyte count rises to 30,000 is acceptable at this point. Occasionally, dramatic long-term remission follows a single course of therapy.

Hydroxyurea is another oral agent that causes a rapid reduction in the white blood cell count but has a shorter effective half-life, mandating frequent monitoring of blood counts. Recently alpha interferon, used in chronic phase CGL, has decreased the percent of Ph[1]-positive cells and restored nonclonal hematopoietic cell growth in some patients, but the overall response rate is lower than with the traditional oral agents.

The duration of the chronic phase does not appear to be prolonged by leukapheresis. This technique can be of considerable help in the management of extremely high initial white counts or for leukostasis, or in unusual clinical situations such as the development of CGL during pregnancy.

Bone Marrow Transplantation

Bone marrow transplantation (see Chapter 31) is the treatment of choice for those patients under age 50 years who have an HLA-compatible match. It represents potentially curative treatment in this otherwise uniformly fatal disease. At the time of diagnosis, patients and their siblings should be HLA typed. If there is an HLA-compatible sibling, transplantation should be done within the first year. Prior to transplantation, leukocytosis should be treated with hydroxyurea rather than with busulfan to avoid potential pulmonary toxicity after transplantation. Allogeneic bone marrow transplantation results in 60 to 70% long-term survival without reemergence of the Ph[1] chromosome. For patients under age 50 without an HLA-compatible sibling, a search for an unrelated donor through the International Bone Marrow Registry should be pursued, although the long-term survival rate is significantly lower with an unrelated donor.

ACCELERATED PHASE

Clinically, this phase is recognized by a rising white cell count refractory to busulfan, decreasing hemoglobin and platelet counts, and increasing numbers of immature granulocytes. The patient may develop adenopathy, extramedullary infiltrates, bone pain, and fever. Once this syndrome occurs, the median survival is usually under 4 months. Accompanying the clinical and peripheral blood findings is a change in the bone marrow morphology and histology, with development of marked reticulin fibrosis and shift to more blasts, promyelocytes, eosinophils, and basophils. These features are usually transient and are quickly replaced by a picture of acute leukemia.

BLAST CRISIS

Blast crisis is characterized by the presence of 30% myeloid blasts and promyelocytes in the bone marrow (myeloid blast crisis) or 20% lymphoblasts (lymphoid blast crisis). About 70% of the cases at this point can be classified as one of the variants of AML (types M1 to M6), 25% as lymphoblastic, and 5% as a mixture of blasts. In many of the ALL-type cases and some of the AML cases, terminal transferase activity has been demonstrated.

The treatment of blast crisis has traditionally involved the use of intensive AML programs, and results have been disappointing. When blast crisis is morphologically lymphoblastic, prednisone and vincristine can produce a reversal to the chronic phase of CGL in about 40% of patients. Another approach is to treat with intensive marrow-ablative therapy, then rescue by reinfusing the patient's own stem cells. This treatment requires harvesting peripheral stem cells by leukapheresis during the chronic phase of the disease. Marrow recovery occurs in all patients, and remissions of up to 1 year have resulted.

REFERENCES

Arlin Z, Silver R, Bennett JM: Blastic phase of clinical myeloid leukemia: A proposal for standardization of diagnostic and response criteria. Leukemia 4:755–757, 1990.

Goldman J: The Philadelphia chromosome: From cytogenetics to oncogenes. Br J Haematol 66:435–437, 1987.

Talpaz M, Kantarjian H, et al: Update on therapeutic options for chronic myelogenous leukemia. Semin Hematol 27:31–36, 1990.

Thomas ED, Clift RA: Indications for marrow transplantation in chronic myelogenous leukemia. Blood 73:861–864, 1989.

CHRONIC LYMPHOCYTIC LEUKEMIA ("B" CLL)

DIAGNOSIS AND STAGING

CLL is a neoplastic disorder of mature lymphoid cells; the vast majority of cases are of B-cell origin. CLL cells are monoclonal and express either kappa or lambda light chains (but not both) on the cell-surface membrane. About 50% of patients have chromosomal abnormalities. CLL is usually associated with hypogammaglobulinemia. CLL must be distinguished from Waldenström's macroglobulinemia (Chap. 11), characterized by hyperviscosity and elevated IgM with a cell type best described as a "plasmacytoid lymphocyte." CLL is rarely diagnosed in patients under 40 years of age.

The diagnosis of CLL requires an absolute peripheral blood lymphocytosis of greater than 5000/mm^3. Most cells resemble normal mature lymphocytes; less than 10% of the cells are immature (contain nucleoli). Bone marrow aspirates reveal infiltration with more than 30% lymphoid cells, and biopsies demonstrate one or more patterns of involvement: interstitial, nodular, or diffuse. A diffuse pattern is associated with a poorer prognosis than the other types. If a lymph node is biopsied, the pathologic picture is usually that of a diffuse well-differentiated lymphocytic lymphoma.

The Rai classification (Table 8–1) defines the stages of CLL. In the early, or indolent, phase of CLL, patients are asymptomatic, have minimal to no adenopathy or splenomegaly, and have only mild anemia. Such patients may require no treatment for many months to years. In "active" CLL, there is significant anemia, thrombocytopenia, progressive adenopathy and splenomegaly, weight loss, and a rise in the lymphocyte count. Hypogammaglobulinemia is frequent, and secondary infections develop. Treatment is indicated when these features are found.

RICHTER'S SYNDROME

In contrast to the regular transformation of CGL to blast crisis, progression of CLL to an acute phase (Richter's syndrome) is unusual (less than 10% of cases). Richter's syndrome, manifested by rapid enlargement of lymph nodes, hepatosplenomegaly, fever, and weight loss, is an acute and usually fatal complication of CLL. The peripheral blood and bone marrow contain large blast cells with basophilic cytoplasm, occasional nuclear indentations, and a prominent nucleolus. The syndrome may be leukemic or may present only as lymphomatous involvement. The therapy of Richter's syndrome should be the same as that recommended for diffuse large cell lymphomas (Chap. 10).

THERAPY

The alkylating agents (chlorambucil, 3 to 6 mg/day orally, or cyclophosphamide, 100 to 200 mg/day orally) have been the mainstay of therapy for most patients with CLL when

Table 8–1. **RAI STAGING SYSTEM FOR CHRONIC LYMPHOCYTIC LEUKEMIA**

STAGE	CLINICAL FEATURES	APPROXIMATE SURVIVAL (MONTHS)
0	Absolute lymphocytosis	150
I	Lymphocytosis plus adenopathy	100
II	Lymphocytosis plus enlarged liver or spleen, or both	70
III	Lymphocytosis plus anemia (nodes, liver, and spleen may or may not be enlarged)	20
IV	Lymphocytosis plus thrombocytopenia (anemia and organomegaly may or may not be present)	20
Overall		70

Adapted from Rai KR, Sawitsky A, Cronkite EP, et al: Clinical staging of chronic lymphocytic leukemia. Blood 46:219–234, 1975.

treatment is required. The leukocyte count can be lowered rapidly with therapy, and clinical symptoms are often controlled. However, relatively few complete remissions occur, and survival is not improved. An alternative program is the use of high-dose chlorambucil, 30 mg/M² orally every 2 weeks, combined with a 5-day course of prednisone, 50 mg/day every 2 weeks. With this schedule almost 20% of patients achieve complete remission. Other combinations using vincristine and cyclophosphamide with prednisone have been tried but probably offer little advantage over the chlorambucil-prednisone regimen. The median survival of patients with advanced CLL is now 4 years with combination chemotherapy.

Within the past few years, three new agents have shown promise in the treatment of refractory CLL. The most active is fludarabine, a fluorinated analogue of arabinosyladenosine. Sixty percent of patients respond, with 15% achieving a complete remission. Other agents under study include deoxycoformycin (pentostatin) and 2-chloro-deoxyadenosine.

REFERENCES

Foon K, Rai KR, Gale RP: Chronic lymphocytic leukemia: New insights into biology and therapy. Ann Intern Med 113: 525–539, 1990.

Keating MJ: Fludarabine phosphate in the treatment of chronic lymphocytic leukemias. Semin Oncol 17:49–62, 1990.

Dighiero G, Travade P, Chevret S, et al: B-cell chronic lymphocytic leukemia: Present status and future directions. Blood 78:1901–1914, 1991.

CHRONIC T-CELL LEUKEMIAS

With the use of immunologic markers, about 10% of the chronic lymphoid leukemias are found to be of thymic, or T-cell, origin. Several morphologic subtypes exist, but only two will be discussed here.

ADULT T-CELL LEUKEMIA/LYMPHOMA (ATLL)

ATLL occurs in clusters in certain geographic regions, including southwestern Japan, the Caribbean, Africa, and southeastern United States. It is caused by a human type C retrovirus, HTLV–I (human T-cell leukemia/lymphoma virus 1). The majority of cases present with high white counts, abdominal pain, skin rashes, hypercalcemia, hepatosplenomegaly, and lymphadenopathy. The malignant cells demonstrate marked polymorphism with bizarre nuclear shapes ("clover-leafed"). Aggressive treatment with combination chemotherapy produces only modest responses.

SÉZARY SYNDROME

Sézary syndrome represents the leukemic counterpart of mycosis fungoides, a cutaneous T-cell lymphoma. Patients with Sézary syndrome have an exfoliative erythroderma with mononuclear cells in the epidermis and circulating in the blood. The leukemic cells have an atypical appearance with a size similar to monocytes and a nucleus with a grooved pattern. The disease has a variable and usually chronic course. Irradiation, including extracorporeal techniques, UVA light with psoralen (PUVA), and a variety of chemotherapeutic agents (bleomycin, vinblastine, pentostatin) are effective. Even nonchemotherapeutic agents, including *cis*-retinoic acid, can produce responses.

REFERENCES

Kim JH, Durack DT: Manifestations of human T-lymphotropic virus type I infection. Am J Med 84:919–928, 1988.

Kuzel TM, Roenigk HH, Rosen ST: Mycosis fungoides and the Sézary syndrome: A review of pathogenesis, diagnosis, and therapy. J Clin Oncol 9:1298–1313, 1991.

Table 8–2. **LABORATORY FINDINGS IN HAIRY CELL LEUKEMIA**

LABORATORY FINDING	PERCENT
Monocytopenia	95
Anemia	85
Thrombocytopenia	80
Neutropenia	75
Bicytopenia or pancytopenia	50–80
Increased marrow reticulin	85
Marrow "dry tap"	50
TRAP	75–95

HAIRY CELL LEUKEMIA (HCL)

Hairy cell leukemia is rare; about 1000 cases are diagnosed each year. The median age at diagnosis is 55 years, and males are affected four times as often as females. Presenting complaints arise as a result of splenomegaly or cytopenias. Splenomegaly is present in 85% of patients and extends below the umbilicus in one-third. Minimal adenopathy is present in 10% of patients. Many patients do well for several years; the median survival is 5 years, similar to CLL. Infections from bacterial, viral, and fungal agents are a major problem, as are anemia and thrombocytopenia.

LABORATORY FEATURES

The hallmark of this disease is a unique mononuclear B cell with agranular, blue-gray cytoplasm, striking cytoplasmic irregularities or projections (hairs), and an indented nucleus with a single nucleolus. The cytoplasm contains a tartrate-resistant acid phosphatase referred to as TRAP. Characteristic hairy cells are present in the peripheral blood, bone marrow, spleen, and lymph nodes. Cytopenias are frequent (Table 8–2).

TREATMENT

The managment of asymptomatic patients consists of observation alone. Patients who develop symptomatic cytopenias or splenomegaly may undergo splenectomy or be treated with alpha interferon. Splenectomy benefits 75% of patients by improving blood counts, but about 50% of patients progress and require further therapy. Recombinant alpha interferon produces significant remissions, with response rates close to 80%. Five to 10% of cases achieve complete remissions with disappearance of hairy cells from the bone marrow. Approximately 40% relapse within 2 years and require retreatment.

Pentostatin, an investigational new agent, achieves an 80 to 90% response rate, with close to 50% complete remissions, and only 20 to 30% of patients relapse within 3 years. Because pentostatin reduces lymphocyte populations (especially T cells), infectious complications may increase. Recently, another new agent, 2-chlorodeoxyadenosine, has achieved a very high complete remission rate after only one course of treatment. Large confirmatory clinical trials are underway.

REFERENCES

Berman E, Heller G, Kempin S, et al: Incidence of response and long-term follow-up in patients with hairy cell leukemia treated with recombinant interferon alfa–2a. Blood 75:839–845, 1990.

Piro LD, Carrera CJ, Carson DA, Beutler E: Lasting remissions in hairy cell leukemia induced by a single infusion of 2-chlorodeoxyadenosine. N Engl J Med 322:1117–1121, 1990.

Cassileth PA, Cheuvart B, Spiers ASD, et al: Pentostatin induces durable remissions in hairy cell leukemia. J Clin Oncol 9:243–246, 1991.

9
HODGKIN'S DISEASE

Pradyumna D. Phatak

Hodgkin's disease is a neoplastic lymphoproliferative disorder of unknown etiology. Remarkable progress has been made in the treatment of this disease over the past 30 years; today the majority of patients presenting with Hodgkin's disease will be cured.

EPIDEMIOLOGY AND ETIOLOGY

Hodgkin's disease accounts for less than 1% of new cancers in the United States; however, its preponderance in young adulthood and its potential curability direct attention to it that is out of proportion to its frequency. The disease follows a bimodal age distribution curve, with the first peak occurring in the early twenties followed by a decline till age 45, and then a gradual increase with advancing age. The two peaks tend to have distinct epidemiologic, histopathologic, and clinical characteristics, suggesting that they represent different disease entities, possibly with different etiologies. Younger patients tend to present with supradiaphragmatic disease of the nodular sclerosis histologic type. The older patients are more likely to have disease below the diaphragm in the absence of mediastinal involvement, and the mixed cellularity subtype is more common.

Despite strong epidemiologic data implicating an infectious or environmental agent, particularly in the younger age incidence peak, no infectious or environmental agent has been conclusively identified. The etiology of Hodgkin's disease remains unknown.

PATHOLOGY

The diagnosis of Hodgkin's disease depends on the pathologic examination of an involved lymph node. Lymph node architecture is effaced by a mixture of cells, including lymphocytes, histiocytes, plasma cells, and eosinophils. The pathognomonic feature is the presence of Reed-Sternberg cells (Fig. 9–1), which typically contain two or more large vesicular nuclei, each with a prominent nucleolus. While the presence of Reed-Sternberg cells is necessary for the diagnosis of Hodgkin's disease, it is not sufficient; Reed-Sternberg–like cells may rarely be seen in non-Hodgkin's lymphomas, solid tumors, and even in viral infections.

The Reed-Sternberg cell and its variants are believed to be the neoplastic cells of Hodgkin's disease. The relative paucity of neoplastic cells in involved tissues makes Hodgkin's disease unique among neoplastic disorders. The origin of the neoplastic cell continues to be debated. Its immunophenotype can have features of B cells, T cells, or occasionally histiocytes, suggesting either an aberrant lineage or the ability to mature along either lymphoid or histiocytic cell lines.

CLASSIFICATION

Hodgkin's disease is classified histologically into four major subtypes depending on histologic appearance of the disease in involved lymph nodes.

Lymphocyte Predominance (LP). About 5% of total cases. Mature lymphocytes are abundant and Reed-Sternberg cells are few. This type usually occurs in young men and presents in an early stage. Prognosis is excellent. Subclassification of this group into nodular and diffuse subtypes has recently been found to be of prognostic significance. The nodular subgroup has features that resemble nodular non-Hodgkin's lymphomas, including an indolent clinical course despite a tendency to relapse.

Nodular Sclerosis (NS). About 50% (30 to 75%) of most series. Annular bands of collagen divide the involved node into large nodules. It predominantly affects young women, the mediastinum is often involved, and the prognosis is good.

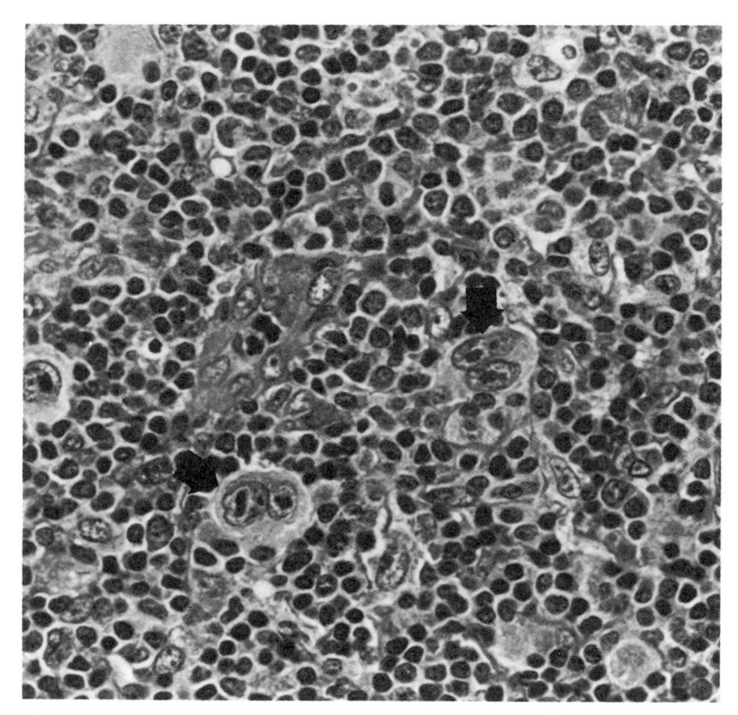

Figure 9–1. Classic Reed-Sternberg cells displaying multiple large nucleoli in each polypoid nucleus. The typical background of mature-appearing small and large lymphocytes, plasma cells, and mononuclear Reed-Sternberg variants is present. (Courtesy of Dr. Michael Briselli.)

Mixed Cellularity (MC). About 40% of most series. A mixed infiltrate of lymphocytes, plasma cells, eosinophils, benign histiocytes, and moderate numbers of Reed-Sternberg cells is seen. It predominantly affects males, patients tend to be older, systemic symptoms are common, the stage may be advanced, and the prognosis is intermediate.

Lymphocyte Depletion (LD). Less than 5%. Few lymphocytes and many Reed-Sternberg cells are present. Microscopically, this type may be mistaken for large cell (histiocytic) lymphoma. LD tends to occur in older patients and is often associated with systemic symptoms and widespread involvement. Prognosis is generally poor.

CLINICAL FEATURES

Patients with Hodgkin's disease usually present with painless lymphadenopathy that may or may not be accompanied by systemic symptoms, including fevers, night sweats, weight loss, malaise, and pruritus. Adenopathy most often involves cervical and mediastinal lymph node groups, with occasional contiguous involvement of para-aortic and inguinal nodes. Only a minority of patients have liver, spleen, bone marrow, or lung involvement at the time of diagnosis. Rarely, Hodgkin's disease presents in an extralymphatic site such as bone, breast, gastrointestinal tract, or endocrine gland. Extralymphatic presentations occur more commonly in the non-Hodgkin's lymphomas (Chap. 10).

When Hodgkin's disease becomes progressive and refractory to treatment, symptoms depend on which organ systems are most extensively involved. Liver infiltration with jaundice and eventually hepatic failure may develop. Pulmonary involvement may result in respiratory failure. Pancytopenia develops as a result of advancing bone marrow invasion and previous myelosuppressive therapy. A syndrome common in advanced Hodgkin's disease consists of anorexia, weight loss, malaise, anemia, and repeated infections with a variety of organisms. Granulocytopenia and immunologic defects due to the disease itself account for the propensity toward infection in patients with advanced Hodgkin's disease.

STAGING EVALUATION

After a pathologic diagnosis of Hodgkin's disease is established by biopsy of an enlarged node, further clinical, radiologic, and laboratory evaluation is directed toward defining the extent of the disease. This process is called clinical staging and is essential for selection of the most appropriate therapy.

The initial evaluation includes a careful history and physical examination with particular attention to lymph node–bearing areas, complete blood count, screening blood chemistries, and chest x-ray. Abnormal blood studies are common but not helpful in indicating stage or prognosis. If the chest x-ray is suspicious for mediastinal node involvement, CT of the chest is indicated. An iliac crest bone marrow biopsy may reveal bone marrow involvement.

An abdominal CT scan is performed to assess retroperitoneal and iliac lymph node involvement and to image the liver and spleen. Lymphangiography may demonstrate abnormal retroperitoneal nodes even if the CT scan does not reveal adenopathy. The lymphangiogram allows assessment of nodal architecture as well as nodal size and may indicate defects suggestive of Hodgkin's involvement in nodes of normal size. CT scanning, on the other hand, allows visualization of upper para-aortic, porta hepatis, mesenteric, and splenic hilar nodes, which are not demonstrated by lymphangiography. The two techniques are therefore complementary, and in many centers a negative CT is routinely followed by a lymphangiogram.

Staging laparotomy (Table 9–1) should be considered after the clinical staging evaluation described above is complete. The purpose of staging laparotomy is to detect disease in retroperitoneal nodes, spleen, or liver that has not been identified by the clinical staging procedures and to confirm the presence of Hodgkin's disease in radiologically abnormal nodes visualized by CT or lymphangiogram. Laparotomy is indicated if its findings will influence the choice of therapy. However, if the finding of occult abdominal or retroperitoneal disease would not influence the choice of therapy, then laparotomy should be omitted. In general, laparotomy is most often required in patients with clinical stages IA or IIA disease, and occasionally in patients with clinical stage IIIA disease. Patients with stage IIIB or IV disease will require chemotherapy regardless of laparotomy findings; therefore, the procedure would be superfluous in this group.

Most series report that laparotomy results in a change in the clinical stage in about 30 to 40% of patients, with most changes in the direction of increasing stage (i.e., from stage I or II to stage III or IV). Reliance on clinical stage in these patients would result in undertreatment and high risk of subdiaphragmatic recurrence. The minority whose clinical stage is decreased by laparotomy are spared the toxicity of inappropriate overtreatment based on clinical stage.

In experienced hands, the morbidity of staging laparotomy is low and the surgical mortality rate is less than 1%. Removal of the spleen predisposes the patient (especially a child) to severe infection; pneumococcal (and possibly meningococcal) vaccine should be given preoperatively. In premenopausal women desiring to preserve fertility, the surgeon should also perform an oophoropexy, tacking the ovaries to the midline where they may be shielded if pelvic radiotherapy is included in the treatment plan.

STAGING SYSTEM

The use of a widely accepted, standardized staging system for Hodgkin's disease is extremely important in comparing results of treatment and predicting prognosis. The

Table 9–1. **STAGING LAPAROTOMY FOR HODGKIN'S DISEASE**

General abdominal exploration	Porta hepatis
Splenectomy	Upper paraaortic
Wedge biopsy of liver, both lobes	Mesenteric
Needle biopsy of liver, both lobes	Lower paraaortic
Lymph node biopsies	Iliac
Celiac	Oophoropexy (selected cases)
Splenic hilar	Open marrow biopsy (iliac crest)*

*If closed marrow biopsy not previously performed.

staging system for Hodgkin's disease, also applied to the non-Hodgkin's lymphomas, is given below:

Stage I. Involvement of a single lymph node region (I) or localized involvement of a single extralymphatic organ or site (I_E).

Stage II. Involvement of two or more lymph node regions on the same side of the diaphragm (II) or localized involvement of a single associated extralymphatic organ or site and its regional lymph nodes on the same side of the diaphragm (II_E).

Stage III. Involvement of lymph node regions on both sides of the diaphragm (III), which may also be accompanied by localized involvement of an associated extralymphatic organ or site (III_E), or by involvement of the spleen (III_S), or both (III_{SE}). Stage III_1 indicates involvement of upper abdominal lymphatic structures: spleen, porta hepatis nodes, celiac nodes, or splenic hilar nodes. Stage III_2 includes involved nodes in the para-aortic, iliac, mesenteric, or inguinal areas, with or without involvement of the upper abdominal lymphatic structures.

Stage IV. Disseminated (multifocal) involvement of one or more extralymphatic organs with or without associated lymph node involvement or isolated extralymphatic organ involvement with distant (nonregional) nodal involvement.

If systemic symptoms of unexplained weight loss in excess of 10% of body weight, fever, or night sweats are present, the letter "B" is added to the stage. The letter "A" denotes absence of systemic symptoms.

TREATMENT

GENERAL PRINCIPLES

The treatment of Hodgkin's disease has improved dramatically in the past 30 years, illustrating the value of coordinated interdisciplinary cooperation consisting of meticulous pathologic classification, careful clinical and surgical staging, and a team approach to therapy by medical oncologists and radiation therapists. Prior to the development of modern radiotherapy and cytotoxic chemotherapy, the median survival of patients with Hodgkin's disease was about 2 years. At present, most patients with localized disease are cured with radiation therapy, and a majority of those with disseminated disease are cured with combination chemotherapy or combined modality treatment.

Nevertheless, the treatment of Hodgkin's disease in any stage is complicated and in transition to some extent. The previous trend to increase the intensity of treatment to obtain higher remission rates with longer durations has been tempered by recognition of the long-term complications of such a therapeutic strategy. Current investigational efforts are directed toward finding treatment programs that maximize remission rates and durations while minimizing immediate and long-term complications.

Several principles are basic to the management of Hodgkin's disease and guide selection of therapy:

- Hodgkin's disease often appears to spread in an orderly fashion from one group of nodes to the next contiguous group.
- Radiation therapy in sufficient dose (about 4000 cGy) is tumoricidal for a mass of Hodgkin's disease.
- Combination chemotherapy is capable of curing patients with Hodgkin's disease too widespread to be treated effectively by tolerable doses of radiation.

Application of these principles has led to the following general guidelines for treatment:

Stages IA and IIA. Radiation therapy (4000 to 4500 cGy) delivered to areas of known involvement as well as adjacent lymph node areas at risk to contain occult disease (extended field irradiation).

Stage IIB. Often treated with both radiation therapy and combination chemotherapy because of a high failure rate following radiation alone.

Stage IIIA. Controversial. Recommendations include radiotherapy alone, chemotherapy alone, and combined modality therapy.

Stages IIIB and IV. Combination chemotherapy, primarily. Low-dose radiation to bulky sites of involvement is sometimes used for "consolidation," particularly in patients with nodular sclerosis.

LOCALIZED HODGKIN'S DISEASE

Radiation therapy is the mainstay of treatment for early-stage Hodgkin's disease. Proper treatment with a locally applied modality such as radiotherapy depends on identification of all involved sites of disease. Obviously, radiotherapy will not be curative if the patient has occult abdominal disease not included in the radiation fields. Accurate clinical and pathologic staging is thus critical to the successful use of radiotherapy in this disease.

Modern megavoltage therapy and experienced personnel can cure localized Hodgkin's disease in 70 to 90% of patients. Megavoltage equipment is required to allow sufficiently high dosages to sterilize tumor masses, reducing the true (in-field) recurrence rate to less than 5%. Megavoltage energies also permit the use of large, complex fields (mantle, inverted Y) that encompass multiple lymph node areas simultaneously. Most patients with localized disease above the diaphragm are treated with extended field radiotherapy, omitting pelvic radiation and sparing pelvic bone marrow. Under some circumstances and in some centers, total lymphoid irradiation is employed.

STAGES IIB AND IIIA

Although patients with stage IIB or IIIA Hodgkin's disease can be treated with radiation therapy alone, the risk of relapse is high, especially in certain high-risk situations. Patients with bulky mediastinal involvement (greater than one-third of the chest diameter on posteroanterior chest x-ray) or extension into lung parenchyma or other extranodal regions have high relapse rates following radiation alone and are best managed by combining chemotherapy and radiation therapy. Most institutions would also treat stage III_2A patients with chemotherapy. No uniform treatment plan can be offered for any of these groups, however, and each patient requires an individually tailored approach by a multidisciplinary team, based on individual characteristics and institutional norms.

ADVANCED HODGKIN'S DISEASE

Almost every chemotherapeutic agent tested has exhibited some activity against Hodgkin's disease. The major active agents are listed in Table 9–2. Single agents, however, produce only partial responses of brief duration.

Combination chemotherapy achieves complete remissions in about 75% of patients with stage IIIB or IV disease who have not previously received chemotherapy, and about two-thirds of those patients in complete remission remain free of disease for 10 years. The design of appropriate multidrug combinations for Hodgkin's disease makes use of the following concepts:

1. A combination of active single agents is used, resulting in additive therapeutic benefit without entirely additive toxicity. From the list of active single agents in Table 9–2, a variety of combinations has been developed. In general, one or more myelosuppressive agents (alkylating agents, vinblastine, nitrosoureas, procarbazine) are combined with one

Table 9–2. **CHEMOTHERAPEUTIC AGENTS ACTIVE IN HODGKIN'S DISEASE**

Alkylating Agents	Etoposide (VP-16)
Nitrogen mustard	Cisplatin
Cyclophosphamide	Cytosine arabinoside
Chlorambucil	Antibiotics
Dacarbazine (DTIC)	Adriamycin (doxorubicin)
Nitrosoureas	Bleomycin
BCNU	Vinca Alkaloids
CCNU	Vincristine
Streptozotocin	Vinblastine
Miscellaneous	Corticosteroids
Procarbazine	

Table 9–3. **MOPP CHEMOTHERAPY FOR ADVANCED HODGKIN'S DISEASE***

AGENT	DOSE
Nitrogen mustard (Mustargen)	6 mg/m^2 IV days 1 and 8
Vincristine (Oncovin)	1.4 mg/m^2 IV days 1 and 8
Procarbazine	100 mg/m^2 PO days 1–14
Prednisone†	40 mg/m^2 PO days 1–14

*Repeat cycle every 28 days, minimum of 6 cycles.
†Cycles 1 and 4 only.

or more drugs with minimal marrow toxicity (vincristine, bleomycin, prednisone). Selecting drugs with differing mechanisms of action and nonoverlapping toxicities enhances the likelihood of complete remissions of prolonged duration.

2. Drugs are given intermittently, permitting bone marrow, gastrointestinal tract, and other tissues to repair damage during a 2- to 4-week drug-free interval during each cycle.

3. Complete remissions occur much more frequently in response to combinations than to single agents. Patients who attain complete remission have a greater likelihood of improved survival than those who achieve only partial remissions, and long-term disease-free survival and cure are possible only in the group achieving complete remissions.

4. Maintenance chemotherapy following achievement of complete remission offers no advantage and may actually be harmful.

MOPP Chemotherapy

The development of MOPP chemotherapy (Table 9–3) by DeVita and associates in the 1960s marked the beginning of curative chemotherapy for advanced Hodgkin's disease. Since that time, several groups of investigators have attempted to improve on the results obtained using MOPP. One approach has been to use variations of the MOPP regimen. Another approach is to use different "non–cross-resistant" regimens such as the ABVD regimen (see below) of Bonadonna et al. More recently, combinations of MOPP and ABVD-like regimens have been used.

MOPP Variants

Numerous regimens have been developed in an attempt to reduce the substantial toxicity of MOPP and improve its results. These regimens for the most part have either substituted agents for one of the MOPP constituents or added additional drugs, or both. For example, the substitution of BCNU (bischloroethylnitrosourea) or chlorambucil for nitrogen mustard appears to reduce nausea and vomiting compared with MOPP, but treatment results are not improved.

The BCVPP regimen (Table 9–4) produces the same complete response rate as MOPP (76% versus 73%) and a similar disease-free survival rate (about 50 to 60% at 5 years) as reported in a randomized prospective study of the two regimens performed by the Eastern Cooperative Oncology Group (ECOG). In previously untreated patients, remission dura-

Table 9–4. **BCVPP CHEMOTHERAPY FOR ADVANCED HODGKIN'S DISEASE***

AGENT	DOSE
BCNU	100 mg/m^2 IV day 1
Cyclophosphamide	600 mg/m^2 IV day 1
Vinblastine	5 mg/m^2 IV day 1
Procarbazine	100 mg/m^2 PO days 1–10
Prednisone	60 mg/m^2 PO days 1–10

*Repeat cycle every 28 days, minimum of 6 cycles.

tions were longer in patients receiving BCVPP. In addition, BCVPP caused far less gastrointestinal and neurologic toxicity. The ECOG concluded that as primary induction therapy for advanced Hodgkin's disease, BCVPP is an effective alternative to MOPP, with equal or superior efficacy and less toxicity.

ABVD Chemotherapy

ABVD (Adriamycin [doxorubicin], bleomycin, vinblastine, and dacarbazine) chemotherapy (Table 9–5) was developed by Bonadonna et al. for patients who progress during MOPP therapy or relapse within 1 year after treatment with MOPP or a MOPP variant. The relative success of ABVD in this setting, with a 52% complete remission rate and a 20% 5-year disease-free survival, led to studies using ABVD or combinations of MOPP and ABVD as initial therapy for patients with advanced Hodgkin's disease or those relapsing after initial radiation therapy.

Several randomized studies have now confirmed the superiority of ABVD or ABVD-containing regimens over MOPP alone. Bonadonna et al. compared ABVD plus radiotherapy to MOPP plus radiotherapy in patients with stages IIB, IIIA, and IIIB disease. The ABVD-treated patients achieved a superior complete remission rate (94% versus 79%, $p<0.01$) and 4-year disease-free survival rate. Overall survival was better in the ABVD group, but this difference did not reach statistical significance.

The same group has also compared MOPP chemotherapy alone with alternating cycles of MOPP and ABVD in patients with stage IV Hodgkin's disease. Seventy-one percent of MOPP-treated patients achieved complete remissions, compared with 92% of patients treated with the alternating regimens ($p=0.02$). Five-year disease-free survival for complete responders was 54% for the MOPP-treated patients and 84% for the patients receiving the alternating cycles ($p<0.005$). Overall survival was also significantly superior in the patients receiving alternating cycles. Preliminary data from a large randomized trial conducted by the Cancer and Leukemia Group B (CALGB), which compared MOPP versus ABVD versus alternating cycles of MOPP and ABVD in advanced Hodgkin's disease, show that both ABVD-containing regimens were superior to MOPP alone.

The overall consensus among oncologists today is that ABVD chemotherapy is the treatment of choice for advanced Hodgkin's disease and must be the standard to which new regimens are compared. Some authorities, however, argue that the randomized trials cited above did not employ MOPP regimens with sufficiently high dose intensity, and therefore the results of these studies should be accepted with caution.

Alternating MOPP/ABVD and the MOPP/ABV Hybrid

Although alternating therapy with MOPP and ABVD has been shown to be superior to MOPP alone, no randomized study so far has demonstrated the superiority of the alternating regimen over ABVD alone. A single institution study by Klimo and Connors in British Columbia has reported on the use of a hybrid regimen that uses the MOPP and ABVD drugs in a single monthly cycle but omits dacarbazine. This MOPP/ABV hybrid resulted in a 97% complete remission rate and a 93.5% overall survival rate at a median follow-up of 4.5 years. Randomized trials are currently under way comparing the hybrid regimen to ABVD and to alternating cycles of MOPP and ABVD.

Salvage Therapy for Relapsed Hodgkin's Disease

The success of salvage therapy for Hodgkin's disease in relapse after an initial attempt at curative therapy depends on the nature of the initial therapy and the duration of the

Table 9–5. **ABVD CHEMOTHERAPY FOR ADVANCED HODGKIN'S DISEASE***

AGENT	DOSE
Adriamycin (doxorubicin)	25 mg/m² IV days 1 and 15
Bleomycin	10 mg/m² IV days 1 and 15
Vinblastine	6 mg/m² IV days 1 and 15
Dacarbazine	375 mg/m² IV days 1 and 15

*Repeat cycles every 28 days, minimum of 6 cycles.

first remission. Relapses after radiation therapy can be effectively treated by chemotherapy, with ABVD achieving superior results compared with MOPP. Relapses that occur more than 12 months after initial therapy can be treated with the same regimen used initially. ABVD is effective salvage therapy in MOPP failures, and achieves a 5 to 10% long-term disease-free survival rate in such patients. Patients who relapse after two or more chemotherapy regimens cannot be cured with conventional chemotherapy. However, judicious use of single-agent chemotherapy in this setting can maintain partial disease control for long periods of time. Preliminary evidence suggests that high-dose chemotherapy with autologous bone marrow rescue or allogeneic bone marrow transplantation may offer hope of long term-disease-free survival, especially in those patients whose disease responds to salvage chemotherapy.

COMPLICATIONS OF TREATMENT

Significant complications may follow any form of therapy for Hodgkin's disease. Experienced personnel and proper equipment in the case of radiation therapy represent the best methods for keeping complications to a minimum.

Potential complications of radiotherapy for Hodgkin's disease include hypothyroidism, pericarditis, pneumonitis, spinal cord injury, infertility, and rarely damage to bone, liver, or kidney. See Chapter 4 for a more detailed discussion of the complications of radiation therapy.

Combination chemotherapy may produce all of the familiar acute side effects (Chap. 5) as well as some serious long-term complications. Chemotherapy with MOPP and its variants produces permanent sterility in almost all men and many young women. ABVD has a lower likelihood of leading to sterility, but the use of Adriamycin and radiation to the heart may cause cardiomyopathy, and increased risk of pulmonary damage occurs in patients treated with both bleomycin and chest irradiation. Greater myelotoxicity is observed in patients receiving combined modality therapy also.

Second malignancies, especially acute nonlymphocytic leukemias (ANLL) and non-Hodgkin's lymphomas, pose a substantial risk for patients treated with combined modality therapy or chemotherapy alone. The actuarial risk of ANLL in these patients is approximately 5 to 10% at 10 years. The risk of ANLL appears to be greater in patients over age 40, in those who received total nodal irradiation plus MOPP, and in those who received maintenance chemotherapy, a practice now obsolete. Patients who received radiotherapy and then required chemotherapy for salvage after relapse have a greater risk than those who received combined modality as initial treatment. ABVD appears to produce fewer second malignancies than MOPP and its variants, but greater follow-up of ABVD-treated patients is required before a firm conclusion on this point can be drawn.

Attempts to reduce the incidence of treatment-related second malignancies by avoiding chemotherapy and combined modality treatment must not jeopardize the potential for curing the underlying disease. The risk of death from inadequately treated Hodgkin's disease generally exceeds the long-term risk of second malignancies. Chemotherapy and combined modality programs should therefore be employed whenever the incidence of relapse following radiation therapy alone is sufficiently high to endanger long-term survival.

SUMMARY

The likelihood of curing patients with Hodgkin's disease, even in stage IV, is so great that carefully monitored intensive chemotherapy and/or radiation therapy should be made available to all patients. The optimal planning of such therapy is best ensured by employing at the outset a multidisciplinary approach involving the medical oncologist, radiation therapist, pathologist, diagnostic radiologist, and surgeon.

REFERENCES

Bonadonna G, Valagussa P, Santoro A: Alternating non–cross-resistant combination chemotherapy on MOPP in Stage IV Hodgkin's disease. Ann Intern Med 104:739–746, 1986.

Coltman CA (ed): Hodgkin's disease. Semin Oncol 17(6):641–772, 1990.
Crnkovich MJ, Leopold K, Hoppe RT, et al: Stage I to IIB Hodgkin's disease: The combined experience at Stanford University and the Joint Center for Radiation Therapy. J Clin Oncol 5:1041–1049, 1987.
Kaplan HS: Hodgkin's disease: Biology, treatment, prognosis. Blood 57:813–822, 1981.
Klimo P, Connors JM: MOPP/ABV hybrid chemotherapy for advanced Hodgkin's disease. Semin Hematol 24(suppl 1):35–40, 1987.
Mauch PM, Canellos GP, Rosenthal DS, Hellman S: Reduction of fatal complications from combined modality therapy in Hodgkin's disease. J Clin Oncol 3:501–505, 1985.
Mauch P, Larson D, Osteen R, et al: Prognostic factors for positive surgical staging in patients with Hodgkin's disease. J Clin Oncol 8:257–265, 1990.
Prosnitz LR: Therapy of IIIA Hodgkin's disease. Int J Rad Oncol Biol Phys 13:1595–1597, 1987.
Santoro A, Bonadonna G, Valagussa P, et al: Long term results of combined chemotherapy-radiotherapy approach in Hodgkin's disease: Superiority of ABVD plus radiotherapy versus MOPP plus radiotherapy. J Clin Oncol 5:27–37, 1987.
Williams SF, Farah R, Golomb HM (eds): Hodgkin's disease. Hematol/Oncol Clin North Am 3:187–368, 1989.

10
NON-HODGKIN'S LYMPHOMAS

Zachary B. Kramer

The non-Hodgkin's lymphomas (NHL) are a heterogeneous group of malignancies with diverse natural histories and clinical presentations. The biological diversity of these cancers parallels that of the normal immune cells (lymphocytes) from which these neoplasms derive. The optimal management of NHL is determined by disease-related variables and by host factors. The former include the histologic subtype of lymphoma and the extent and anatomic sites of disease. The latter include the age of the patient and the presence of comorbid conditions. Appropriate and timely therapy can cure a significant proportion of NHL patients, especially those with localized, higher-grade tumors.

INCIDENCE AND ETIOLOGY

In developed nations such as the United States, the age-adjusted incidence of NHL has steadily increased over the last few decades. NHL now accounts for 3 to 5% of all cancer deaths. The National Cancer Institute (NCI) estimates that 37,200 new cases were diagnosed in 1991 in the United States, and men were affected slightly more often than women. The incidence of NHL increases with age, peaking in the seventh and eighth decades for males and females, respectively. Most epidemiologic studies demonstrate a second incidence peak in childhood.

The etiology of most types of NHL remains somewhat obscure. However, understanding of the pathogenesis of these neoplasms has been advanced by developments in molecular biology, cytogenetics, and virology, and by epidemiologic observations. Environmental factors have some etiologic role, as evidenced by the marked variation in the geographic distribution of lymphomas and by the greater risk of NHL after exposure to ionizing radiation and herbicides. Congenital and acquired immunodeficiency states definitely predispose to NHL; for example, immunosuppressed renal allograft recipients experience a 40- to 100-fold increased risk. Epstein-Barr virus (EBV) infection appears to be important in the pathogenesis of NHL in the immunodeficient. Owing to the absence of normal cytotoxic/suppressor T-cell function, EBV-induced B-cell proliferation proceeds unchecked, allowing somatic mutations such as gene rearrangements and malignant transformation of lymphocytes.

Molecular genetic changes imposed by acquired chromosomal translocations represent critical oncogenic events in lymphoma. Clonal cytogenetic abnormalities can be identified in most cases of NHL, and certain chromosomal aberrations are specific for given subtypes of lymphoma. Examples include the t(14:18) (q32:q21) translocation characteristic of follicular B-cell lymphomas and the t(8:14) (q24:q32) translocation seen in Burkitt's lymphoma. These translocations typically involve oncogenes—genes that regulate normal cell growth and proliferation. The dysregulation or increased expression of oncogenes produced by these translocations contributes to the neoplastic transformation of the affected lymphocytes.

CLASSIFICATION

The histologic classification of the NHL has evolved considerably, along with advances in immunology and hematopathology. Efforts continue toward the development of a comprehensive, universally accepted schema that is both reproducible and clinically meaningful. Although a multitude of classification systems has been proposed over the years, only the two most durable and popular will be discussed (Table 10–1). The older Rappaport system, developed while immunology was in its scientific infancy, distinguishes between lymphomas with nodular (follicular) and diffuse growth patterns. This distinction offers considerable prognostic value. Lymphomas are further identified by their predominant cell population, i.e., lymphocytes, histiocytes, or undifferentiated cells. (The histiocyte-

Table 10–1. **WORKING FORMULATION OF NON-HODGKIN'S LYMPHOMAS FOR CLINICAL USAGE**

WORKING FORMULATION	RAPPAPORT-RELATED TERMS
Low Grade	
A. Malignant lymphoma, diffuse	Lymphocytic, well-differentiated
Small lymphocytic consistent with CLL	
B. Malignant lymphoma, follicular	Nodular, poorly differentiated
Predominantly small cleaved	
C. Malignant lymphoma, follicular	Nodular, mixed
Mixed, small cleaved, and large cell	
Intermediate Grade	
D. Malignant lymphoma, follicular	Nodular, histiocytic
Predominantly large cell	
E. Malignant lymphoma, diffuse	Diffuse, poorly differentiated
Small cleaved cell	
F. Malignant lymphoma, diffuse	Diffuse, mixed
Mixed, small, and large cell	
G. Malignant lymphoma, diffuse	Diffuse, histiocytic
Large cell	
Cleaved cell	
Noncleaved cell	
High Grade	
H. Malignant lymphoma	Diffuse, histiocytic
Large cell, immunoblastic	
I. Malignant lymphoma	Lymphoblastic
Lymphoblastic	
Convoluted cell	
Nonconvoluted cell	
J. Malignant lymphoma	Diffuse undifferentiated
Small noncleaved cell	
Burkitt's	Burkitt's
	Non-Burkitt's
Miscellaneous	
Composite	(Same terms)
Mycosis fungoides	
Histiocytic	
Extramedullary plasmacytoma	
Unclassifiable	

Modified from Burke JS: The histopathologic classification of non-Hodgkin's lymphomas: Ambiguities in the Working Formulation and two newly reported categories. Semin Oncol 17:3–10, 1985.

like cells of the Rappaport system were subsequently shown to be large lymphocytes.) The Rappaport system gained wide acceptance by clinicians because it identified the more indolent nodular lymphomas and thereby stratified NHL based on clinical behavior.

In 1982, the NCI published the Working Formulation for Clinical Usage, based on the NHL Pathologic Classification Project. The Working Formulation integrates the clinically useful features of its predecessors with features of lymphoma immunology. The Working Formulation is fairly easy to apply, since it is based solely on light microscopic features of the lymphoma. Lymphomas are subdivided into low-, intermediate-, and high-grade categories based on their natural histories and into follicular (nodular) and diffuse categories based on architecture.

CLINICAL PRESENTATION

The clinical features of NHL are highly variable and depend on the grade, immunophenotype, and anatomic site. Lymphadenopathy is a common presentation, and involvement of multiple noncontiguous nodes is not unusual. Low-grade lymphomas generally produce gradual nodal enlargement, whereas rapid nodal growth is typical of intermediate- or high-grade tumors. Unlike Hodgkin's disease, extranodal involvement predominates in one-third of NHL cases and is especially characteristic of the higher-grade NHL. Enlarging lymph nodes may impinge on adjacent organs, producing airway obstruction, superior vena cava syndrome, pericardial effusion, spinal cord compression, or obstructive uropathy. Gastrointestinal tract lymphomas may present with visceral obstruction or perforation, whereas primary central nervous system (CNS) lymphomas produce focal neurologic deficits or symptoms of elevated intracranial pressure.

Patients with NHL often suffer from constitutional symptoms such as anorexia, fever, night sweats, and weight loss. Sometimes rapidly growing lymphomas present with metabolic complications, e.g., lactic acidosis or hypercalcemia, or with pancytopenia due to marrow infiltration. To some extent, the immunophenotype of the lymphoma is predictive of its clinical behavior. For example, cutaneous lymphomas are typically of T-cell origin. Primary CNS lymphomas are almost exclusively B-cell neoplasms.

DIAGNOSIS AND STAGING

The diagnosis and accurate classification of NHL requires examination of an adequate lymph node biopsy by a skilled pathologist. An appreciation of the overall architecture of involved nodes is necessary for precise categorization. For this reason, lymph node biopsies are preferred, when feasible, over other tissues. At times, light microscopic examination of biopsy specimens must be supplemented by more sophisticated techniques, such as cell marker studies or tumor cytogenetics. Marker studies are usually performed on fresh tissues and employ monoclonal antibodies to lymphocyte differentiation antigens, in conjunction with flow cytometry or immunohistochemistry methods. Cell marker studies help determine the immunophenotype of the lymphoma, i.e., T or B cell, lymphoblast versus mature lymphocyte, and distinguish reactive polyclonal lymphoid hyperplasia from monoclonal lymphoid neoplasms. Cytogenetic studies, if available, can identify clonal chromosomal abnormalities that are characteristic of certain lymphomas.

The above techniques are also useful in distinguishing variants of NHL from atypical Hodgkin's disease or anaplastic carcinoma. The immunophenotype and cytogenetics of the NHL subclasses will be discussed more extensively in subsequent sections.

After the diagnosis of NHL is confirmed, systematic assessment of the bulk and anatomic extent of disease (staging) is essential. The objectives of staging are manifold: (1) determination of prognosis; (2) recognition of impending complications; (3) treatment planning, if radiotherapy or surgery are contemplated; and (4) establishment of a baseline for evaluation of treatment response. Required staging procedures are delineated in Table 10–2.

The process of staging begins with a meticulous history and physical examination, with attention to constitutional symptoms, adenopathy, hepatosplenomegaly, and abdominal masses. Routine laboratory studies should include a serum lactate dehydrogenase (LDH) level and examination of the peripheral blood for circulating lymphoma cells. In virtually all patients computed tomography (CT) scans of the abdomen and pelvis and bone marrow aspirate and biopsy are indicated. Additional staging procedures may be warranted based on clinical findings or the underlying histology. Meningeal involvement is common in

Table 10–2. **STAGING PROCEDURES FOR PATIENTS WITH NON-HODGKIN'S LYMPHOMAS**

Required
Careful history and physical examination
Blood chemistries, including liver function tests, electrolytes, calcium, uric acid
Complete blood counts
Bone marrow biopsy
Chest x-ray
Abdominal image (CT, ultrasound)
Additional procedures as needed
Specific x-rays of gastrointestinal tract, CNS, if symptoms present
Chest CT scan if plain chest x-ray is abnormal
Bone scan if symptoms present
Lumbar puncture if symptoms present or if lymphoblastic, Burkitt's or large cell with bone marrow involvement

Burkitt's lymphoma, lymphoblastic lymphoma, and NHL of the paranasal sinuses; therefore lumbar puncture for cerebrospinal fluid (CSF) cytology is indicated. CSF examination may also be indicated for patients with diffuse large cell lymphoma involving bone marrow. Patients with Waldeyer's ring lymphomas often have concomitant small bowel lymphoma; upper gastrointestinal contrast studies are recommended in these cases.

The Ann Arbor staging system, originally designed for Hodgkin's disease, is also used for adult NHL (Table 10–3). Alternative systems have been formulated for the high-grade pediatric lymphomas. The majority of adults with NHL have advanced disease at presentation, and stage is often underestimated by noninvasive studies. The Ann Arbor system has shortcomings when used in isolation to define prognosis. Other factors such as histology, tumor bulk, involvement of multiple extranodal sites, and patient performance status may have great prognostic significance independent of stage.

TREATMENT AND OUTCOME

The prognosis and therapy of the NHL, organized by grade, are discussed in the sections that follow. The terminology of the Working Formulation is used exclusively. In addition, the clinical, cytogenetic, and immunologic features specific to the NHL subtypes will be reviewed. Certain rare lymphomas and those associated with human immunodeficiency virus (HIV-1) infection (Chap. 29) are considered separately.

LOW-GRADE LYMPHOMAS

The low-grade lymphomas account for approximately 50% of NHL in adults. These "indolent" lymphomas are usually stage III or IV at presentation, and the diagnosis may follow years of asymptomatic lymphadenopathy. Bone marrow involvement occurs commonly, especially with small lymphocytic (SL) or follicular, small cleaved cell (FSC) lymphomas, and a leukemic phase is seen in 10 to 20% of cases. Virtually all low-grade lymphomas express B-cell markers and variable amounts of surface immunoglobulin. The immunophenotype of SL lymphoma is identical to that of chronic lymphocytic leukemia. Most follicular lymphomas express the common acute lymphoblastic leukemia antigen (CALLA) and exhibit a specific cytogenetic abnormality—t(14:18) (q32:q21). This chromosomal translocation involves the immunoglobulin heavy chain locus on chromosome 14 and the *BCL*-2 oncogene on chromosome 18.

The natural history of the low-grade NHL is fascinating. Spontaneous regression of disease occurs in 15 to 30% of patients and may last months or years. In addition, histologic transformation to intermediate or high-grade NHL may occur. This phenomenon becomes more likely each subsequent year after diagnosis, with a 5 to 10% risk of transformation each year.

The median survival of patients with low-grade NHL is 5 to 7 years, and there is no "plateau" in disease-related survival over time. Most patients with low-grade lymphomas cannot be cured of their disease. A number of factors, including histology, affect the

Table 10–3. **STAGING SYSTEM FOR NON-HODGKIN'S LYMPHOMAS**

STAGE	DEFINITION
I	Involvement of a single lymph node region or of a single extranodal organ or site (I_E)
II	Involvement of two or more lymph node regions on the same side of the diaphragm or localized involvement of an extranodal site or organ (II_E) and one or more lymph node regions on the same side of the diaphragm
III	Involvement of lymph node regions on both sides of the diaphragm, which may also be accompanied by localized involvement of an extranodal organ or site (III_E) or spleen (III_S) or both (III_{SE}).
IV	Diffuse or disseminated involvement of one or more distant extranodal organs with or without associated lymph node involvement

Fever >38°C, night sweats, and/or weight loss >10% of body weight in the 6 months preceding admission are defined as systemic symptoms and denoted by the suffix "B." Other patients are denoted by the suffix "A." The same staging system is used in Hodgkin's disease (Chapter 9).

prognosis of low-grade NHL. In one large study of follicular lymphoma, the degree of nodularity in biopsy specimens predicted outcome. Patients with purely follicular patterns survived significantly longer than those with mixed diffuse and follicular histology. Most reviews have found advanced age, elevated LDH, constitutional symptoms, and abnormal liver function to impact negatively on survival. As expected, patients who enter complete remission after treatment fare better than partial responders.

The appropriate management of patients with low-grade lymphoma is a bit controversial. Treatment decisions should be individualized dependent on patient age, comorbid illness, and the presence or absence of lymphoma-related symptoms. Patients with localized lymphomas—stages I and II—are candidates for "curative" extended field radiotherapy. Approximately 50 to 60% will be disease free 10 years after such treatment. Given the indolent nature of the low-grade lymphomas and their tendency for subclinical dissemination, it remains uncertain whether radiotherapy is truly curative in this setting.

The optimal approach to patients with stage III or IV low-grade NHL is debated. No definitive evidence indicates that these patients are curable with standard treatment, and many remain relatively asymptomatic for years. The Stanford group has followed a large series of newly diagnosed, asymptomatic, low-grade lymphoma patients without treatment. Treatment was given only when demanded by symptoms or bulky disease, and the median time to progression requiring therapy was 3 years. The overall survival of these patients was not compromised by this "watch and wait" approach. Moreover, many patients were spared the acute and delayed toxicities of treatment, and several enjoyed spontaneous regressions of disease. Given these observations, expectant management seems appropriate for selected patients. An exception to this approach may be warranted for asymptomatic patients with follicular, mixed small and large cell (FM) lymphoma, in whom the NCI reported excellent long-term results with C-MOPP (cyclophosphamide, Oncovin [vincristine], procarbazine, and prednisone) chemotherapy. Stages III and IV FML patients achieved a 72% complete remission rate with treatment, and remission durations averaged 6 years. However, the curability of FML with chemotherapy has not been confirmed by other groups.

Chemotherapy is clearly indicated for symptomatic, advanced low-grade NHL. The choice of treatment (Table 10–4) is dictated by the clinical situation. Patients with modest symptoms and no impending complications are treated with single agents such as chlorambucil or oral cyclophosphamide. More severely ill patients should receive combination chemotherapy (Table 10–5) because of the rapidity of response with these regimens. Chemotherapy produces complete remissions in 50 to 80% of patients, but often remissions are not durable. Less than 10% of patients with FSCL remain in remission 5 years after initial chemotherapy. To date, comparative studies show no overall survival advantage for combination chemotherapy or combined modality treatment over single-agent chemotherapy.

INTERMEDIATE-GRADE LYMPHOMAS

The intermediate-grade NHL are rapidly growing neoplasms that differ substantially from their low-grade counterparts. Paradoxically, a sizable fraction of these aggressive lymphomas are stage I or II at diagnosis, but up to one-third present at extranodal sites. Initial bone marrow involvement is encountered in only 10 to 30% of cases. Within the intermediate-grade category considerable clinical and immunologic heterogeneity exists. Follicular large cell (FLC) and diffuse, small cleaved cell (DSCC) lymphomas are always B-cell tumors, whereas the others may be either T- or B-cell malignancies. DSCCL uniquely shares the clinical, histologic, and immunologic features of SL and FSC lymphomas.

Table 10–4. **SUGGESTED APPROACHES TO TREATMENT OF LOW-GRADE NON-HODGKIN'S LYMPHOMAS**

Stages I and II
- Regional field irradiation

Stages III and IV
- Asymptomatic (low risk): deferred initial therapy
- Modest symptoms (low risk): single-agent chemotherapy
- Major symptoms (high risk to vital organs): combination chemotherapy or chemotherapy plus irradiation

Table 10–5. **COMBINATION CHEMOTHERAPY FOR FAVORABLE HISTOLOGY NON-HODGKIN'S LYMPHOMAS**

REGIMEN	DRUGS	INTERVAL
CVP	Cyclophosphamide, 400 mg/m^2 PO days 1–5 Vincristine, 1.4 mg/m^2 IV day 1 Prednisone, 100 mg/m^2 PO days 1–5	q21 days
COP	Cyclophosphamide, 800 mg/m^2 IV day 1 Vincristine (Oncovin), 2 mg IV day 1 Prednisone, 60 mg/m^2 PO days 1–5	q14 days
CP	Cyclophosphamide, 1000 mg/m^2 IV day 1 Prednisone, 100 mg PO days 1–5	q4 weeks
CHOP	Cyclophosphamide, 750 mg/m^2 IV day 1 Adriamycin (doxorubicin), 50 mg/m^2 IV day 1 Vincristine (Oncovin), 2 mg IV day 1 Prednisone, 100 mg PO days 1–5	q3 weeks

The intermediate-grade NHL are inherently chemosensitive; combination chemotherapy cures 30 to 60% of patients with advanced disease. Diffuse large cell lymphoma (DLCL) accounts for one-third of NHL in adults and is the focus of most therapeutic trials. The first cures of diffuse aggressive lymphomas were accomplished with the C-MOPP regimen. The subsequent introduction of Adriamycin (doxorubicin) resulted in major therapeutic gains. One of the original doxorubicin-based regimens—CHOP (cyclophosphamide, hydroxydaunomycin [doxorubicin], Oncovin [vincristine], and prednisone)—is still widely used today. Multi-institutional trials of CHOP chemotherapy demonstrate that about 50% of patients with DLCL enter complete remission, and 30% become long-term disease-free survivors. The efficacy of Adriamycin led to the development of increasingly intensive "generations" of multiagent chemotherapy regimens, which use additional cytotoxic drugs, sometimes in alternating sequences (Table 10–6). "Improved" results with the newer generations of chemotherapy regimens have been reported in uncontrolled trials, but a recent large prospective randomized study revealed no advantage for any of the more intensive regimens over standard CHOP chemotherapy.

With the exception of CNS lymphoma, radiation therapy has a very limited role in the initial treatment of intermediate-grade NHL. Although one study reported a 70% disease-

Table 10–6. **TREATMENT PROGRAMS FOR DIFFUSE AGGRESSIVE LYMPHOMAS**

CHEMOTHERAPY REGIMENS	NUMBER OF PATIENTS	COMPLETE REMISSION RATE (%)	LONG-TERM SURVIVAL (%)
First Generation			
MOPP/C-MOPP	24	46	37
BACOP	32	48	34
CHOP (SWOG)	418	53	30
COMLA	48	40	32
Second Generation			
COP/BLAM	33	72	61
M-BACOD	101	77	57
ProMACE-MOPP	79	73	65
Third Generation			
M-BACOD	80	75	58
ProMACE d1, MOPP d8	54	76	60
ProMACE/CytaBOM	57	79	68
MACOP-B	61	84	75

From Gaynor R, Fisher RI: Diffuse aggressive lymphomas in adults. *In* Magrath IT (ed): The Non-Hodgkin's Lymphomas. Baltimore, William & Wilkins, 1990.

free survival for stage I patients treated with radiotherapy, these results were achieved only in laparatomy-staged patients with low tumor burdens. The combination of involved field radiotherapy plus short-course chemotherapy is highly effective in low-risk stages I and II patients, but the contribution of radiotherapy in this setting is undefined.

The prognosis of patients with intermediate-grade NHL depends on many variables, and in some studies, Ann Arbor stage has not proved especially useful. Multivariate analysis of large clinical trials suggests that poor performance status, bulky disease (elevated LDH or tumors greater than 7 to 10 cm), and multiple extranodal sites of disease predict for lower response rates and decreased survival. Increasing patient age and T-cell phenotype are also associated with a worse prognosis.

Relapses of intermediate-grade NHL usually occur within 2 years of complete remission, although 20% of patients relapse later. The management of patients with relapsing or initially resistant disease is very difficult. Second-line chemotherapy offers little chance for cure, although high response rates are seen in patients with long initial remissions and low tumor burdens. Contemporary salvage regimens frequently contain cisplatin, ifosfamide, etoposide, and high-dose cytosine arabinoside and produce formidable toxicity.

The only potentially curative procedure for relapsed patients is high-dose chemoradiotherapy with autologous bone marrow transplantation (Chap. 31). Thirty to 40% of patients who respond to conventional salvage chemotherapy or have minimal residual lymphoma at the time of transplant will be cured.

HIGH-GRADE LYMPHOMAS

The high-grade NHL are virulent malignancies with diverse clinicopathologic features. The highly proliferative nature of diffuse small noncleaved cell (DSNCCL) and lymphoblastic lymphomas (LBL) is such that urgent staging and treatment are required. With the exception of lymphoblastic lymphoma, these neoplasms often arise in immunodeficient hosts and in extranodal tissues. Immunoblastic lymphomas may be of B- or T-cell lineage, and their natural history and management are similar to DLCL.

Lymphoblastic lymphomas develop predominantly in children and young adults, and males are more often affected. Between 50 and 70% of patients present with a mediastinal mass, which may be complicated by the superior vena cava syndrome or airway obstruction. Bone marrow infiltration, peripheral adenopathy, and "B" symptoms are common at diagnosis. Eight-five percent of LBL are early T-cell malignancies and are histologically and immunophenotypically identical to T-cell ALL. Lymphoblastic lymphoma may evolve into overt ALL, and the clinical differentiation between the two is somewhat artificial. Cytogenetic studies of LBL often show abnormalities of 14q11, which correlate with T-cell receptor gene rearrangements. Treatment of these patients with pediatric ALL chemotherapy protocols, including CNS prophylaxis, has been highly successful. These regimens can cure 85 to 90% of patients with stages I and II LBL and 60 to 80% of those with more advanced disease. Prognosis is adversely affected by an elevated serum LDH (greater than 300), white blood cell count greater than 30,000, initial CNS or bone marrow involvement, and delayed achievement of remission after induction chemotherapy.

The diffuse small noncleaved cell lymphomas (DSNCCL) are fulminant B-cell tumors that predominate in childhood and account for 30 to 50% of pediatric NHL. These lymphomas also arise in the setting of severe immunodeficiency, i.e., acquired immune deficiency syndrome (AIDS) (Chap. 29). The DSNCCL are categorized into Burkitt's and non-Burkitt's subtypes; the latter exhibits more cellular pleomorphism. Burkitt's lymphoma is endemic to regions of Africa and arises only sporadically in the United States and Europe. Epstein-Barr virus (EBV) infection has an etiologic role in Burkitt's lymphoma, especially the endemic variety. EBV DNA can be isolated from 95 and 15% of endemic and sporadic lymphomas, respectively. Most DSNCCL of childhood have a cytogenetic abnormality resulting in a translocation between the immunoglobulin heavy chain gene on chromosome 8 and the c-myc oncogene on chromosome 14, t(8:14) (q24:q32). The DSNCCL uniformly express B-cell markers, including CALLA and surface immunoglobulin.

The sporadic form of this lymphoma usually presents as an abdominal mass, and the ileum is involved in half the cases. African Burkitt's lymphoma typically presents as a rapidly enlarging jaw tumor or as an orbital or paraspinal mass. Prior to treatment, precautions must be taken to prevent chemotherapy-induced tumor lysis syndrome (Chap. 23), including forced diuresis, urinary alkalinization, and allopurinol administration. The treatment of DSNCC lymphomas requires multiagent chemotherapy regimens that include high-dose cyclophosphamide, high-dose methotrexate, vincristine, and prednisone. With adequate treatment, remissions are achieved rapidly, and the total duration of therapy depends on the initial stage of disease. Prophylactic intrathecal chemotherapy is routinely given to prevent CNS relapse. Prognosis is a function of stage and of tumor burden as assessed by LDH level.

Patients with localized or resected abdominal DSNCC lymphomas have a 90% chance of cure with timely treatment, whereas only 60 to 80% of those with unresectable abdominal disease are cured. Patients with initial CNS or marrow involvement do relatively poorly; durable remissions are realized in 20 to 50% of cases. Patients who relapse and those who are at high risk for relapse are potential candidates for bone marrow transplantation.

ADULT T-CELL LEUKEMIA/LYMPHOMA (ATCLL)

ATCLL is a very aggressive malignancy caused by infection with HTLV–1, the human T-cell leukemia virus. HTLV–1 is a retrovirus endemic to regions of southern Japan, Africa, the Caribbean, and the southeastern United States. Approximately 0.01 to 0.1% of infected individuals ultimately develop lymphoma. ATCLL usually presents abruptly with cutaneous lesions, adenopathy, organomegaly, lytic bone lesions, hypercalcemia, and pulmonary infiltrates. Eosinophilia, peripheral blood involvement, and meningeal spread at diagnosis are common findings. Some patients exhibit a lengthy prodromal illness characterized by rash, lymphocytosis, and hypergammaglobulinemia.

The cells of ATCLL have the phenotype of mature T4 (helper) lymphocytes and express large amounts of interleukin 2 (IL-2) receptor. Serum levels of the IL-2 receptor correlate with tumor burden and disease activity. The appearance of ATCLL cells in blood is diagnostic; the cells have multilobulated or convoluted nuclei. The histopathology of affected lymph nodes is variable and nonspecific, e.g., immunoblastic or diffuse mixed lymphoma. The treatment of this disorder is very unsatisfactory, and only brief remissions are attained with chemotherapy. Opportunistic infections occur frequently and are often fatal.

CUTANEOUS T-CELL LYMPHOMAS (Mycosis Fungoides, Sézary Syndrome)

The cutaneous T-cell lymphomas (CTCL) are rare disorders with predominantly dermal manifestations. Mycosis fungoides (MF) is a slowly progressive lymphoma that initially resembles benign dermatitides. Rashes may exist for several years before a definitive diagnosis of MF is established. The cutaneous lesions of MF evolve over time from eczematoid patches to indurated plaques and finally to tumorous nodules; all types of lesions may exist concurrently. The entire skin may be infiltrated, and diffuse erythroderma develops in some cases. The Sézary syndrome (SS) is a closely related condition manifested by diffuse erythroderma and circulating lymphoma cells in peripheral blood. SS may arise de novo or develop after long-standing MF.

Involvement of peripheral nodes occurs in 50% of patients with CTCL and correlates with the extent of cutaneous disease. Visceral lymphoma develops late in the course of MF, and the liver, spleen, and lungs are commonly affected. The histology of CTCL is best appreciated in biopsies of skin lesions. Characteristically, lymphoid cells densely infiltrate the upper dermis, and groups of cells are noted in the epidermis (Pautrier's microabscesses). MF and SS are mature T-cell cancers with a helper-cell phenotype.

The prognosis of patients with CTCL is related to the degree of skin and nodal involvement and to the presence of visceral disease, and these variables also guide therapy. Patients with skin-only disease benefit from topical nitrogen mustard, PUVA phototherapy, or total skin electron beam radiotherapy. The Sézary syndrome and visceral CTCL are treated with chemotherapy, and several agents are active. Patients with SS may also respond to extracorporeal photopheresis; interferons are also effective in CTCL. The median survival of patients with limited disease is 9 to 10 years, compared with 2.5 years and 1 year for patients with erythroderma or visceral disease, respectively.

REFERENCES

Armitage JO, Cheson BD: Interpretation of clinical trials in diffuse large cell lymphoma. J Clin Oncol 6:1335–1347, 1988.
Coleman CN, Picozzi VJ, Cox RS: Treatment of lymphoblastic lymphoma in adults. J Clin Oncol 4:1628–1637, 1986.
Connors JM, Klimo P, Fairey RN, et al: Brief chemotherapy and involved field radiation therapy for limited stage histologically aggressive lymphoma. Ann Intern Med 107:25–30, 1987.
Hopper RT, Wood GS, Abel EA: Mycosis fungoides and the Sézary syndrome: Pathology, staging and treatment. Curr Probl Cancer 14:295–361, 1990.
Kessinger A, Nademanee A, Forman SJ, et al: Autologous marrow transplantation for Hodgkin's and non-Hodgkin's lymphoma. Hematol Oncol Clin North Am 4:577–591, 1990.
Kim JH, Drack DT: Manifestations of human T-lymphotropic virus type 1 infection. Am J Med 84:919–928, 1988.
Magrath IT (ed): The Non-Hodgkin's Lymphomas. Baltimore, William & Wilkins, 1990.
Morrison WH, Hoppe RT, Weiss LM, et al: Small lymphocytic lymphoma. J Clin Oncol 7:598–606, 1989.
Pollack IF, Lunsford D, Flickinger JC, et al: Prognostic factors in the diagnosis and treatment of primary CNS lymphoma. Cancer 63:939–947, 1989.
Velasquez WS, Cabanillas F, Salvador P, et al: Effective salvage therapy for lymphomas with cis-platinum combination with high dose ara-C and dexamethasone (DHAP). Blood 71:117–121, 1988.
Williams SF, Golomb HM (eds): Non-Hodgkin's lymphoma. Semin Oncol 17:1–136, 1990.

11
MULTIPLE MYELOMA

John P. Olson

INCIDENCE AND ETIOLOGY

Multiple myeloma is second only to non-Hodgkin's lymphoma as the most common hematologic malignancy in the U.S. population. It is the most common hematologic malignancy in African Americans, in whom the annual incidence is about twice that of Caucasians. Approximately 12,000 new cases, or 4 to 5 per 100,000 population, were diagnosed in the United States in 1990. This represents 1% of all new cancers and 15% of all new hematologic malignancies. The peak incidence is in the seventh decade, and fewer than 10% of patients are under 50 years of age. The cause is unknown.

PATHOLOGY AND PATHOGENESIS

Multiple myeloma is a malignant disorder of the plasma cell, the terminally differentiated cell of the B-lymphocyte lineage. The myeloma stem cell is a B lymphocyte at the stage where commitment to specific heavy and light globulin chains has occurred.

Multiple myeloma is characterized by diffuse proliferation of neoplastic plasma cells throughout the hematopoietic marrow. Occasional plasma cells may be found in the peripheral blood of patients with myeloma, but the presence of large numbers—plasma cell leukemia—is uncommon. Plasma cell infiltrates are present in many organs at autopsy, but unlike other B-cell malignancies such as chronic lymphocytic leukemia and non-Hodgkin's lymphoma, the clinical features, therapeutic problems, and complications in myeloma usually are not due to extramedullary disease. Instead, the clinical manifestations result from involvement of bone and bone marrow, from inappropriate secretion of monoclonal proteins and other cell products, and from the impaired immune function of the residual nonneoplastic plasma cells.

In multiple myeloma, the marrow plasmacytosis exceeds 10% in most specimens. Patients with minimal or equivocal plasmacytosis but other suspicious clinical or laboratory features may require examination of marrow from another site or direct biopsy of a bone lesion. The relative proportion of mature and immature plasma cells varies considerably from case to case, but generally cells of intermediate maturity predominate.

A benign reactive marrow plasmacytosis of 10 to 20% accompanied by a polyclonal globulin elevation occurs commonly in a diverse group of disorders, including collagen-vascular disease, chronic liver disease, and chronic infection. Clinical differentiation from multiple myeloma usually is not difficult.

Monoclonal proteins (M-proteins), either the entire immunoglobulin molecule or the light chain fragment (Bence Jones protein), are present in over 95% of patients with myeloma. The other 1 to 3% have "nonsecretory" myeloma. The frequency with which one of the four immunoglobulin classes is found in the monoclonal protein spike is proportional to the fraction of nonneoplastic cells programmed to produce that immunoglobulin class under normal circumstances: IgG > IgA > IgD > IgE. In about 70% of patients, the malignant plasma cells produce monoclonal kappa or lambda light chains in excess. In about 15 to 20% of patients, only light chains are produced. Light chains have a relatively low molecular weight and are rapidly filtered by the renal glomeruli. In these patients, the serum protein electrophoresis (SPEP) usually reveals hypogammaglobulinemia and the M-protein (light chain) is found only in the urine. This occurrence is often called "light chain" myeloma.

Most patients with multiple myeloma show a decrease in the serum concentration of normal immunoglobulins due to decreased production and often increased catabolism. Table 11–1 summarizes the sensitivity, usefulness, and limitations of tests for detecting abnormalities of immunoglobulin secretion.

Production of M-proteins is not limited to malignant plasma cells. Other cells in the B-cell lineage produce immunoglobulins, and therefore other B-cell malignancies may be associated with monoclonal immunoglobulin elevations. About 5% of patients with diffuse

Table 11–1. **TESTS FOR MONOCLONAL IMMUNOGLOBULINS**

SERUM TESTS

Serum Protein Electrophoresis (SPEP)

- Useful screening test.
- Useful to quantitate therapeutic response or progressive disease.
- Does not identify immunoglobulin (Ig) classes (IgG, IgA, IgM, IgD, IgE).
- May not detect monoclonal Ig in low concentration.

Serum Immunofixation

- Identifies Ig class and light chain type.
- More sensitive than SPEP in detecting low concentrations of monoclonal Ig.
- Does not provide quantitative data.

Serum Quantitative Immunoglobulins by Nephelometry

- Useful for quantitating level of specific Ig classes and light chain types.
- Useful for serial studies.

URINE TESTS

Albustix

- Insensitive to light chains (Bence Jones protein).

Heat Test

- Requires 150 mg light chains/dL urine—positive in 40–50% of patients.
- "False" positives in 20% because it does not distinguish polyclonal (kappa *and* lambda) from monoclonal (kappa *or* lambda) light chains.

Sulfosalicyclic Acid Test (SAT)

- More sensitive than heat test—detects 35–40 mg light chains/dL urine.
- Not specific for light chains—positive test with albumin.
- Positive SAT and negative Albustix suggest presence of light chains.

Urine Electrophoresis

- Positive in 70–80% of myeloma patients.
- Concentration of urine may be required.
- Useful for demonstrating monoclonal urinary protein.

Urine Immunofixation

- Defines polyclonal versus monoclonal light chain—identifies light chain type.
- Positive in 70–80% of myeloma patients.
- Concentration of urine may be required.
- Not quantitative.

Urine Quantitative Immunoglobulins by Nephelometry

- Useful for quantitating level of specific urinary light chain type.
- Useful for serial studies.

Total Protein, 24-Hour Urine

- Useful for quantitating response to therapy in patients with monoclonal light chain excretion.

non-Hodgkin's lymphoma or chronic lymphocytic leukemia have M-proteins. Amyloidosis occurs in about 10% of patients with multiple myeloma, and about 25% of patients with amyloidosis have multiple myeloma. The other 75% usually have a serum or urinary M-protein. A fragment of the monoclonal light chain produced in such patients interacts with tissues and becomes part of the amyloid fibril.

CLINICAL FEATURES AND NATURAL HISTORY

The clinical features of multiple myeloma are summarized in Table 11–2. Most patients present with bone pain and are found to have anemia, proteinuria, diffuse osteoporosis

Table 11–2. **CLINICAL AND LABORATORY FINDINGS AT PRESENTATION**

FREQUENCY	FINDING
Usually present (>50% of cases)	Bone pain
	Anemia
	Monoclonal serum protein spike
	Osteoporosis and lytic bone lesions
	Bence Jones proteinuria
	Marrow plasmacytosis >10%
Frequently present (25–50% of the cases)	Hypercalcemia
	Renal insufficiency
	Hyperuricemia
Occasionally present (10–25% of cases)	Light chain myeloma
	Hepatomegaly
	Leukopenia
	Thrombocytopenia
	Amyloidosis
Uncommonly present (<10% of cases)	Splenomegaly
	Lymphadenopathy
	No serum or urinary M-protein (nonsecretory myeloma)
	Hyperviscosity syndrome

with or without multifocal lytic bone lesions, and a monoclonal serum protein. Symptoms and signs related to hypercalcemia, renal failure, or infection may be present. Occasionally, detection of proteinuria or hypergammaglobulinemia in an asymptomatic patient may be the first sign of the disease.

The clinical course is characterized by bone destruction, hypercalcemia, nerve root or spinal cord compression, and hypoproliferative anemia. Abnormalities of immunoglobulin production contribute to the increased risk of infection, may be associated with a renal tubular lesion that predisposes to renal insufficiency, and occasionally trigger the development of amyloidosis. Progressive myeloma is the most common underlying cause of death, but infection and renal failure are the most common direct causes. More importantly, these complications are responsible for most of the early deaths that occur at a rate of 10 to 20% in the first 3 months, often before an adequate trial of chemotherapy is administered.

A response to chemotherapy has a substantial effect on the natural history of myeloma. Responders live up to 2 to 3 years longer than nonresponders. Most of the latter die within a year or so after diagnosis. Like other indolent lymphoid malignancies, multiple myeloma is probably incurable by present means, although the long-term results of bone marrow transplantation are as yet unknown. The median survival is 2.5 to 3 years. Long-term survival of 5 and 10 years is limited to 15 and 2% of patients, respectively. Most patients die during the chronic progressive phase of myeloma. However, about 25% have a more acute terminal course characterized by various combinations of pancytopenia, fever, extramedullary disease, rising LDH, rapidly progressive myeloma cell proliferation, immunoblastic lymphomatous transformation, and/or plasma cell leukemia.

STAGING AND PROGNOSIS

Staging systems ideally should provide prognostic information, therapeutic guidance, and criteria for comparing results of therapeutic trials. Several important categories and stages of plasma cell proliferative disorders generally and multiple myeloma in particular have been identified (Table 11–3). These include (1) monoclonal gammopathy of undetermined significance (MGUS), also termed benign or essential monoclonal gammopathy; (2) smoldering and asymptomatic myeloma; (3) localized plasmacytoma; and (4) several stages of frank multiple myeloma.

Monoclonal gammopathy of undetermined significance (MGUS) describes the occurrence of an M-protein in a patient who does not have the diagnostic features of multiple myeloma, other lymphoplasmacytic proliferative disorders, or amyloidosis. The prevalence of MGUS rises sharply with advancing age: 0.5–1.0% in the entire population, 3% in those over 70 years of age, and about 20% in those over 95 years of age. The high frequency of MGUS in the elderly guarantees that it will frequently occur coincidentally with other diseases.

Table 11–3. **PLASMA CELL PROLIFERATIVE DISORDERS**

	MGUS	SMOLDERING MYELOMA	MYELOMA
M-protein	<3 g/dL	>3 g/dL	>3 g/dL
Plasmacytosis	<5%	>10%	>10%
Urinary light chain	Uncommon	Often; Small amount	Usually
Other immune globulins decreased	Rarely	Occasionally	Usually
Clinical features of myeloma	Absent	Absent	Present

Osteoporosis, mild anemia, and renal insufficiency are common in this group. Diagnostic difficulty may ensue. Careful evaluation, therapeutic delay, and serial clinical and laboratory observation are indicated.

About one-third of patients with MGUS die within 10 years of unrelated diseases. Many patients have a stable monoclonal gammopathy after 10 years—over one-third of the total group and over half those not dying of unrelated diseases. Multiple myeloma, macroglobulinemia of Waldenström, amyloidosis, or other lymphoproliferative disorders develop in 20 to 30% of patients followed for 10 years. Those patients whose monoclonal globulin rises more than 50% above the initial level are at highest risk.

Smoldering myeloma describes a group of asymptomatic patients with M-protein and marrow plasma cell levels compatible with myeloma but lacking other clinical features. Asymptomatic myeloma describes patients with minimal stage I disease as defined below. These two groups of patients should be followed closely with regular clinical and laboratory evaluation so that progression can be detected early. Several years may ensue before treatment is required.

Localized plasmacytomas of bone or extramedullary tissue (usually the paranasal sinuses, oronasopharynx, or regional lymph nodes) comprise about 5% of plasma cell malignancies. Monoclonal serum or urinary proteins are present in about 25% and often disappear or decrease after surgical excision or local radiation therapy. The natural history and prognosis differ depending upon the site of the plasmacytoma. Progression—usually the development of multiple myeloma—occurs in 75% of those with bone involvement, compared with only 5 to 10% of those with extramedullary soft tissue plasmacytomas. Radiation therapy usually provides good local control. The risk of myeloma requires long-term follow-up. Most transformations occur within 3 to 5 years and are rare after 10 years.

A staging system for multiple myeloma was developed 10 to 15 years ago utilizing readily available laboratory and x-ray measurements that correlate with the tumor cell burden (Table 11–4). The addition of subgroups based on renal function provides a staging system with prognostic significance, particularly in defining poor-risk patients. Other patient variables have prognostic significance independent of stage (Table 11–5). These variables appear to correlate with the biologic behavior of the malignant plasma cells rather than with tumor cell number. The serum $beta_2$-microglobulin level is the single most important measurement for assessing prognosis at the time of diagnosis. This small protein forms part of the HLA complex on all nucleated cells. It is shed into the blood,

Table 11–4. **CLINICAL STAGING SYSTEM**

CRITERIA	STAGE I*,‡ LOW TUMOR BURDEN	STAGE III†,‡ HIGH TUMOR BURDEN
Hemoglobin	>10 g/dL	<8.5 g/dL
Serum calcium	<11.5 mg/dL	>11.5 mg/dL
Myeloma protein		
IgG	<5 g/dL	>7 g/dL
IgA	<3 g/dL	>5 g/dL
Urinary light chains	<4 g/24 hr	>12 g/24 hr
Skeletal status	≤3 lytic lesions or mild osteoporosis	>4 lytic lesions

*Stage I requires that all criteria be met.

†Stage III requires only one of the criteria. Stage II (intermediate cell burden) is present if the findings fit neither stage I nor stage III criteria.

‡Subgroups A and B for each of the three stages are defined by a creatinine of <2 mg% or >2 mg%, respectively.

Table 11–5. **PROGNOSTIC VARIABLES**

		MEDIAN SURVIVAL (MONTHS)
Stage	I	61
	IIA and IIB	54
	IIIA	30
	IIIB	15
Creatinine	<2 mg/dL	34
	>2 mg/dL	14
Serum $beta_2$-microglobulin	<4 mg/L	43
	>4 mg/L	12
Plasma cell labeling	<0.4%	38
	>0.4%	18
Age	<63 years	42
	>63 years	14

and its level is proportional to the myeloma cell burden, proliferative activity, and renal function. Patients with levels exceeding 4 to 6 mg/L have a shorter survival. The development of elevated levels after a therapeutic response and during the plateau phase of the disease predicts for early relapse.

The occurrence of an objective response to chemotherapy, particularly in poor-risk patients, has significant prognostic impact, with a two- to threefold increase in median survival rates. A rapid response, presumably reflecting a higher fraction of cells in active cell cycle, often predicts for a short remission and survival.

TREATMENT

The physician responsible for the care of a patient with myeloma faces a number of decision points during the course of the disease. These include (1) when to treat and when to delay treatment; (2) the choice of initial chemotherapy; (3) the duration of therapy and the role of maintenance therapy; (4) when to change therapy and the management of relapsing or refractory disease; (5) the role of surgery and radiation therapy; (6) management of complications; and (7) the role of new therapies, including hematopoietic growth factors, interferon, and high-dose chemotherapy with or without bone marrow or stem cell support.

WHEN TO TREAT—WHEN TO DELAY

The need for treatment is evident in most patients who present with symptoms and signs of painful bone disease, anemia, hypercalcemia, renal failure, or infection. However, in three groups of patients, therapeutic delay or limited local therapy with careful follow-up observation is appropriate. Patients with only a monoclonal serum or urinary protein who appear to have MGUS and patients with smoldering or asymptomatic myeloma should be followed closely without therapy. Initial management of patients with plasmacytoma consists of surgical biopsy, or excision, and local radiation therapy. Staging studies should include metastatic bone survey, bone marrow aspiration, complete blood count, and blood chemistries, including LDH, serum $beta_2$-microglobulin, serum immunofixation, and protein electrophoresis. Careful follow-up is indicated.

CHOICE OF INITIAL TREATMENT

Chemotherapy is the major treatment modality in multiple myeloma. Surgery and radiation therapy have limited adjuvant roles. The combination of oral melphalan and prednisone (MP) administered over 4 to 7 days every 4 to 6 weeks has been a standard of therapy for 20 years. An objective response, defined as a decrease in serum or urine M-protein by >50%, occurs in 50 to 60% of patients, and an additional 10 to 20% show disease stabilization and symptomatic improvement. The absorption of oral melphalan is quite variable. The effective dose is that which produces mild leukopenia of 3000 to 4000/mm^3. It is advisable to monitor mid-cycle white blood cell counts and increase the daily dose of melphalan by 2 mg with similar increments in subsequent cycles until a leukopenic effect is achieved. Most patients improve with this regimen, but nearly half experience no, brief, or only symptomatic benefit, and all responding patients eventually relapse. Efforts to improve response rates and survival have produced other active treatment programs.

Three combinations of active drugs (Table 11–6)—the five-drug M2 regimen, the six-drug alternating regimen, and the three-drug vincristine, Adriamycin (doxorubicin], dexamethasone (VAD) regimen—have been widely used and compared with MP or similar regimens in randomized trials. The results have been disappointing; median survival has shown no, equivocal, or only modest improvement despite increase in the frequency of objective response, complete remission rate, and percent reduction in tumor bulk. Cost, inconvenience, and toxicity are higher with these alternative regimens. At present, there is no consensus that MP should be replaced as initial therapy. Some evidence suggests that a subgroup of patients with poor prognostic features may benefit from these alternative regimens, and they are often used in this setting, occasionally in combination with intermittent high-dose glucocorticoids (HDGC).

High-dose glucocorticoids, both as single agents and in combination regimens such as VAD, weekly cyclophosphamide with every other day prednisone, and interferon plus dexamethasone, are effective and useful. They are used most in relapsed or refractory patients. Infection is a major toxicity, and prophylactic ciprofloxacin or trimethoprim-sulfa and oral antifungals should be considered.

Recombinant alpha interferon, a biologic response modifier, has activity in myeloma and other chronic B-cell malignancies. It is incorporated in several current cooperative group trials. Neither the optimum dose and schedule nor the patients that will benefit have been defined fully. One randomized trial indicated that interferon was effective in delaying relapse when used as a single agent during the plateau phase. Interferon also may increase the complete response rate and median survival when used in conjunction

Table 11–6. **COMBINATION CHEMOTHERAPY REGIMENS**

DRUGS	DOSAGE*	SCHEDULE
M2 REGIMEN (VBMCP)*		**Every 4–5 weeks**
Vincristine	1.2 mg/M^2 IV (2 mg max)	Day 1
BCNU	20 mg/M^2 IV	Day 1
Melphalan	8 mg/M^2 PO	Days 1–4
Cyclophosphamide	400 mg/M^2 IV	Day 1
Prednisone	40 mg/M^2 PO	Days 1–7
	20 mg/M^2 PO (first cycle only)	Days 8–14
ALTERNATING REGIMEN* (VMCP-VBAP)		**Alternate every 3 weeks**
Vincristine	1 mg IV	Day 1
Melphalan	5.5 mg/M^2 PO	Days 1–4
Cyclophosphamide	110 mg/M^2 PO	Days 1–4
Prednisone	60 mg/M^2 PO	Days 1–4
Vincristine	1 mg IV	Day 22
BCNU	30 mg/M^2 IV	Day 22
Doxorubicin	30 mg/M^2 IV	Day 22
Prednisone	60 mg/M^2 PO	Days 22–25
VAD		**Every 4 weeks**
Vincristine	0.4 mg IV infusion	Over 24 hr; days 1–4
Doxorubicin	9 mg/M^2 IV infusion	Over 24 hr; days 1–4
Dexamethasone	40 mg PO	Every morning for 4 days; repeat days 9–12 and days 17–20 on odd-numbered cycles; days 1–4 only on even-numbered cycles

*Initial doses of myelosuppressive drugs often reduced by 25–50% in selected poor-risk patients.

with other common regimens in the initial treatment of myeloma and when used in combination with high-dose glucocorticoids in refractory disease.

DURATION OF TREATMENT AND MAINTENANCE THERAPY

Most responding patients show symptomatic improvement and a downward trend in their M-protein within the first 2 to 4 months of treatment. The rate of response may be more rapid with the multidrug regimens than with MP. A slow or equivocal response in the first few months may be worrisome, but as long as patients are stable as judged by clinical and M-protein measurements, they should be continued on initial therapy.

The M-protein level reaches a plateau in most responding patients and may disappear in up to 20 to 30%. The continuation of chemotherapy for more than 4 to 6 months after the M-protein disappears or plateaus carries no benefit in terms of survival and may increase complications, including the risk of treatment-related leukemia. The leukemogenic risk is proportional to the total alkylator dose and exceeds 10 to 15% of those surviving 8 to 10 years.

The median duration of unmaintained remission is about 1 year. Remission may be a few months longer when maintenance chemotherapy is continued. Several prognostic features predict for length of remission whether maintenance therapy is continued or not (Table 11–7). It is important to monitor all patients regularly during the plateau phase. Relapses can be rapid and should be treated before symptoms develop. Recommendations against maintenance treatment may change if preliminary evidence of benefit for interferon during the plateau phase is confirmed.

THERAPY OF RELAPSING OR RESISTANT MYELOMA

Each of four subgroups of patients with relapsing/resistant disease requires a different therapeutic approach:

- Patients who are symptomatically improved but with stable or less than 50% reduction in M-protein should be continued on initial therapy for at least 1 year unless progression occurs sooner. Consideration should then be given to careful follow-up without therapy or, perhaps, to maintenance with interferon.
- Patients who relapse from complete remission or from the plateau phase while off therapy (unmaintained remission) should be treated with the regimen that was successful initially. A second response occurs in about half the patients and is more likely if therapy is begun when laboratory evidence of relapse occurs before symptoms appear.
- Patients who respond initially and then relapse while still on therapy (secondary resistance) and those who do not respond but progress on initial therapy (primary resistance) have low response rates (20 to 30%) to alternative alkylating drug combinations with or without doxorubicin. HDGC-based regimens produce objective responses in up to 60% of patients and are probably the appropriate choice. Some evidence suggests that infusional vincristine and doxorubicin combined with HDGC (VAD regimen) improve response rates in patients exhibiting secondary resistance. However, the exact contribution of infusional vincristine and doxorubicin or weekly cyclophosphamide or interferon in combination with HDGC is far from defined. In patients who progress on VAD, the options include interferon, which has about 20% response rate in resistant patients, or high-dose melphalan or cyclophosphamide. The responses tend to be short. Hemibody radiation may be helpful for multifocal bone pain in advanced, refractory myeloma.

Table 11–7. **DURATION OF UNMAINTAINED REMISSION**

OFTEN LESS THAN 1 YEAR	OFTEN MORE THAN 1 YEAR
Stage III disease	Stage I disease
Light chain myeloma	Loss of monoclonal protein
Renal insufficiency	Slow response
Rapid response	Serum beta$_2$-microglobulin <4–6 mg/L
Serum beta$_2$-microglobulin >4–6 mg/L	

SOME NEW TREATMENT DIRECTIONS

Recombinant alpha interferon is an active agent in the early stage, plateau phase, and resistant phase of myeloma. It may be particularly promising as a relatively nontoxic adjuvant in initial chemotherapy programs and as a nonleukemogenic single agent in the plateau phase. Current drug trials should clarify uncertainties regarding dose, schedule, and favorable patient groups.

Consolidation therapy for responding but poor-prognosis patients in the plateau phase is under study. Regimens include combinations of VAD or high-dose chemotherapy with interferon.

High-dose IV melphalan, often combined with hematopoietic growth factors, autologous or allogeneic marrow transplantation, or stem cell infusion, has been used both in advanced, refractory myeloma and in early disease after a good response to chemotherapy. Several studies in the latter favorable patient group reveal complete remission rates of up to 50% and a projected increased survival, but a substantial relapse rate. Follow-up is short in most studies.

SUPPORTIVE CARE AND THE MANAGEMENT OF COMPLICATIONS

Median survival in myeloma has tripled over the past 3 to 4 decades from less than 1 year to about 3 years. Infection and renal failure are the most common causes of death. Bone pain and fractures are the most common causes of morbidity. Increased understanding and better management tools for these complications have had a major impact on survival.

Infection often occurs in the setting of refractory and progressive myeloma or in the first 1 to 3 months after diagnosis. Bronchopulmonary and urinary tract infections are most common. Death may occur before an adequate trial of chemotherapy. Patients with poor prognostic features are at increased risk. Empiric broad-spectrum antibiotic regimens are indicated, with attention to the potential for enhanced nephrotoxicity of some antibiotics. Intermittent courses of IV gamma globulin have had prophylactic value in some small series, and this agent is recommended for several months in patients who have had a major infection.

Renal failure is present at diagnosis in 20% of patients and occurs in 50% at some time during the course of their disease. Most instances occur in patients with a high tumor burden. The presence of azotemia is the single most important clinical factor affecting prognosis. Median survival is one-third to one-half that of patients without renal failure, and this increased mortality is independent of stage. Slowly progressive renal failure is most common, but acute renal failure occurs in 5% of all patients. Urinary secretion of free light chains is the underlying cause of renal tubular damage. Some combination of additional renal insults, such as dehydration, infection, hypercalcemia, nephrotoxic antibiotics, contrast media, or other agents usually precipitates or aggravates renal dysfunction. Management of renal failure consists of treating or preventing the precipitating factors. Plasmapheresis may be useful in acute renal failure.

Bone destruction occurs in most patients. X-rays reveal diffuse osteoporosis with or without focal lytic lesions and fractures in 80% of patients. Analgesics, back supports, internal fixation of long bone fractures, and local radiation are the mainstays of therapy. Many patients experience a substantial reduction in pain following the first cycle or two of chemotherapy. Local radiotherapy should be delayed if possible in anticipation of this response. Moderate dose (1500 to 2000 cGy) local radiotherapy in conjunction with chemotherapy may relieve severe pain, prevent new fractures, hasten bone healing after surgical fixation, and reverse impending cord compression. Field sizes should be limited to decrease damage to hematopoietic marrow and the consequent reduction in tolerance to chemotherapy.

Despite a good response to chemotherapy, remineralization of bone is not common. Efforts to stimulate bone formation with combinations of fluoride, vitamin D, calcium, and androgens are usually not helpful. Trials with diphosphonates are underway.

Hypercalcemia occurs in about 20% of patients initially. Moderate elevations may be corrected or prevented by adequate hydration and diuresis, by ambulation even if limited to movement from bed to chair, and by the glucocorticoid therapy that is part of most chemotherapy regimens. Marked hypercalcemia requires aggressive therapy. Prompt correction is critical in preventing rapidly progressive renal failure (see Chap. 23).

The hyperviscosity syndrome is a relatively uncommon complication of multiple myeloma. Visual changes, hemorrhagic phenomena, fluctuating neurologic symptoms, and evidence of cardiovascular failure may be present. Macroglobulinemia of Waldenström is responsible for over 85% of cases. Multiple myeloma associated with IgG levels greater than 5 g/dL or IgA polymer formation is responsible for most of the remainder. Plasmapheresis is indicated.

MACROGLOBULINEMIA

Monoclonal proteins of the IgM class (macroglobulins) are responsible for 10 to 15% of the occurrences of monoclonal gammopathy. A diverse group of disorders are included. Some patients have typical non-Hodgkin's lymphoma (NHL) or chronic lymphocytic leukemia (CLL). A few have lytic bone disease and other features of multiple myeloma. Most patients have no other evidence of a lymphoplasmacytic proliferative disorder and are examples of monoclonal macroglobulinemia of undetermined significance. The remainder have a disorder—Waldenström's macroglobulinemia—characterized by various combinations of anemia, mucocutaneous bleeding, retinal vascular changes, polyneuropathy, and enlargement of lymph nodes, spleen, and liver. A pleomorphic infiltrate consisting of small lymphocytes, plasma cells, and plasmacytoid lymphocytes is present in the marrow and enlarged organs. Some patients have lymphocytosis in the peripheral blood. Differentiation from CLL or NHL may be difficult and arbitrary.

Bone disease and hypercalcemia in macroglobulinemia are rare, Bence Jones proteinuria occurs with almost equal frequency as in myeloma, and renal failure is less common. Morbidity and mortality are consequences of bleeding, infection, and the hyperviscosity syndrome. The median survival is 3 to 4 years with a wide range.

Macroglobulinemia is often an indolent, slowly progressive disorder more closely comparable to chronic lymphocytic leukemia or nodular lymphoma than to multiple myeloma. Except in the presence of the hyperviscosity syndrome, therapy is rarely urgent. The distinction between nonprogressive monoclonal macroglobulinemia and progressive malignant disease may be difficult initially. In many patients, it is best to delay chemotherapy and carefully assess disability and progression with serial observations.

The hyperviscosity syndrome is uncommon at relative serum viscosity levels less than 6 and IgM levels less than 4 g/dL. The presence and severity of symptoms and signs are the best guides to the use of plasmapheresis. Patients who require plasmapheresis usually should receive chemotherapy also.

Drug therapy for macroglobulinemia is not based on the controlled, comparative trials that can be cited for multiple myeloma. Low-dose alkylating therapy produces objective responses in most patients. Chlorambucil is used most often. A dose of 0.025 to 0.1 mg/kg/day is adjusted to achieve mild leukopenia of 3000 to 4000/mL. Glucocorticoids are usually omitted, but selective use for short periods should be considered in symptomatic patients with bulky organ enlargement, anemia, and thrombocytopenia. The M-2 regimen, alpha interferon, or fludarabine may be effective in patients with disease resistant to chlorambucil and glucocorticoids.

REFERENCES

Barlogie B, Epstein J, Selvanayagam P, Alexanian R: Plasma cell myeloma—new biological insights and advances in therapy. Blood 73:865–879, 1989.

Bataille R, Durie BGM, Grenier J, Sany J: Prognostic factors and staging in multiple myeloma: A reappraisal. J Clin Oncol 4:80–87, 1986.

Bergsagel DE: Use a gentle approach for refractory myeloma patients. J Clin Oncol 6:757–758, 1988.

Bergsagel DE, von Wussow P, Alexanian R, et al: Interferons in the treatment of multiple myeloma. J Clin Oncol 8:1444–1445, 1990.

Buzaid AC, Durie BGM: Management of refractory myeloma: A review. J Clin Oncol 6:889–905, 1988.

Cuzik J, DeStavola BL, Cooper EH, et al: Long term prognostic value of serum beta 2-microglobulin in myelomatosis. Br J Haematol 75:506–510, 1990.

Jagannath S, Barlogie B, Dicke K, et al: Autologous bone marrow transplantation in multiple myeloma: Identification of prognostic factors. Blood 76:1860–1866, 1990.

Knowling MA, Harwood AR, Bergsagel DE: Comparison of extramedullary plasmacytomas with solitary and multiple plasma cell tumors of bone. J Clin Oncol 1:255–262, 1983.
Kyle RA: New approaches to the therapy of multiple myeloma. Blood 76:1678–1679, 1990.
Kyle RA, Lust JA: Monoclonal gammopathies of undetermined significance. Semin Hematol 26:176–200, 1989.

12
BREAST CANCER

Susan Rosenthal

Breast cancer is the most common malignant disease of women and the second leading cause of cancer deaths (after lung cancer) among women in the United States. It currently accounts for 32% of new cancers in American women and 18% of cancer deaths in this group. In 1992, 181,000 new cases of breast cancer and 46,300 deaths from this disease will occur in this country. About one in every nine American women will develop breast cancer at some time during her life.

EPIDEMIOLOGY AND ETIOLOGY

Breast cancer incidence becomes appreciable at about age 30, and the incidence rate increases with each succeeding decade. No American woman is at "low risk" for this malignancy, but epidemiologic studies have identified women with higher than average risk and have yielded tantalizing clues to the etiology of the disease. Women with early menarche, late menopause, and nulliparity or first childbirth after age 30 are at higher risk, hinting that prolonged estrogen stimulation of breast tissue can lead to breast cancer (Table 12–1). Some studies indicate that prolonged use of postmenopausal estrogens or of oral contraceptives increases breast cancer risk, but these data are controversial.

Circumstantial evidence suggests that diet influences breast cancer risk. Breast cancer is relatively rare in Africa and Asia but quite common in industrialized nations. Internationally, breast cancer incidence bears a linear relationship to dietary fat intake. Descendents of immigrants from low-incidence countries to high-incidence areas acquire the high breast cancer rates of their new homelands, further supporting the etiologic role of environmental factors such as diet. However, it is unclear whether American women can alter their risk of breast cancer by dietary modification. Several studies of American

Table 12–1. **RISK FACTORS FOR BREAST CANCER**

FACTOR	RELATIVE RISK*
Family History	
First-degree relative with breast cancer	1.2–3.0
Premenopausal	3.1
Premenopausal and bilateral	8.5–9.0
Postmenopausal	1.5
Postmenopausal and bilateral	4.0–5.4
Menstrual History	
Age at menarche <12 years	1.3
Age at menopause >55 years with >40 menstrual years	1.48–2.0
Pregnancy	
First child after 35 years	2.0–3.0
Nulliparous	3.0
Other Neoplasms	
Contralateral breast cancer	5.0
Cancer of a major salivary gland	4.0
Cancer of the uterus	2.0
Benign Breast Disease	
Atypical lobular hyperplasia	4.0
Lobular carcinoma in situ	7.2
Previous breast biopsy	1.86–2.13

From Love SM, Gelman RS, Silen W: Fibrocystic "disease" of the breast—A nondisease? N Engl J Med 307:1013–1019, 1982.

*General population risk = 1.0.

women with relatively low dietary fat intake have failed to demonstrate a corresponding lower risk of breast cancer.

Studies of survivors of the atomic bombings in Japan, of women having multiple fluoroscopies for tuberculosis, of women treated with radiotherapy for mastitis, and of children treated with thymic irradiation demonstrate that large doses of radiation increase breast cancer risk. Radiation exposure from current mammography equipment and routine chest radiography is too low to cause concern. The role of alcohol consumption in the etiology of breast cancer is controversial. Women with fibrocystic changes in the breasts are not at increased risk, unless atypical hyperplasia is recognized in a biopsy specimen. Women who have a first-degree relative with breast cancer have a risk two to three times that of the general population, and this risk increases further if the relative had breast cancer at an early age or had bilateral disease.

PATHOLOGY

The great majority of breast cancers are adenocarcinomas. Seventy to 80% are infiltrating ductal carcinomas. Medullary (4 to 5%) and tubular carcinomas also arise from ductal sources but differ because of their characteristic pathologic appearance and better prognosis. Another important histologic variety is infiltrating lobular carcinoma (8 to 10%), which is often multifocal or bilateral and associated with in situ disease. Paget's disease of the breast consists of eczematoid changes of the nipple with underlying carcinoma. Inflammatory carcinoma (1 to 2%) presents with a breast that appears inflamed (red, warm, and painful) due to obstruction of the dermal lymphatics with carcinoma cells. These patients have a poor prognosis and require systemic treatment. Sarcomas and primary lymphomas of the breast occur rarely .

The time required for breast tumors to double in volume (doubling time), estimated both clinically and in vitro, ranges from a few days to more that a year (median 100 days). In comparison to many other cancers, these relatively slow growth rates help explain the long interval between diagnosis and recurrence in many breast cancer patients.

Tumor stage (Table 12–2), histologic grade, hormone receptor levels, proliferative index (measured by DNA flow cytometry), and other factors (HER–2/*neu* oncogene amplification, ploidy, cathepsin D levels) correlate with survival. The pathologist should measure tumor size carefully, examine axillary lymph nodes meticulously, and send fresh tissue for hormone receptor analysis in every case of breast cancer. Flow cytometry, which can be performed on fixed, embedded material, is available for difficult cases (especially certain node-negative cases; see below). The value of other more sophisticated analyses is yet to be confirmed.

SCREENING FOR BREAST CANCER

The goal of cancer screening is to detect early, potentially highly curable cancers in asymptomatic individuals in the general population and in high-risk groups. Screening for breast cancer using the combination of physical examination of the breasts and mammography has clearly proved effective in several large prospective studies. These studies demonstrate that screening can detect smaller and lower-stage breast cancers with a consequent improvement in survival. The effects of physician examination, self-examination by the patient, and mammography are hard to separate, but all contribute to the early detection of breast cancer. For women in the general population, the American Cancer Society currently recommends the following:

- Women over age 20 should perform breast self-examination every month.
- Women between ages 20 and 40 should have a breast examination by a physician every 3 years, and yearly after age 40.
- Women between the ages of 35 and 40 should have an initial screening mammogram.
- Women between the ages of 40 and 50 should have annual or biannual mammography, and women over 50 should have annual mammography.

High-risk women (family history of breast cancer in a first-degree relative, previous breast cancer, previous breast biopsy with atypical hyperplasia) require more intensive screening.

Table 12–2. **TNM STAGING OF BREAST CANCER**

Primary Tumor (T):	
T1S	Carcinoma in situ: intraductal carcinoma, lobular carcinoma in situ, or Paget's disease of the nipple with no tumor
T1	Tumor 2 cm or less in greatest dimension
T2	Tumor 2–5 cm in greatest dimension
T3	Tumor more than 5 cm in greatest dimension
T4	Tumor of any size with direct extension to chest wall or skin
T4a	With fixation to chest wall
T4b	With edema, infiltration, or ulceration of skin of breast (including peau d'orange), or satellite nodules confined to the same breast
T4c	Both of above
T4d	Inflammatory carcinoma
	Dimpling of the skin, nipple retraction, or any other skin change except those in T4b may occur in T1, T2, or T3 without affecting the classification.
Regional Node Involvement (N):	
N0	No regional lymph node metastasis
N1	Metastasis to movable ipsilateral axillary lymph node(s)
N2	Metastasis to ipsilateral axillary lymph node(s) fixed to one another or to other structures
N3	Metastasis to ipsilateral internal mammary lymph node(s)
Distant Metastases (M):	
M0	No evidence of distant metastases
M1	Distant metastases present

STAGE GROUPING FOR INVASIVE CANCER

Stage 0	Tis	N0	M0
Stage I	T1	N0	M0
Stage IIA	T0, T1	N1	M0
	T2	N0	M0
Stage IIB	T2	N1	M0
	T3	N0	M0
Stage IIIA	T0–2	N2	M0
	T3	N1–2	M0
Stage IIIB	Any T	N3	M0
	T4	Any N	M0
Stage IV	Any T	Any N	M1

From Beahrs OH, Henson DE (eds): Manual for Staging of Cancer. 3rd ed. Philadelphia, JB Lippincott, 1988.

CLINICAL PRESENTATION

Breast cancer usually presents as a painless mass detected either by the patient herself or by the physician during the course of a routine physical examination. All breast masses must be biopsied (or aspirated if cystic), but certain characteristics—hardness, immobility, fixation to skin, satellite lesions, peau d'orange skin changes, axillary adenopathy—are highly suggestive of malignancy. Bloody discharge from the nipple may be an initial complaint; an underlying mass is usually present. A swollen, tender, inflamed breast is usually caused by acute mastitis but may be due to inflammatory carcinoma. Neglected breast cancers may occasionally present as large, malodorous masses with ulceration of the skin and sometimes with destruction of the entire breast.

With increased use of screening mammography, more breast cancers are being detected without a palpable mass. These smaller tumors have a lower rate of axillary node involvement and a better long-term prognosis.

Occasionally, patients first present with signs and symptoms of metastatic disease. Bone pain or pathologic fracture and malignant pleural effusion are most common. Axillary adenopathy, hepatomegaly with or without liver failure, brain metastases (focal signs, personality change, seizure, decreased level of consciousness), skin nodules, respiratory symptoms, and other manifestations may also be presenting complaints. Careful physical examination of the breasts and mammography should be the first steps in the evaluation of any woman presenting with metastatic adenocarcinoma of unknown primary origin.

The course of breast cancer is variable. The disease may progress rapidly with widespread dissemination to vital organs, or it may follow an indolent course with slowly progressive local growth. In some cases, particularly in elderly women with bone metastases, progression may be slow and survival duration relatively long.

DIAGNOSIS AND INITIAL EVALUATION

Diagnosis of breast cancer is made by biopsy of the breast mass and microscopic examination of the biopsy specimen. Excisional biopsy, needle aspiration, or core needle biopsy may be done on an outpatient basis, allowing confirmation of the diagnosis and discussion of therapeutic options before definitive therapy is undertaken.

Initial workup of a patient with breast cancer includes a careful history and physical examination, chest x-ray, complete blood count, and screening liver chemistries. Mammography localizes the tumor prior to biopsy and detects other suspicious areas, but a negative mammogram does not alter the requirement to biopsy (or aspirate) any palpable breast mass.

A bone scan may detect subclinical bone metastases, but this study is rarely positive in asymptomatic individuals. The incidence of positive bone scans in patients with stages I and II breast cancer is less than 5%. In patients with stage III disease and in those with any complaint of bone pain, the yield from bone scanning is sufficiently high to make the procedure worthwhile. Some oncologists and surgeons recommend a baseline bone scan in all breast cancer patients for the purpose of comparison with any future examinations.

If the history or physical examination points to problems involving a specific organ system, that system requires evaluation with appropriate diagnostic tests. For example, if hepatomegaly is present or the liver function tests are abnormal, then the workup should include a liver scan or abdominal CT scan. If the patient complains of headache or develops focal neurologic signs, then a CT scan of the brain is indicated. In the absence of specific signs and symptoms, these diagnostic studies are unnecessary.

Table 12–2 summarizes the TNM staging classification for breast cancer.

HORMONE RECEPTORS

Hormone receptors are proteins present in the cytosol of many breast cancer cells. These receptors (estrogen receptor [ER], progesterone receptor [PR]) mediate the effects of estrogen and progesterone on the cellular level. The hormone enters the cell, binds to the receptor, and the hormone-receptor complex then translocates to the nucleus and ultimately alters DNA synthesis, RNA synthesis, and cell division. If the receptor is lacking, these events do not take place, and the tumor is not hormonally dependent.

Receptor proteins are markers of cellular differentiation and are more often present in histologically well-differentiated tumors or those with lower proliferative indices. Estrogen receptor correlates poorly with tumor size and only weakly with nodal status (more ER-positive stage I patients and more ER-negative stage II patients).

Accurate, quantitative hormone receptor determinations depend on careful handling of the specimen. Tumor tissue obtained for hormone receptor analysis must be frozen immediately after removal. Delay in freezing, premature thawing during transport, lack of tumor in the assay specimen, and poor assay methodology contribute to falsely negative results. Recently developed immunohistochemical techniques allow quantitative determination of hormone receptor status in fixed, embedded tissue (see Chap. 2).

CLINICAL IMPLICATIONS

ER is present in 40 to 50% of premenopausal breast cancers and in 60 to 70% of postmenopausal breast cancers. Generally, postmenopausal women have higher receptor levels (usually measured as femtomoles [fmol] of receptor per milligram of cytosol protein) than premenopausal women. Seventy-five percent of ER-positive tumors are also PR positive. PR-positive tumors that are ER negative occur infrequently. With disease evolution, cellular dedifferentiation and loss of receptor protein may occur. Nevertheless, receptor status remains remarkably constant in most patients, and the result obtained from receptor analysis of the primary tumor reliably predicts the responsiveness to endocrine therapy for metastatic disease that may develop many years later.

High circulating estrogen levels may bind to cytosol ER and contribute to the lower levels of receptor found in premenopausal women and to the receptor-negative status commonly seen in breast cancers in pregnant women. Women on estrogen replacement therapy for menopausal symptoms are also often receptor negative. This phenomenon may also explain the occurrence of ER-negative, PR-positive tumors.

Many studies correlate the presence of hormone receptors in the original breast cancer with a longer survival. It is unclear if the longer survival in receptor-positive patients is due to delay in time to first relapse or increased survival following first recurrence, or both. The presence of receptors also predicts a different pattern of relapse. Receptor-positive tumors are less likely to relapse in viscera and brain than are receptor-negative tumors. The greatest clinical use of receptor status, however, is to predict the responsiveness of metastatic disease to hormonal interventions.

THERAPEUTIC IMPLICATIONS

Hormone receptor positivity predicts responsiveness to all forms of endocrine therapy, but the assay is most reliable in identifying those patients unlikely to respond. Since breast cancers are heterogeneous, the amount of receptor protein is probably proportional to the number of positive cells. Receptor status is a continuum, and a dose-response effect is clearly observed. The response rate to hormonal therapy is 40% for tumors that contain 10 to 100 fmol ER/mg cytosol protein and 70 to 80% for tumors that contain more than 100 fmol ER/mg cytosol protein. However, no significant correlation exists between duration of remission and amount of estrogen receptor.

Several investigators have combined chemotherapy and hormonal therapy in the treatment of receptor-positive advanced breast cancer. Theoretically, the combination of chemotherapy and hormonal therapy could be counterproductive: the cytotoxic drugs could cause a decrease in receptor protein synthesis, impairing the therapeutic efficacy of the hormones. Conversely, the hormones could slow cell-cycle progression, interfering with the impact of chemotherapy. In addition, hormones and cytotoxic agents might compete for cellular uptake carriers. Alternatively, combined chemohormonotherapy might produce enhanced effectiveness. Since receptor-positive breast cancers contain both hormone-sensitive and autonomous (receptor-negative) cells, combined therapy would affect a greater proportion of cells than either modality alone. The two modalities work by differing mechanisms, so maximum effective doses of each can be administered without overlapping toxicities.

Clinical results from studies exploring these questions have been difficult to interpret. Several adjuvant studies have shown benefit from the addition of tamoxifen to chemotherapy. Other studies have failed to demonstrate a difference. In advanced disease, results with chemohormonotherapy have been conflicting. Further evaluation of the role of combined chemohormonotherapy in receptor-positive breast cancer is necessary.

LOCAL-REGIONAL THERAPY

The goal of local therapy is to ensure local control of disease. Traditionally, the initial management of breast cancer has been surgical, with removal of the breast and draining lymph nodes (radical mastectomy, modified radical mastectomy, or total mastectomy with axillary lymph node dissection). In the past, breast cancer was thought to spread from the primary site to regional lymph nodes in a well-defined, orderly sequence, and only subsequently to disseminate widely. This concept of the natural history of breast cancer justified the use of increasingly radical local procedures in the hope of preventing dissemination.

The failure of radical local procedures to improve the cure rate for breast cancer stimulated a new understanding of the natural history of this disease. The current model considers breast cancer a systemic disease at the time of diagnosis: in many cases, tumor has disseminated prior to detection of the primary, and local modalities, no matter how radical, cannot be expected to cure those patients in whom systemic micrometastasis has already taken place.

MASTECTOMY

Numerous clinical trials from both the United States and Europe demonstrate that radical surgery does not improve the prognosis of stages I and II breast cancer when compared with less radical procedures. In perhaps the most well-known of these trials, the National Surgical Adjuvant Breast Project (NSABP) showed no difference between radical mastectomy, simple mastectomy plus radiation, and simple mastectomy alone in overall survival or incidence of distant metastases in patients with clinically negative axillary lymph nodes. In patients with clinically positive axillary nodes, there was no difference between radical mastectomy and simple mastectomy plus radiation. These studies, and many others like them, support the hypothesis that breast cancer is a systemic disease and that variations in local-regional therapy are unlikely to affect survival substantially. These studies also suggest that treatment of the axillary nodes is neither harmful nor beneficial with regard to survival.

The use of postoperative radiation therapy following mastectomy results in a lower incidence of local-regional recurrences within the treated area but does not alter survival. Irradiation at the first sign of local recurrence will also achieve local control and avoid the unnecessary treatment of a large number of patients who will never develop this problem. In most centers, routine postoperative radiation is no longer given to breast cancer patients unless special circumstances (positive surgical margins, stage III disease) require it.

BREAST CONSERVATION

Randomized, controlled studies show that local excision of a breast cancer (lumpectomy, segmentectomy, or quadrantectomy) followed by radiation therapy to the breast offers comparable 5-year survival to more extensive surgery, with a much better cosmetic result. European data with 20-year follow-up also support the use of breast conservation surgery.

Breast conservation surgery may be recommended safely to most women with early breast cancer if high-quality radiation therapy is available. Patients who are poor candidates for breast conservation include those with multifocal disease, extensive intraductal disease in addition to infiltrating ductal disease, positive surgical margins, large tumor size, and small breasts in which tumor excision would give a poor cosmetic result.

LOCALLY ADVANCED DISEASE

Locally advanced breast cancers have a very poor prognosis when treated with surgery alone. These tumors, considered inoperable for cure (Table 12–3), present difficult management problems. They are often treated with radiation therapy, with or without limited surgery, and systemic therapy. Radiotherapy achieves a better local control rate, but both local control and freedom from distant relapse may be improved with chemotherapy. The optimal systemic therapy, the best local modality, and the proper sequencing of treatments remain to be determined.

PROGNOSIS

Despite advances in early diagnosis and primary treatment with surgery, radiation therapy, or both, close to half of all breast cancer patients develop systemic metastases and ultimately die of their cancer. The single most important prognostic factor in primary breast cancer is the presence or absence of metastases to the axillary nodes (Table 12–4);

Table 12–3. **CRITERIA FOR INOPERABILITY OF BREAST CANCER***

Distant metastases	Extensive local disease
Supraclavicular adenopathy	Edema of the breast
Edema of the arm	Satellite skin nodules
Inflammatory carcinoma	Ulceration
Very large, fixed axillary nodes	Fixation of the tumor to chest wall

*Criteria are relative and refer to surgery with expectation of a reasonable chance of cure.

Table 12–4. **SURVIVAL IN BREAST CANCER AS A FUNCTION OF PATHOLOGIC NODE STATUS**

NODAL STATUS	PERCENT SURVIVAL	
	5-Year	**10-Year**
All patients	63.5	45.9
Negative axillary nodes	78.1	64.9
Positive axillary nodes	46.5	24.9
1–3	62.2	37.5
4+	32.0	13.4

an axillary node dissection is always necessary, whatever the primary modality selected, to obtain this prognostic information. Table 12–5 lists other important prognostic factors.

ADJUVANT (SYSTEMIC) THERAPY

The long-term outlook for women with breast cancer correlates with the extent of axillary nodal involvement at the time of surgery (see Table 12–4). Patients with positive axillary nodes are likely to have micrometastatic disease at the time of diagnosis. Adjuvant therapy is early systemic therapy for patients at high risk of harboring micrometastatic disease. Axillary nodal involvement identifies those patients at the greatest risk of subsequent recurrence, and therefore those with the most to gain from successful adjuvant therapy.

Data from animal tumor model systems provide several principles applicable to adjuvant chemotherapy for human tumors:

- The greater the tumor burden, the less likely that any form of therapy, local or systemic, will be successful. Micrometastatic disease may be eradicated by the same agents that fail to cure macroscopic metastatic disease.
- The greater the delay between removal of the primary tumor and commencement of adjuvant chemotherapy, the worse the outcome.
- High doses of chemotherapy administered intermittently are more effective than low doses given continuously.
- Limited duration of treatment minimizes toxicity. Prolonged treatment does not improve the cure rate.
- Use of combination chemotherapy should minimize the emergence of drug-resistant tumor cell clones.

Over the past 30 years, and particularly during the past decade, a tremendous amount of clinical experience has been gained with the use of adjuvant chemotherapy in various

Table 12–5. **PROGNOSTIC FACTORS IN EARLY BREAST CANCER**

Prognostic factors
Involved axillary lymph nodes
Tumor size
Histologic type
Nuclear grade
Hormone receptor levels
Lymphatic or blood vessel invasion
Aneuploidy
DNA flow cytometry
Proliferative rate
Mitotic rate
S phase fraction
Thymidine labeling index
Cathepsin D level*
HER2/*neu* oncogene amplification and/or overexpression*
Levels of several growth factors and/or growth factor receptors*

*Indicates that the value of this prognostic factor has not been confirmed.

categories of patients with breast cancer. Also, the development of reliable hormone receptor assays and an effective antiestrogenic hormone (tamoxifen) has made adjuvant hormonal therapy feasible and attractive. Hundreds of clinical trials describe adjuvant systemic therapy in patients with breast cancer. The results are frequently conflicting and the conclusions contradictory. Therefore, in September 1985 and again in June 1990, the National Institutes of Health convened Consensus Development Conferences on the Adjuvant Therapy of Breast Cancer. After a thorough review of all the data from worldwide clinical trials, the consensus panelists reached several conclusions regarding the use of adjuvant systemic therapy, which are summarized below.

ADJUVANT CHEMOTHERAPY FOR PREMENOPAUSAL PATIENTS

The efficacy of adjuvant chemotherapy in node-positive premenopausal women is highly reproducible in multiple controlled prospective clinical trials, and such therapy is standard for these patients. Adjuvant chemotherapy provides a highly significant increase in both disease-free survival and overall survival in this group. Adjuvant chemotherapy with a CMF-like regimen (Table 12–6) in node-positive women under age 50 reduces the 5-year mortality from about 36% to about 27%, preventing approximately one-fourth of the early deaths. While survival advantages are evident, they are far from ideal, and the optimal regimen and duration of therapy have not yet been defined.

The same combinations of drugs and schedules used for advanced disease are used in the adjuvant setting. Table 12–6 lists several standard regimens. Short courses of chemotherapy (perhaps 3 to 6 months) are as effective as longer treatment durations. Dose reductions may compromise the efficacy of adjuvant chemotherapy; full doses should be administered to the degree possible. Regardless of whether primary breast cancer is managed by conservative surgery and breast irradiation or by mastectomy, adjuvant systemic therapy should be given in full doses to all appropriate patients. The integration and sequencing of chemotherapy and breast irradiation are not standardized; a variety of schedules are employed.

The role of adjuvant hormonal therapy (ovarian ablation, antiestrogens, or gonadotropin-releasing hormone agonists) either alone or in addition to chemotherapy for premenopausal women is under study in clinical trials and remains unresolved at present.

A discussion of systemic adjuvant therapy for node-negative breast cancer in premenopausal women appears in a later section of this chapter.

ADJUVANT CHEMOTHERAPY FOR POSTMENOPAUSAL PATIENTS

The role of adjuvant chemotherapy for postmenopausal women is less clear. Many adjuvant chemotherapy trials fail to demonstrate an increase in disease-free or overall survival for postmenopausal patients with positive axillary nodes. In a systematic overview of 61 randomized trials involving almost 30,000 women treated with systemic adjuvant therapy, cytotoxic chemotherapy demonstrated a clear reduction in mortality for women under 50 but not for those over 50 (Table 12–7). Tamoxifen, on the other hand, reduced

Table 12–6. **COMBINATION CHEMOTHERAPY OF BREAST CANCER**

Regimen	Drugs	Schedule
CMF* (original)	Cyclophosphamide, 100 mg/m² PO every day for 14 days Methotrexate, 40 mg/m² IV day 1, day 8 5-Fluorouracil, 600 mg/m² IV day 1, day 8	Repeat every 28 days as tolerated
CMF* (iv)	Cyclophosphamide, 600 mg/m² IV day 1 Methotrexate, 40 mg/m² IV day 1 5-Fluorouracil, 600 mg/m² IV day 1	Repeat every 21 days as tolerated
CAF*	Cyclophosphamide, 500 mg/m² IV day 1 Adriamycin (doxorubicin), 50 mg/m² IV day 1 5-Fluorouracil, 500 mg/m² IV day 1	Repeat every 21 days as tolerated
AC*	Adriamycin (doxorubicin), 60 mg/m² IV day 1 Cyclophosphamide, 600 mg/m² IV day 1	Repeat every 21 days as tolerated

*Doses are modified for leukopenia, thrombocytopenia, impaired renal and liver function. Maximum tolerated dose should be used.

Table 12–7. **MORTALITY EFFECTS OF ADJUVANT THERAPY**

AGE (YEARS)	THERAPY	EFFECT
Under 50	Chemotherapy	+ + +
Over 50	Chemotherapy	0
Under 50	Tamoxifen	0
Over 50 (ER$^+$)	Tamoxifen	+ +

mortality only in the over 50 age group. A large recent study from the NSABP indicates that a 3-month course of cyclophosphamide and Adriamycin (doxorubicin) plus 5 years of tamoxifen produces superior disease-free survival and overall survival to tamoxifen alone, but these results await confirmation.

Given this information and the known toxicity, inconvenience, and expense of adjuvant chemotherapy, what recommendations can be made for the treatment of postmenopausal node-positive patients? Clearly, further research is necessary to improve results, and, whenever possible, postmenopausal patients should enter appropriate clinical trials. If such entry is not possible, the therapeutic decision must balance the toxicity and cost of treatment against its expected benefit. For patients (particularly the elderly) with positive hormone receptor levels, this choice is relatively straightforward: tamoxifen has proven effectiveness and minimal toxicity. Outside a clinical trial, tamoxifen is preferred in this subset of patients (see below).

For younger postmenopausal patients with positive receptors and many positive nodes and for patients with positive nodes but negative hormone receptors, the choice is difficult and controversial. For some patients, a possible advantage in disease-free and overall survival may outweigh the side effects and expense of treatment. For these individuals, adjuvant chemotherapy is appropriate, especially for patients with four or more positive nodes. However, adjuvant chemotherapy cannot be considered standard treatment for this group of patients. Until more information is available from clinical trials, these patients will require individualized management.

ADJUVANT ENDOCRINE THERAPY FOR POSTMENOPAUSAL PATIENTS

Numerous studies have demonstrated a highly significant benefit of tamoxifen on disease-free survival in postmenopausal patients with hormone receptor–positive tumors and positive axillary nodes. Pooling the results of all the randomized tamoxifen studies in node-positive patients over age 50, adjuvant tamoxifen appears to reduce the 5-year mortality from about 30% to about 24 to 25%, thus avoiding approximately one-fifth of the early deaths. This benefit of tamoxifen in women over 50 is even more worthwhile because it can be achieved without serious toxicity. Adjuvant tamoxifen (10 mg b.i.d.) is the standard therapy in postmenopausal, node-positive, receptor-positive women. The optimal duration of adjuvant tamoxifen therapy remains undefined; most patients receive at least 2 to 5 years of treatment. Current trials are evaluating the role of tamoxifen given for longer periods. Doses of tamoxifen higher than 20 mg daily are not indicated.

The therapeutic benefit of tamoxifen correlates with increasing levels of hormone receptors (especially PR), but further investigation on this point is required. The role of tamoxifen combined with cytotoxic chemotherapy for patients with positive axillary nodes and positive receptors remains controversial. The recent NSABP study combining 3 months of cyclophosphamide and Adriamycin with 5 years of tamoxifen (see above) is very encouraging, however.

Patients receiving adjuvant tamoxifen develop fewer contralateral primary breast cancers. This tantalizing finding led to the possibility of breast cancer prevention in high-risk patients. The NSABP is currently conducting a randomized, placebo-controlled trial of preventive tamoxifen use in the elderly and in first-degree relatives of patients with premenopausal breast cancer. The results of this trial are eagerly awaited.

ADJUVANT CHEMOTHERAPY FOR NODE-NEGATIVE BREAST CANCER

Until recently, routine administration of adjuvant systemic therapy in women with histologically negative axillary nodes was not recommended. Such women have a relatively low relapse rate (25 to 30% at 10 years, compared with 75% for patients with node-positive tumors) and a correspondingly good survival. However, in 1988, the National Cancer Institute issued a "Clinical Alert," releasing preliminary results of three clinical trials demonstrating an improved disease-free survival for patients with negative nodes who received systemic adjuvant therapy. Since that time, systemic adjuvant therapy either with cytotoxic chemotherapy or tamoxifen or both has come into widespread use. Which regimen to use, when to combine chemotherapy with endocrine therapy, and whether patients with very small tumors (less than 1.0 cm) require adjuvant therapy remain topics of debate.

A variety of prognostic indicators helps predict the risk of relapse in patients with negative nodes. Relapse rate is clearly a function of tumor size, and patients with very small tumors have a 5-year disease-free survival rate in excess of 90%. Hormone receptor positivity also signals a better prognosis. DNA flow cytometry with measurement of tumor cell ploidy and fraction of cells in S phase correlates with prognosis in several studies. The greater the degree of aneuploidy and the higher the proliferative rate (as measured by S phase percentage or thymidine labeling index), the greater the risk of subsequent dissemination. Table 12–5 lists additional risk factors under investigation. Ultimately, careful analysis of multiple risk factors may identify those patients at high risk of dissemination, so that only those patients most likely to benefit receive systemic adjuvant therapy. Conversely, risk-factor analysis should allow patients with an excellent prognosis following local modalities alone to avoid costly and potentially toxic systemic therapy.

ADVERSE EFFECTS OF ADJUVANT THERAPY

The acute toxicity of adjuvant chemotherapy includes varying degrees of leukopenia, nausea and vomiting, fatigue, and hair loss. Amenorrhea frequently occurs as a result of cytotoxic therapy and is rarely reversible in women over 40 years of age. Weight gain is common, especially with prednisone-containing regimens. The acute physical side effects are usually tolerable with symptomatic treatments and rarely result in hospitalization or death. The psychological, social, and economic costs are less well studied and may be equally significant. Long-term studies show a small increase in the incidence of acute leukemia in some series, but no greater risk for the development of solid tumors or second breast cancers.

The side effects of tamoxifen are relatively minor. Some patients develop hot flashes, and others may have a small amount of vaginal discharge. Because of the estrogen agonist activity of the drug, thromboembolic complications may occur in a small percentage of patients. Increased osteoporosis and a higher incidence of cardiovascular disease were both feared consequences of widespread tamoxifen use, but more recent data reveal that tamoxifen appears to protect against both complications, probably on the basis of its estrogenic activity. This same activity, however, may increase the risk of endometrial carcinoma in patients taking tamoxifen, but the number of cases encountered has been very small and the validity of this association is uncertain.

SUMMARY

Established adjuvant programs improve disease-free and overall survival in certain subgroups of breast cancer patients. The toxicity of these programs is acceptable and in most cases readily controlled with simple measures. Ongoing clinical trials are addressing additional questions regarding the systemic management of early breast cancer, including the interaction of breast conservation surgery (less than mastectomy) and radiation with systemic therapy; the efficacy of adjuvant chemotherapy and/or endocrine therapy in patients with negative axillary nodes; refinements of staging and prognostic subgroups; the development of innovative and more effective chemotherapy programs, including dose intensification and bone marrow transplantation; changes in the timing and scheduling of drugs, including pre- and perioperative treatment; optimal duration of chemotherapy and tamoxifen administration; accurate assessment of the psychological, social, and economic impact of adjuvant therapy; and continued assessment of the late effects of adjuvant therapy.

METASTATIC DISEASE

To date, no curative therapy for metastatic breast cancer has been developed. Regardless of how limited or innocent seeming, recurrent breast cancer is invariably fatal. Therefore, outside of a clinical trial, the goal of therapy is palliation using the least toxic methods available.

Generally, patients with localized disease should receive a local form of therapy. Local treatment may be excision in the case of a cutaneous or nodal recurrence in order to verify the pathology and to reexamine the receptor status. Local radiation therapy is indicated for control of painful bone lesions and chest wall recurrences. Radiation therapy is mandatory for brain metastases, along with dexamethasone to control cerebral edema. Many oncologists recommend systemic therapy in addition to local treatment for limited disease, recognizing that widespread dissemination will soon follow. Nevertheless, there is no evidence from randomized trials that early systemic therapy in the setting of limited metastatic disease improves outcome when compared with a strategy of local treatment alone and systemic therapy only when symptoms of advancing disease require it.

Most patients with metastatic breast cancer require systemic therapy at some time during the course of their disease. Systemic therapy often induces clinically worthwhile responses, but they are rarely complete and virtually never permanent. Many oncologists prefer to treat only patients with measurable or evaluable metastatic disease to allow objective evaluation of the response to systemic therapy and avoid prolonged ineffective treatment. However, patients with severe symptoms from bone involvement, for example, rarely have measurable disease but frequently require systemic therapy nonetheless. The choice of systemic treatment depends on the site(s) and extent of recurrence, the severity of the symptoms, the tempo of disease progression, and, most importantly, the hormone sensitivity of the tumor. Figure 12–1 outlines a suggested schema for the management of metastatic breast cancer with sequential systemic therapies.

HORMONAL THERAPY

Hormonal manipulation is the oldest effective systemic treatment for breast cancer. Traditional treatments range from ablative endocrine procedures such as oophorectomy, adrenalectomy, and hypophysectomy (now obsolete), to additive hormonal therapies using pharmacologic doses of estrogens (rarely used today), androgens, progestins, and glucocorticoids. Tamoxifen, an antiestrogen with minimal side effects, is the first hormonal manipulation for most endocrine-responsive patients. Table 12–8 lists the major hormonal alternatives.

Tumors lacking hormone receptors are unlikely to respond to any hormonal manipulation, and metastases in ominous visceral sites (bone marrow, liver, and lymphangitic lung involvement) are usually unresponsive to hormonal therapy even if ER positive. Response to hormonal therapy may be slow in onset, so it is inappropriate for rapidly progressing or life-threatening disease, regardless of the receptor status. While the absence of hormone receptors reliably predicts for failure of hormonal manipulation, only about 60% of patients with positive receptors will respond to endocrine therapy (Table 12–9). The median duration of response to hormonal therapy is 9 to 15 months.

The clinical features that predict for response to hormonal therapy include a long disease-free interval from mastectomy to first recurrence, predominantly osseous and soft tissue metastases, and older age. Response to an initial hormone therapy (e.g., tamoxifen) increases the likelihood of response to a second hormone therapy (e.g., aminoglutethimide or progestin). Estrogen receptor positivity correlates with these clinical features. The presence of progesterone receptor increases the probability of response. Randomized trials comparing hormonal therapies have failed to demonstrate a clearcut advantage for any one form of treatment over the others. Therefore, the choice of initial hormonal therapy and the sequence of subsequent hormonal maneuvers depend on tradition and on the relative toxicities of the various modalities. In almost all cases, tamoxifen is the initial hormonal agent of choice.

Tamoxifen

Antiestrogens block the uptake of estrogens in target tissues by binding to the estrogen receptor. The only antiestrogen currently approved as safe and effective is tamoxifen. The

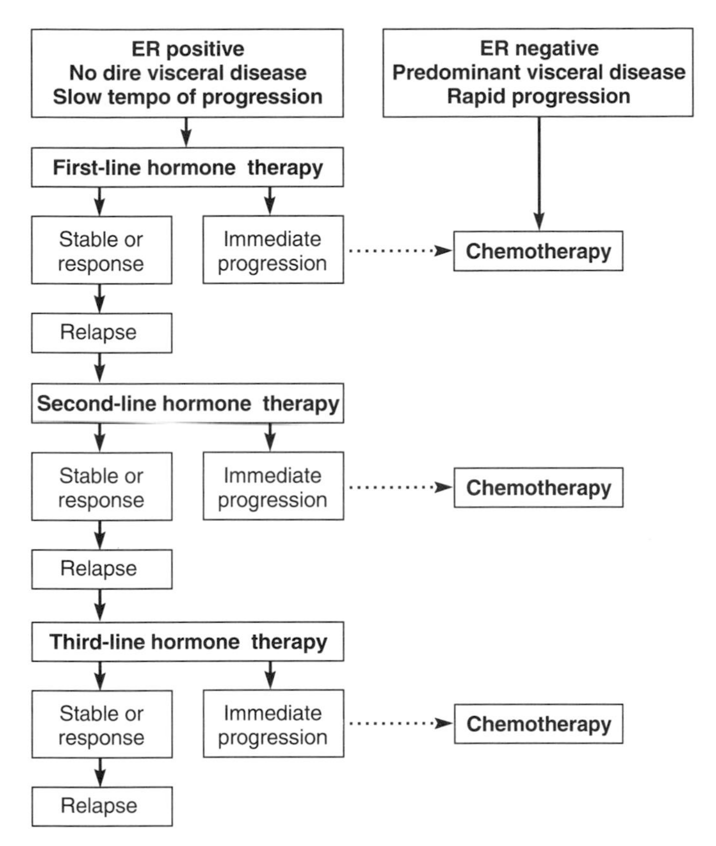

Figure 12–1. Suggested flow diagram for the management of metastatic breast cancer. Patients with only a solitary site of metastatic disease (e.g., chest wall, single bone metastasis) are usually treated with local radiotherapy. Visceral disease includes bulky liver metastases, lymphangitic lung disease, and extensive bone metastases. Patients who respond to treatment are usually continued on that treatment until disease progression. At that point, the next therapy is instituted.

overall response rate of tamoxifen in ER-positive patients is about 50 to 60%, and patients with higher ER levels have a greater likelihood of response. As with all hormonal therapies, responses are most common when disease is limited to soft tissue and bone. The median duration of response is about 12 to 16 months, with a range of 4 to more than 40 months. Side effects are rare except for hot flashes.

In postmenopausal patients, tamoxifen is the preferred initial hormonal agent. Patients who respond to tamoxifen and then relapse retain the capacity to respond to progestins, androgens, aminoglutethimide, and diethylstilbestrol. Preliminary data in premenopausal patients suggest that tamoxifen is as effective as oophorectomy. Most oncologists recommend the use of tamoxifen as the initial hormonal treatment in premenopausal as well as postmenopausal women. Premenopausal patients who respond to tamoxifen and then relapse are likely to respond to subsequent oophorectomy.

Oophorectomy

Bilateral oophorectomy in premenopausal women was one of the earliest forms of systemic therapy for breast cancer and is still in use today. Oophorectomy will induce a regression of metastatic tumor in 50 to 60% of ER-positive patients with a median duration of 9 to 12 months. Radiation castration produces similar results, but the onset of response may be delayed for up to 2 months. The recent development of gonadotropin-releasing

Table 12–8. **HORMONAL THERAPY FOR METASTATIC BREAST CANCER**

METHOD	COMMENT
Premenopausal	
Ablative	
Oophorectomy	Surgery or radiation therapy
Tamoxifen	10 mg b.i.d.
LHRH agonist	Leuprolide or goserelin, injected monthly
Additive	
Androgen	Fluoxymesterone, 10 mg b.i.d.
Postmenopausal	
Ablative	
Tamoxifen	10 mg b.i.d.
Additive	
Estrogen	Diethylstilbestrol, 5 mg t.i.d.
Androgen	Fluoxymesterone, 10 mg b.i.d.
Additional Choices in Prior Hormone Responders of Any Age	
Adrenalectomy	
Surgical	Requires adrenal hormone replacement
Medical	Aminoglutethimide, 250 mg q.i.d.; hydrocortisone replacement, 20 mg b.i.d.
Progestins	Megestrol acetate, 40 mg q.i.d.
Glucocorticoids	Prednisone or dexamethasone

hormone analogues (i.e., leuprolide, goserelin) now offers a third alternative; namely, medical castration. These agents initially stimulate but ultimately deplete pituitary secretion of gonadotropins with the consequent suppression of ovarian hormone synthesis. About 40 to 50% of oophorectomy responders will subsequently respond to a second hormonal maneuver. Patients responding to a succession of hormone treatments survive longer than nonresponders by 20 to 24 months.

Androgens and Progestins

Androgens are comparable in efficacy to other hormonal manipulations in the treatment of osseous metastases. Androgen therapy is complicated by virilization and increased libido, and also by erythrocytosis, which can improve the sense of well-being. Progestational agents (medroxyprogesterone acetate or megesterol acetate) are often effective in women who have previously responded to other additive regimens. Side effects are few and include fluid retention and weight gain. The mechanism of action is unknown. Appetite improvement and weight gain due to megesterol acetate may warrant continuation of this agent even in the absence of an antitumor response, particularly if additional therapeutic options are limited.

Adrenalectomy and Aminoglutethimide

Since the second major source of estrogens is the adrenal gland, surgical or medical adrenalectomy is another ablative choice. Because of the substantial morbidity and

Table 12–9. **ESTROGEN RECEPTOR STATUS AND RESPONSE TO ENDOCRINE THERAPY**

	PERCENT RESPONSE	
TREATMENT	ER+	ER−
Additive	35–60	5–10
Ablative	40–65	5–10
Tamoxifen	50–60	5–10

mortality of surgical adrenalectomy and the permanent requirement for replacement hormones, medical adrenalectomy is preferable. Aminoglutethimide blocks adrenal steroid synthesis and also inhibits the extra-adrenal conversion of androstenedione to estrone and estradiol. Adequate replacement hydrocortisone must be given with aminoglutethimide to suppress any compensatory rise in pituitary ACTH release; synthetic glucocorticoids such as dexamethasone are ineffective because aminoglutethimide accelerates their metabolism.

Aminoglutethimide is usually administered initially in a dose of 250 mg twice a day for 2 weeks, and then increased to the full dose of 250 mg four times daily. This regimen reduces the severity of the initial drug-induced neurologic symptoms. Hydrocortisone replacement (40 mg) in any of a variety of schedules is given as well. Aminoglutethimide may cause significant adverse effects, including neurologic abnormalities (lethargy, ataxia, weakness), fever, and a pruritic maculopapular rash. A low-dose regimen (250 mg twice daily without hydrocortisone supplementation) limits side effects and is apparently as effective as the original high-dose regimen. In prospective randomized studies, medical adrenalectomy is as effective as either hypophysectomy or surgical adrenalectomy and represents a more acceptable alternative for most patients.

Following discontinuation of aminoglutethimide and hydrocortisone, the adrenals recover the ability to secrete steroids at a basal level and in response to stress within 1 to 2 days. Therefore, gradual tapering of these drugs is unnecessary.

Estrogens

Diethylstilbesterol (DES) is the estrogen most commonly used in the treatment of breast cancer. The usual dose is 5 mg t.i.d. Nausea, vomiting, and anorexia accompany DES treatment in close to 50% of patients; many are unable to tolerate continuation of therapy. Urinary incontinence, fluid retention, and withdrawal bleeding can be troublesome side effects as well. Tamoxifen has almost entirely replaced DES in the management of ER-positive metastatic breast cancer. DES is occasionally used as the final hormonal option for patients who have responded and then progressed on all other hormones and who are still candidates for hormonal therapy.

Disease "Flare" and Withdrawal Response

With any additive hormonal therapy, particularly tamoxifen, patients with extensive bone metastases may develop a flare of disease immediately after the onset of treatment. The flare consists of increased bone pain, sometimes associated with hypercalcemia. Treatment should be continued, if possible, while symptomatic measures (analgesia and calcium-lowering medications) are instituted to control the flare. After several days to a week, the flare subsides and the patient usually manifests an excellent response.

Patients who have responded to a hormonal agent and have then progressed will sometimes have a "withdrawal response" to the abrupt cessation of the hormone. This rebound regression produces responses in up to 30% of treated cases and may predict for response to subsequent hormonal therapy. Many oncologists therefore delay further therapy long enough to allow a withdrawal response to occur, provided symptoms are not so severe that such a delay would endanger the patient.

CYTOTOXIC THERAPY

Cytotoxic chemotherapy is the treatment of choice for patients with symptomatic metastatic breast cancer that is (1) hormonally nonresponsive, (2) manifested by significant liver or lung involvement, and (3) severe or life threatening, requiring rapid relief. At some point during the course of her disease, almost every woman with metastatic breast cancer will require chemotherapy. Cytotoxic chemotherapy is the most dependable treatment of metastatic breast cancer; response rates of 50 to 75% are consistently obtained with modern combination regimens. There is no way to determine in advance which patients will respond to cytotoxic chemotherapy; a therapeutic trial is necessary.

In controlled trials in the 1960s, combination chemotherapy proved superior to single agent therapy in response rates and duration of response. Many different combinations (several listed in Table 12–6) have been developed for advanced breast cancer, relying heavily on the four most active agents—cyclophosphamide, Adriamycin, methotrexate, and 5-fluorouracil. No one regimen can be recommended as standard; differences in effectiveness among the different regimens in comparable patient groups are small. Adriamycin-containing regimens produce modestly higher response rates, but response durations with all regimens are virtually identical. Median response durations range from 6 to 12 months, and median survival from the initiation of chemotherapy from 12 to 30 months.

Attempts to improve results using alternating non–cross-resistant chemotherapy regimens (as used in Hodgkin's disease) have failed. Several new active agents have been developed in recent years, including mitoxantrone, vindesine, cisplatin, and others, but none produces improved complete response rates or response durations. The addition of immunotherapy has provided no benefit, but the use of biological response modifiers (e.g., monoclonal antibodies, interferons, interleukins) is currently under investigation. High-dose chemotherapy followed by autologous bone marrow transplantation is also being studied, both in advanced breast cancer and in high-risk patients (more than 10 positive lymph nodes) in the adjuvant setting.

Several pretreatment variables predict the likelihood of objective response to combination chemotherapy and longer duration of survival. A small number of involved sites (or limited tumor bulk), good performance status, and lack of extensive liver involvement all predict for a better outcome. However, responses to combination chemotherapy may occur in all sites, including bone, soft tissue, liver, and other viscera.

In patients previously treated with adjuvant CMF who relapse more than 1 year after completion of adjuvant therapy, CMF retreatment results in an equivalent response rate and duration of response to those of previously untreated patients. In patients with early relapse following CMF adjuvant therapy, use of another combination, preferably including an anthracycline, is indicated.

Following response and subsequent progression after treatment with an initial chemotherapeutic regimen, a second-line regimen is usually given. Most salvage programs have response rates in the 20 to 40% range, and response durations rarely exceed several months. No one salvage regimen appears superior to the others. Toxicity is often substantial in this group of pretreated patients with fairly extensive disease, and treatment results are frequently disappointing. Nevertheless, the sequential use of several chemotherapeutic regimens occasionally achieves prolonged relief of symptoms and control of disease.

Studies comparing the use of chemotherapy alone with chemohormonotherapy have yielded conflicting results. Some show improved response rates with the combined approach, but most fail to demonstrate improved survival. It is often assumed that chemotherapy has a substantial impact on the survival of patients with advanced breast cancer. However, data to support this assumption are difficult to find. Studies from several institutions comparing the interval from first recurrence to death over several decades, encompassing the prechemotherapeutic era and the period of modern combination chemotherapy, show little overall improvement. Chemotherapy undoubtedly prolongs the survival of some subgroups of patients, and regardless of its effects on survival, chemotherapy clearly improves the quality of life of patients with metastatic breast cancer, even considering the side effects of treatment.

OTHER MEASURES

Regardless of which forms of systemic therapy are employed, patients with breast cancer often require additional modalities of treatment. Local radiation to painful bone lesions is particularly important. Orthopedic consultation and prophylactic pinning of impending fracture sites can produce pain relief and improve function in selected cases. Adequate analgesic therapy (see Chapter 25) is a cornerstone of cancer management. Narcotic analgesics, used properly, successfully control pain for most patients, but nerve blocks and neurosurgical procedures should be considered for severe and refractory problems. Attention to nutritional needs, psychosocial problems, patient and family education, and institutional and home nursing services is important for all patients and especially for those with advanced disease.

SPECIAL ISSUES IN BREAST CANCER

CANCER OF THE MALE BREAST

Carcinoma of the breast in males is rare, accounting for about 1% of all breast cancers. The median age at diagnosis in men is almost 10 years greater than in women. Breast cancer in males appears to be associated with hyperestrogenism and may also be increased in patients with Klinefelter's syndrome. Estrogen receptors have been found in 84% of male breast cancers in some series.

Male breast cancer usually presents in a more advanced stage, and because of the limited amount of breast tissue, often involves the pectoral muscles. Stage for stage, however, the prognosis is similar to that for female breast cancer. The pattern of metastases is also similar. In males as in females, axillary lymph node involvement at the time of diagnosis is the most important prognostic factor.

The standard therapy for metastatic disease is orchiectomy, which produces an objective remission rate of 50 to 60%; tamoxifen achieves equivalent responses and represents a popular alternative to surgery. Estrogens, progestins, antiandrogens, and adrenalectomy (medical or surgical) are also effective, and patients who fail to respond to hormonal therapies are treated with the same chemotherapy regimens used in female breast cancer. The median survival after first recurrence is between 1.5 and 2.0 years, similar to that in female breast cancer. The role of systemic adjuvant therapy for node-positive male breast cancer is unknown, but many authors recommend its use based on analogy with female breast cancer.

BREAST CANCER DURING PREGNANCY

Breast cancer occurs during pregnancy and lactation in 2 to 3% of patients. In the past, this combination was considered to have an ominous prognosis. Part of the apparent poor prognosis was related to delayed detection and consequent advanced stage (75 to 80% stage II) at diagnosis owing to the difficulty in palpating the breast and the contraindication to x-ray mammography during pregnancy. In addition, the endocrine changes during pregnancy (the high estrogenic state that may support proliferation of malignant cells) and the suppression of the immune system during the first half of pregnancy may also enhance tumor growth. Nevertheless, if corrected for stage and estrogen receptor status (usually negative during pregnancy and positive during lactation, in very small series), the outcome is only slightly worse than in the nonpregnant patient.

As many as 7% of fertile women have one or more pregnancies after mastectomy for breast cancer. There is no evidence that pregnancy promotes the recurrence of the cancer, although most oncologists counsel their patients to defer pregnancy for several years after the initial diagnosis, since this is the period of highest recurrence rate. Conversely, there is no evidence that subsequent pregnancy protects against the recurrence of cancer.

INFLAMMATORY BREAST CANCER

Inflammatory carcinoma is both a clinical description of an erythematous, warm, "inflamed"-looking breast and a pathologic diagnosis, denoting the presence of tumor cells in dermal and subdermal lymphatics. The lymphatic obstruction and disrupted flow patterns that result are responsible for the lymphedema of the breast and the tendency for disseminated systemic and chest wall recurrences. Inflammatory carcinoma accounts for about 2% of all breast cancers and carries a median survival with local therapy alone of 1 year; a combined modality approach including aggressive chemotherapy results in median survivals of more than 2 years. Regardless of age, hormone receptor status, or the presence of axillary node involvement, inflammatory carcinoma requires treatment with chemotherapy combined with local measures consisting of radiotherapy to the breast, mastectomy, or both.

BREAST RECONSTRUCTION

Advances in plastic surgical techniques have made breast reconstruction readily available for nearly all women with mastectomies. Steadily increasing numbers of women elect this procedure because of the excellent cosmetic results, improved convenience, and psychologic advantages. No firm data exist concerning the appropriate waiting period between initial mastectomy and breast reconstruction, but most plastic surgeons defer reconstruction for 6 to 12 months. This allows completion of adjuvant chemotherapy, opportunity to detect early recurrence, adequate healing following mastectomy, and time for psychologic adjustment. Alternatively, immediate reconstruction, performed at the time of mastectomy, avoids much of the psychologic trauma of breast amputation and produces excellent cosmetic results.

If possible, breast reconstruction should be discussed with the original surgeon prior to mastectomy. Consultation with the plastic surgeon at that time allows anticipation of any technical problems that might arise, and if the patient chooses, permits immediate reconstruction concurrent with mastectomy. However, breast reconstruction may be performed even many years following mastectomy, and advanced planning is not mandatory. Many women worry that reconstruction will impair early recognition of locally recurrent disease, but no evidence indicates that this is likely.

REFERENCES

Bonadonna G: Conceptual and practical advances in the management of breast cancer. J Clin Oncol 7:1380–1397, 1989.
Bostwick J: Breast reconstruction after mastectomy. Cancer 66:1402–1411, 1990.
Donegan WL: Cancer of the breast in man. CA 41:339–354, 1991.
Early Breast Cancer Trialists' Collaborative Group: Effects of adjuvant tamoxifen and of cytotoxic therapy on mortality in early breast cancer. N Engl J Med 319:1681–1692, 1988.
Harris JR, Hellman S, Henderson IC, Kinne DW (eds). Breast Diseases. 2nd ed. Philadelphia, JB Lippincott, 1991.
Harris JR, Recht A, Connolly J, et al: Conservative surgery and radiotherapy for early breast cancer. Cancer 66:1427–1438, 1990.
Henderson IC, Garber JE, Breitmeyer JB, et al: Comprehensive management of disseminated breast cancer. Cancer 66:1439–1448, 1990.
Henderson IC, Hayes DF, Parker LM, et al: Adjuvant systemic therapy for patients with node-negative tumors. Cancer 65:2132–2147, 1990.
McGuire WL, Tandon AK, Allred DC, et al: How to use prognostic factors in axillary node negative breast cancer patients. J Natl Cancer Inst 82:1006–1015, 1990.
Nayfield SG, Karp JE, Ford LG, et al: Potential role of tamoxifen in prevention of breast cancer. J Natl Cancer Inst 83:1450–1459, 1991.
NIH Consensus Conference: Treatment of early stage breast cancer. JAMA 265:391–395, 1991.
Shapiro S: Determining the efficacy of breast cancer screening. Cancer 63:1874–1880, 1989.
Swain SM, Lippman ME: Systemic therapy of locally advanced breast cancer. Review and guidelines. Oncology 3:21–34, 1989.

13
LUNG CANCER

Martin Brower

INCIDENCE

The National Cancer Institute estimates that in 1992, 168,000 cases of lung cancer were newly diagnosed in the United States, and 143,000 Americans died of this disease, including 93,000 men and 53,000 women. Thirty-four percent of all men and 21% of all women who died of cancer in 1992 died from bronchogenic carcinoma. Lung cancer has been the leading cause of cancer death in men since 1955, and in women since 1985. Cigarette smoking became common among American men after World War I, and after a 20-year lag period, the incidence of lung cancer among men exploded, increasing sevenfold between 1940 and 1975. Women began smoking in large numbers in the 1940s, and the epidemic of lung cancer in women began about 1960, with a quadrupling of the death rate between 1960 and 1985. Fortunately, the proportion of American adults who smoke has declined from half the population in the 1960s to about one-third in the 1990s, and the incidence of lung cancer has plateaued in the last several years.

ETIOLOGY

Cigarette smoking is directly responsible for approximately 85% of cases of lung cancer. Cigarette smoke is a complex mixture of multiple mutagens, carcinogens, and procarcinogens. Procarcinogens are metabolized in the body into active carcinogens, and individual variation in the metabolism of such procarcinogens as benzo(a)pyrene may be responsible for differing susceptibilities to lung cancer.

Clinicians noted a relationship between cigarette smoking and lung cancer as early as 1940. Multiple prospective and retrospective studies have proven that smokers have up to a 14-fold greater lung cancer risk than lifetime nonsmokers. This risk is proportional to the number of cigarettes smoked per day. Discontinuation of cigarette smoking gradually lessens the risk of lung carcinoma, but it may take as long as 30 years for the incidence to be reduced to that of nonsmokers. Passive smoking—that is, exposure of nonsmokers to the cigarette smoke of others—may also lead to an increased risk of lung cancer. The relative risk of lung cancer in nonsmokers whose spouses or parents smoke more than one to two packs per day may be as high as three times that of persons without household cigarette smoke exposure.

Radon appears to cause several thousand cases of lung cancer annually. This radioactive gas is a natural product found in underground mines and in homes in some parts of the United States. Radon decays into short-lived alpha-emitting radon daughters that when inhaled deliver a carcinogenic dose of radioactivity to the lungs. Statistical extrapolation from the incidence of lung cancer in uranium and iron miners with a very high level of exposure to radon suggests that many cases of lung cancer in nonsmokers can be attributed to exposure to low levels of radon.

Exposure to asbestos increases the risk of lung cancer and acts synergistically with smoking, resulting in an incidence that is 60 times higher than that of nonsmokers. Asbestos exposure is also the primary cause of the rare pleural malignancy mesothelioma. Occupational exposure to arsenic, chromium, nickel, and chloromethyl ethers also increases the risk of lung cancer. Lung cancer incidence is higher in urban industrialized areas than in rural areas, possibly related to air pollution. Vitamin A intake is inversely associated with lung cancer risk, especially among smokers. Patients with chronic obstructive pulmonary disease (COPD) appear to be at higher risk for lung cancer than patients with identical smoking histories without COPD.

PATHOLOGY

The four major histologic types of lung cancer are squamous cell carcinoma, adenocarcinoma, large cell carcinoma, and small cell carcinoma. Collectively, squamous cell cancer, adenocarcinoma, and large cell carcinoma are called non-small cell lung cancer (NSCLC). The most common lung cancer in nonsmokers and in women is adenocarcinoma. In recent series, adenocarcinoma exceeds squamous cell lung cancer in overall frequency as the proportion of female lung cancer patients increases.

The most important task for the pathologist after making a diagnosis of lung cancer is to differentiate between small cell lung cancer (SCLC) and NSCLC. SCLC is characterized morphologically by cells that are about two to four times the size of a lymphocyte with inconspicuous nucleoli and scant cytoplasm. Nuclear molding is a characteristic cytologic feature. Morphologic evidence of squamous differentiation (e.g., keratinization or intracellular bridges) or of adenocarcinoma differentiation (e.g., gland formation or intracellular mucin) is absent. The diagnosis of SCLC by bronchoscopy can be quite difficult owing to the characteristic crush artifact on bronchial biopsy specimens of this tumor.

Although the four major types of lung cancer differ morphologically, they may arise from a common bronchial epithelial stem cell. Mixed tumors such as small cell/large cell carcinomas and adeno/squamous carcinomas are not rare. At autopsy, one-third of small cell cancers have a significant component of NSCLC.

SCLC tumors appear "undifferentiated" under the light microscope but in fact are neuroendocrine tumors, secreting over 30 different peptide products. They possess other properties of neuroendocrine tumors, including dense core granules on electron microscopy and markers such as chromogranin A, neuron-specific enolase, and synaptophysin, which can be detected with immunohistochemical techniques. However, some NSCLC tumors also have neuroendocrine markers, so immunohistochemistry alone cannot infallibly distinguish between SCLC and NSCLC.

Basic scientists have discovered characteristic abnormalities in oncogenes and tumor suppressor genes in lung cancer cells. Most SCLC cells have abnormal or absent expression of the products of the retinoblastoma and of the p53 tumor suppressor genes, and a characteristic deletion of a portion of the short arm of chromosome 3 in SCLC also suggests deletion of a tumor suppressor gene. Point mutations in *ras* oncogenes are common in NSCLC and may be associated with a poor prognosis.

CLINICAL PRESENTATION

Lung cancer can present with signs and symptoms of intrathoracic tumor, but commonly distant metastases or paraneoplastic syndromes are symptomatic while the primary tumor is silent. Squamous cell carcinoma has the greatest tendency to remain localized, and small cell carcinoma is most likely to metastasize; adenocarcinoma and large cell carcinoma have intermediate tendencies to metastasize.

Patients with central, endobronchial lesions often present with cough, dyspnea, hemoptysis, wheezing, stridor, or postobstructive pneumonia. Obtaining a chest radiograph 6 weeks after an episode of pneumonia in a smoker is mandatory. Failure of a pneumonia to clear is an indication for bronchoscopy. Peripheral tumors may present with cough or dyspnea or with pain due to pleural or chest wall invasion, but peripheral neoplasms are frequently asymptomatic and discovered on chest radiographs obtained for other purposes. A peripheral pulmonary neoplasm is most likely adenocarcinoma or large cell cancer, whereas squamous cell and SCLC most commonly cause endobronchial obstruction.

The superior sulcus (Pancoast) syndrome occurs when a slowly growing tumor in the apex of the lung produces severe shoulder pain, sometimes radiating down the arm in an ulnar distribution. Persistent shoulder pain in a smoker should be investigated with an apical lordotic chest radiograph to detect an apical mass or rib erosion.

Bronchioloalveolar carcinoma is a subtype of adenocarcinoma that can cause severe dyspnea due to diffuse multinodular or extensive end-airspace lung involvement. These tumors have an increased incidence in patients with interstitial pulmonary fibrosis.

Mediastinal involvement from lung cancer very commonly produces symptoms. Tumors of the right lung and left lower lung can metastasize via the lymphatics to right paratracheal lymph nodes, causing the superior vena cava syndrome (see Chap. 23). Metastases to left-sided mediastinal lymph nodes can paralyze the left recurrent laryngeal nerve, causing hoarseness. Phrenic nerve invasion within the mediastinum can paralyze the diaphragm. Dysphagia may result from extrinsic compression of the esophagus. Tracheoesophageal fistulas are occasionally encountered in such patients as well.

Metastatic presentations of lung cancer include headaches, seizures, confusion, or hemiparesis due to brain metastases; pain due to bone metastases; back pain and paraparesis sometimes accompanied by bladder and bowel dysfunction due to spinal cord compression from extradural metastases; and anorexia and right upper quadrant pain from liver metastases. Lung cancer should be a leading diagnostic consideration in any middle-aged or elderly smoker presenting with evidence of metastatic disease. Lymphadenopathy, soft tissue or skin nodules, and cytopenias from bone marrow involvement can also be initial presentations.

Paraneoplastic syndromes may represent the initial manifestation of lung cancer. Hypercalcemia, most commonly seen with squamous cell lung cancer, causes nausea, vomiting, dehydration, constipation, and confusion. Inappropriate secretion of antidiuretic hormone is common, particularly in SCLC, and can lead to severe hyponatremia. In SCLC, clinically evident ectopic ACTH secretion occurs in 1 to 2% of patients. Ectopic ACTH syndrome tends to be more fulminant than classic Cushing's syndrome. Patients develop profound muscle weakness, hypokalemia, metabolic alkalosis, and moderate elevations of blood glucose, but the characteristic truncal obesity of Cushing's disease is not prominent. Small cell lung cancer is also associated with the myasthenic (Eaton-Lambert) syndrome. Hypertrophic pulmonary osteoarthropathy is common in patients with adenocarcinoma of the lung and occasionally in those with other histologies. This syndrome produces pain, tenderness, and swelling involving the wrists and ankles and may be confused with other rheumatologic conditions. Dermatomyositis can be seen, and hypercoagulable states and marantic endocarditis are not unusual, particularly in patients with adenocarcinoma. Neurologic paraneoplastic syndromes associated with lung cancer include dementia, subacute cerebellar degeneration, and peripheral neuropathy.

DIAGNOSIS

Intensive screening of high-risk asymptomatic individuals with chest x-rays and sputum cytologies every 4 months has not been demonstrated to reduce lung cancer mortality. Randomized studies comparing intensive screening with a control population are in progress. At this time, the American Cancer Society does not recommend any screening program for early detection of lung cancer.

For the patient with suspected lung cancer, the goal is to obtain a tissue diagnosis as quickly as possible and to determine if the patient is curable by surgery. Central lesions require a different approach than peripheral "coin" lesions. With central lesions, although sputum cytology is occasionally rewarding, fiberoptic bronchoscopy is the technique most likely to yield a tissue diagnosis. In addition to tissue samples, bronchoscopy provides information regarding the patency of the airways and helps to assess operability. Specimens are obtained by bronchial brushings, washings, and direct biopsy, and in patients with subcarinal adenopathy a transbronchial biopsy of the lymph node(s) can be performed.

The procedure of choice for small solitary peripheral nodules is surgical removal. If multiple peripheral nodules are present or if the patient is not a surgical candidate, a tissue diagnosis can be made by percutaneous transthoracic needle aspiration. This is a safe, outpatient procedure; pneumothorax occurs in about 25% of patients (requiring a chest tube in about 5%) and hemoptysis occurs in 10 to 20% of patients but is rarely severe. A negative needle aspiration does not rule out malignancy.

If sputum cytology, bronchoscopy, and/or needle aspiration fail to yield a diagnosis, and a search for readily accessible sites of metastatic disease (lymph nodes, skin) is unproductive, then an invasive surgical procedure will be required to obtain tissue. Such procedures include (1) blind scalene node biopsy on the appropriate side; (2) mediastinoscopy, which is ideal for evaluating the right upper mediastinum but is not useful for left upper lobe lesions; (3) mediastinotomy performed with a left anterior incision; and (4) thoracotomy.

STAGING

The new TNM staging classification of lung cancer (Table 13–1), adopted in 1986, is used primarily for NSCLC. In general, stages I and II lung cancers are curable by surgery. Stage IIIa cancers are technically resectable, but stages IIIb and IV cancers are unresectable. In population-based series, fewer than one-quarter of NSCLC patients have stages I

Table 13–1. **TNM STAGING OF LUNG CANCER**

PRIMARY TUMOR (T)

T1 A tumor 3 cm or less in greatest dimension, surrounded by lung or visceral pleura, and without evidence of invasion proximal to a lobar bronchus at bronchoscopy.

T2 A tumor more than 3 cm in greatest dimension, or a tumor of any size that either invades the visceral pleura or has associated atelectasis or obstructive pneumonitis extending to the hilar region. At bronchoscopy, the proximal extent of demonstrable tumor must be within a lobar bronchus or at least 2 cm distal to the carina. Any associated atelectasis must involve less than an entire lung.

T3 A tumor of any size with direct extension into the chest wall (including superior sulcus tumors), diaphragm, or mediastinal pleura or pericardium without involving the heart, great vessels, trachea, esophagus, or vertebral body, or a tumor in the main bronchus within 2 cm of the carina without involving the carina.

T4 A tumor of any size with invasion of the mediastinum or involving heart, great vessels, trachea, esophagus, veterbral body, or carina, or the presence of malignant pleural effusion.

NODAL INVOLVEMENT (N)

N0 No demonstrable metastasis to regional lymph nodes.

N1 Metastasis to lymph nodes in the peribronchial or the ipsilateral hilar region, or both, including direct extension.

N2 Metastasis to ipsilateral mediastinal lymph nodes and subcarinal lymph nodes.

N3 Metastasis to contralateral mediastinal lymph nodes, contralateral hilar lymph nodes, ipsilateral or contralateral scalene or supraclavicular lymph nodes.

DISTANT METASTASIS (M)

M0 No known distant metastasis

M1 Distant metastasis present

Stage Grouping

Stage	Grouping
Stage I	T1 N0 M0, T2 N0 M0
Stage II	T1 N1 M0, T2 N1 M0
Stage IIIa	T3 N0 M0, T3 N1 M0, T1–3 N2 M0
Stage IIIb	T4 or N3, M0
Stage IV	M1

Adapted from Mountain CF: A new international staging system for lung cancer. Chest 89(suppl 4):225S–233S, 1986.

and II disease, about a third have locally advanced disease (stage III), and nearly half have metastatic disease (stage IV) at presentation.

SCLC is staged as limited (chest only) or extensive (chest and extrathoracic disease). TNM staging is rarely used. The exact definition of limited stage varies among institutions and investigators. Patients with ipsilateral supraclavicular nodal disease or ipsilateral pleural effusion are considered limited in some series and extensive in others. Over two-thirds of SCLC patients have extensive stage disease at presentation.

TREATMENT OF NON-SMALL CELL LUNG CANCER

SURGERY

Surgery is the treatment of choice for stage I and stage II lung cancer. Careful preoperative evaluation is mandatory in order to select only potentially curable patients for surgery. With better selection of surgical candidates, the 5-year survival rate following surgical resection has increased in recent years. The 5-year survival of patients with stage I lung cancer is more than 50%, and the 5-year survival of patients with T1N0M0 tumors (coin lesions less than 3 cm in diameter) is 70 to 80%. Five-year survival with stage II disease is 25 to 40%. With modern surgical techniques operative mortality should be about 6% for pneumonectomy and 3% for lobectomy.

The criteria in Table 13–2 determine operability. A chest computed tomography (CT) scan is invaluable, commonly detecting abnormalities such as hilar or mediastinal adenopathy, additional pulmonary nodules, or extrapulmonary metastatic disease not visible on a plain chest radiograph. Pulmonary function testing is mandatory. Assessment of operability must be individualized. An otherwise healthy patient with an asymptomatic coin lesion on chest film and CT needs only a careful physical examination with particular attention to lymph nodes, liver, and central nervous system, followed by a complete blood

Table 13–2. **STANDARD CRITERIA OF INOPERABILITY IN LUNG CANCER**

1. Stage IIIb and stage IV disease, including distant metastases, supraclavicular or scalene nodal metastases, pleural effusion due to malignancy
2. Bulky mediastinal disease
   a. Superior vena cava syndrome
   b. Vocal cord paralysis
   c. Phrenic nerve paralysis
   d. Mediastinal tumor visible on preoperative chest radiograph, confirmed histologically
3. Predicted postoperative FEV_1 less than 800–1000 mL

Direct extension to the chest wall and small cell histology are not necessarily contraindications to surgery.

count and serum chemistries. If this evaluation is negative, the patient should proceed directly to thoracotomy and resection with curative intent. Extensive diagnostic imaging in such a patient has a very low yield. Conversely, patients with evidence of metastatic disease discovered on history and physical examination and patients who are marginal candidates for surgery based on age, pulmonary function, or coexisting medical problems should be carefully studied with appropriate diagnostic tests in order to avoid a needless thoracotomy. Patients who have lost weight prior to the diagnosis of lung cancer also merit extensive work-up for occult metastatic disease prior to surgery.

Chest CT scans should be extended to the upper abdomen to include the liver and adrenal glands, since these are common sites of metastases. As a general rule, if an abnormality on CT represents the only contraindication to performing curative surgery in patients with lung cancer, biopsy confirmation of the suspicious lesion should be obtained before denying potentially curative therapy. Many adrenal abnormalities on CT are benign adenomas or cysts. Enlarged mediastinal lymph nodes on CT may be reactive rather than malignant.

Patients with stage IIIa disease on the basis of direct tumor extension to the chest wall, diaphragm, pleura, or pericardium should not necessarily be rejected for surgery with curative intent. Substantial sections of the chest wall and other structures can be removed and replaced with a Marlex mesh. Innovative reconstruction techniques can permit surgical removal of some stage IIIa tumors with involvement of a mainstem bronchus; such tumors were formerly considered inoperable. The role of surgery in patients with stage IIIa tumors on the basis of mediastinal lymph node involvement, however, is very controversial. Patients with evidence of mediastinal involvement on preoperative chest films have virtually zero 5-year survival after surgical intervention, even when combined with postoperative radiotherapy. Clinical trials combining surgery with chemotherapy in these patients with "bulky N2" disease are ongoing, but subjecting such patients to thoracotomy outside of a clinical trial cannot be recommended. On the other hand, 10 to 15% of patients with clinically unsuspected mediastinal adenopathy whose lymph node involvement is diagnosed only at the time of surgery survive 5 years. Therefore, most thoracic surgeons will proceed with lobectomy or pneumonectomy in such patients, even in the presence of mediastinal lymph node involvement

RADIATION THERAPY

Radiation therapy is an invaluable treatment modality for NSCLC. Radiotherapy can be used with curative intent, either alone or with other modalities, and it is often the most effective palliative modality for incurable patients. Patients with stage I or II disease who are not surgical candidates owing to medical problems or who refuse surgery can be treated with radiotherapy with curative intent. Results are inferior to those achievable with surgery, but as many as 25% of such patients may achieve long-term survival.

Superior sulcus tumors can be treated successfully with radiation therapy. Some surgeons follow radiation therapy with an en bloc resection including involved ribs and chest wall as long as there is no evidence of mediastinal or scalene node involvement or vertebral body extension. Twenty to 40% of such patients may be long-term survivors. Similar results have been achieved with radiation therapy alone.

Patients with inoperable stage IIIa and stage IIIb disease are conventionally treated with radiotherapy. Five-year survival for such patients is about 6%. Although local control is achieved more frequently with higher doses of radiotherapy (6000 vs 4000 cGy), ultimate survival is not improved by the higher dose, since most patients with locally advanced lung cancer ultimately develop distant metastases. Some physicians have advocated careful observation of asymptomatic patients with inoperable, locally advanced lung cancer rather than immediate institution of radiotherapy.

No controlled study has shown any survival benefit for the use of either preoperative or postoperative radiation in conjunction with complete surgical resection of lung cancer. However, most surgeons and radiotherapists recommend postoperative mediastinal irradiation for patients with lymph node involvement demonstrated at thoracotomy. The Lung Cancer Study Group found that local recurrences could be greatly reduced in resected node-positive squamous cell lung cancer patients with the use of postoperative radiotherapy, although no survival benefit followed.

Radiation therapy is an invaluable tool for the palliation of incurable lung cancer. Cough, hemoptysis, and dyspnea due to airway obstruction can be alleviated in 60 to 80% of patients. Radiotherapy is also essential in the treatment of brain metastases and painful bone metastases. Radiation is less successful, however, in restoring airflow to a totally atelectatic lobe or lung.

Radiation therapy for lung cancer is usually well tolerated. Most patients do experience dysphagia and fatigue during treatment, and radiation pneumonitis, pericarditis, and spinal cord injury also represent potential complications.

CHEMOTHERAPY

Until recently, chemotherapy was rarely used in NSCLC. Response rates to single agents in stage IV disease are less than 20%; the most active agents are cisplatin, etoposide, the vinca alkaloids, mitomycin C, and ifosfamide. Although innumerable combination chemotherapy regimens have been tested in metastatic NSCLC, and promising results have often been obtained in small single-institution pilot studies, no regimen reproducibly achieves objective responses in more than 40% of patients with metastatic disease. Commonly used regimens are listed in Table 13–3.

Cisplatin-based regimens produce higher response rates. Dosages of cisplatin in excess of 100 mg/m^2 require inpatient administration, can cause severe toxicity, and to date have not shown survival benefit when compared with outpatient cisplatin regimens in metastatic disease. Several randomized trials have recently compared cisplatin-based combination

Table 13–3. **SELECTED CHEMOTHERAPY REGIMENS FOR METASTATIC NON–SMALL CELL LUNG CANCER**

DRUGS, DOSE, AND SCHEDULE (IV)	RESPONSE RATE (%)	MEDIAN SURVIVAL (WEEKS)*	LETHAL TOXICITY (%)
Cyclophosphamide, 300 mg/m^2, days 1, 8 Adriamycin, 20 mg/m^2, days 1, 8 Methotrexate, 15mg/m^2, days 1, 8 Procarbazine, 100 mg/m^2, days 2–11 PO Repeat every 28 days	17	25	0
Mitomycin C, 10 mg/m^2, day 1 Vinblastine, 6mg/m^2, day 1 Cisplatin, 40 mg/m^2, day 1 Repeat every 21 days	31	22	6
Vindesine, 3 mg/m^2 weekly × 5, then every other week† Cisplatin, 120 mg/m^2, day 1, 29, then every 6 weeks	25	26	7
Etoposide, 120 mg/m^2, days 4, 6, 8 Cisplatin, 60 mg/m^2, day 1 Repeat every 21 days	20	27	4

From Ruckdeschel JC, et al: A randomized trial of the four most active regimens for metastatic non–small cell lung cancer. J Clin Oncol 4:14–22, 1986.

*There was no significant survival difference between regimens.

†Vinblastine, 6 mg/m^2, is commonly substituted for vindesine, 3 mg/m^2.

Table 13–4. **CRITERIA FOR USE OF CHEMOTHERAPY IN METASTATIC NON–SMALL CELL LUNG CANCER OUTSIDE OF INVESTIGATIONAL PROTOCOLS**

Criteria
Symptomatic disease; symptoms cannot be palliated with radiation therapy
Patient physically able to tolerate therapy
Patient fully ambulatory or spending less than 50% of time in bed
No uncontrolled brain metastases
Evaluable disease to permit early discontinuation of therapy if ineffective
Patient understands treatment is noncurative and potentially toxic and gives informed consent

therapy with "best supportive care" for patients with NSCLC. These studies have shown a modest prolongation of median survival with chemotherapy, ranging from 7 to 17 weeks, and in one study the survival benefit reached statistical significance. Whether such results justify routine use is debated. Certainly, otherwise healthy patients who wish a trial of chemotherapy after full discussion of the risks and toxicities of treatment as well as the relatively modest potential benefits should be treated. On the other hand, elderly, severely ill, and bedridden patients and those who are reluctant to consider chemotherapy in any case are best served by a regimen of supportive measures.

Response to combination chemotherapy in NSCLC is likely only in patients with a relatively good performance status. It is highly unusual for a bedridden patient to achieve any benefit from combination chemotherapy, and toxicity is much greater in such patients than in those who are ambulatory. Suggested criteria for the use of combination chemotherapy in NSCLC are given in Table 13–4. It is important to recognize that many patients with incurable lung cancer have a pattern of metastatic spread (e.g., bulky mediastinal nodes, brain or bone metastases) in which radiotherapy is the best palliative modality, whereas other patterns of metastatic disease (e.g., liver metastases, lymphangitic lung disease) might best be approached with chemotherapy.

The response rate to chemotherapy is higher in locally advanced disease than in metastatic disease. Response rates in stage III approach 50%. Because the eventual development of distant metastases is the leading cause of death in patients with seemingly localized lung cancer, interest has grown recently in combining chemotherapy with local treatment modalities for stages II and III lung cancer. The Lung Cancer Study Group demonstrated a slight (though not statistically significant) survival benefit with cisplatin-based combination chemotherapy after resection of stage II and stage III adenocarcinomas and large cell carcinomas. The Cancer and Leukemia Group B demonstrated a 4-month increase in median survival in patients with unresectable stage III lung cancer using high-dose cisplatin induction chemotherapy prior to standard radiotherapy, with an increase in the number of 3-year survivors from 12 to 23% with early follow-up. The use of "neoadjuvant" chemotherapy prior to surgery in patients with mediastinal lymph node involvement with NSCLC is being tested. Further follow-up and detailed cost-benefit analyses will be required before the use of chemotherapy in localized NSCLC can be considered standard practice.

LASER THERAPY

Laser therapy can provide palliation of malignant airway obstruction after all other treatment modalities have failed. The neodymium:yttrium aluminum garnet (Nd:YAG) laser is most commonly used, sometimes with intravenous hematoporphyrin derivative, which selectively concentrates in tumor cells and causes cell death by producing a toxic oxygen radical when the tumor is irradiated with red light. Complications of laser therapy occur in up to half of the cases and include hemorrhage, sepsis, aspiration, respiratory failure, and fistula formation. The risk is especially great in patients with total obstruction of an airway. Nonetheless, temporary palliation is achieved in over 50% of patients treated with laser therapy.

TREATMENT OF SMALL CELL LUNG CANCER

SCLC differs from NSCLC by its propensity for early metastatic spread. It was shown in the early 1970s that 63% of patients resected for "cure" but dying within 30 days of surgery had distant metastases at autopsy. The most common sites of metastatic disease at initial presentation are bone (40%), liver (20 to 25%), bone marrow (20 to 25%), and brain (10 to 15%). In patients with disease limited to the chest by initial physical examination and laboratory studies, it may be worthwhile to obtain liver, bone, and CT brain scans as well as a bone marrow aspiration and biopsy, since a significant proportion will be found to have extrathoracic disease. The prognosis of SCLC is substantially worse in the presence of extrathoracic metastases. Conventional study of bone marrow biopsies and aspirates may understate the true percentage of patients with bone marrow involvement. Studies from the Veterans Administration Lung Group indicate that the survival of untreated SCLC averages 4 months in patients with limited disease and 6 weeks in those with extensive disease.

SURGERY

An occasional patient with SCLC presents with a peripheral coin lesion. These patients should probably undergo surgical resection, applying the same criteria for resectability as in NSCLC. Because of the propensity of even apparently localized SCLC to undergo occult metastasis, these patients should receive combination chemotherapy postoperatively. The long-term survival of such patients is greater than 50%, particularly if no mediastinal lymph node involvement is found at thoracotomy. On the other hand, a randomized study of the Lung Cancer Study Group failed to demonstrate any benefit for the addition of surgery to chemotherapy and radiotherapy in patients with radiographic evidence of mediastinal adenopathy, and these patients make up the vast majority of limited stage SCLC cases.

CHEMOTHERAPY

SCLC can be palliated and occasionally even cured with combination chemotherapy. The median survival of all treated patients is now approximately 1 year: 7 to 9 months for patients with extensive stage and 12 to 18 months for patients with limited stage disease. Common treatment regimens are listed in Table 13–5. All can produce significant myelosuppression, alopecia, nausea, vomiting, and mucositis. Regimens containing Adriamycin (doxorubicin) also carry the risk of cardiotoxicity. Many patients with SCLC have additional cardiac and pulmonary problems related in part to their smoking histories; their ability to tolerate chemotherapy may be limited. With chemotherapy, most patients achieve at least a partial response that is usually associated with substantial subjective improvement. Approximately 50% of patients with limited disease and 20 to 30% of those with extensive disease achieve a complete clinical response. However, the vast majority will eventually relapse. In most studies, only 15% of limited-stage patients and 2% of

Table 13–5. **REPRESENTATIVE CHEMOTHERAPY REGIMENS FOR SMALL CELL LUNG CANCER**

DRUGS	DOSE*	SCHEDULE
Cyclophosphamide Adriamycin Vincristine	750–1000 mg/m², day 1 50 mg/m², day 1 2 mg, day 1	IV every 3 weeks
Cyclophosphamide Etoposide Vincristine	750–1000 mg/m², day 1 75–100 mg/m², days 1–3 2 mg, day 1	IV every 3 weeks
Cyclophosphamide Adriamycin Etoposide	750–1000 mg/m², day 1 40–50 mg/m², day 1 75–100 mg/m², days 1–3	IV every 3 weeks
Etoposide Cisplatin	80–120 mg/m², days 1–3 60–80 mg/m², day 1	IV every 3 weeks
Oral etoposide	50 mg/m², days 1–21	PO every 4 weeks

*Doses are given for patients with good performance status without significant renal, hepatic, or cardiac dysfunction. Dose reductions may be needed for less fit patients.

Table 13–6. **PROGNOSTIC GROUPS IN SMALL CELL LUNG CANCER**

FAVORABLE (?CURABLE)	UNFAVORABLE (?INCURABLE)
Performance status 0–1	Performance status 2–4
Limited disease (chest, supraclavicular nodes, pleural effusion)	Two or more sites of metastatic disease
One site of extrathoracic disease	Liver metastases
No liver or brain metastases	Brain metastases

extensive-stage patients are alive 2 years after diagnosis, and even the long-term survivors are at risk for late relapse. Virtually all long-term survivors fall into the favorable prognosis group described in Table 13–6. Patients in the unfavorable prognosis group almost never live more than 2 years after diagnosis, and the goal of therapy for these patients should be palliation. Very intense chemotherapy regimens add little benefit to the results achieved with easily tolerated outpatient regimens.

RADIATION THERAPY

Multiple randomized trials have addressed the issue of adding thoracic radiotherapy to combination chemotherapy in limited-stage SCLC. Most of the more recent studies using aggressive chemotherapy and radiotherapy techniques have demonstrated a slight survival benefit using combined modality therapy. One commonly used approach combining cisplatin and etoposide chemotherapy with simultaneous thoracic irradiation has produced 2-year survival rates of 30 to 50% in selected patients. It must be recognized that combined modality therapy is inherently more toxic than single modality therapy, and many SCLC patients are unable to tolerate such therapy owing to concurrent medical or psychologic problems.

SCLC has a propensity for central nervous system metastases. The actuarial probability of brain metastases in a patient who survives 2 years may be as high as 70%. Prophylactic cranial irradiation (PCI) was introduced in the 1970s in an attempt to lower the incidence of brain metastases. Recent data suggest that PCI should be reserved for patients who achieve complete clinical responses. The use of PCI must be weighed against the possibility of late cerebral dysfunction, which has been demonstrated in a high proportion of long-term survivors who had received PCI. Although PCI in complete responders lowers the incidence of brain metastases, no survival benefit has been observed. Randomized trials testing the use of PCI in complete responders are ongoing.

REFERENCES

Lung Cancer, General

Bunn PA (ed): Lung cancer. Semin Oncol 15:197–318, 1988.
Eddy DM: Screening for lung cancer. Ann Intern Med 111:232–237, 1989.
Loeb LA, Ernster VL, Warner KE, et al: Smoking and lung cancer, an overview. Cancer Res 44:5940–5958, 1984.

Non–Small Cell Lung Cancer

Bitran JD (ed): Non–small cell lung cancer. Hematol/Oncol Clin North Am 4:1027–1199, 1990.
Dillman RO, Seagren SL, Propert KJ, et al: A randomized trial of induction chemotherapy plus high-dose radiation versus radiation alone in stage III non–small cell lung cancer. N Engl J Med 323:940–945, 1990.
Johnson DH, Einhorn LH, Bartolucci A, et al: Thoracic radiotherapy does not prolong survival in patients with locally advanced, unresectable non–small cell lung cancer. Ann Intern Med 113:33–38, 1990.
Lung Cancer Study Group: Effect of postoperative mediastinal radiation on completely resected stage II and stage III epidermoid cancer of the lung. N Engl J Med 315:1377–1381, 1986.
Rapp E, Pater JL, Willan A, et al: Chemotherapy can prolong survival in patients with advanced non–small cell lung cancer—report of a Canadian multicenter randomized trial. J Clin Oncol 6:633–641, 1988.

Vokes EE, Vijayakumar S, Bitran JD, et al: Role of systemic chemotherapy in advanced non–small cell lung cancer. Am J Med 89:777–786, 1990.

Small Cell Lung Cancer

Fleck JF, Einhorn LH, Lauer RC, et al: Is prophylactic cranial irradiation indicated in small cell lung cancer? J Clin Oncol 8:209–214, 1990.
Johnson BE, Grayson J, Makuch RW et al: Ten-year survival of patients with small cell lung cancer treated with combination chemotherapy with or without radiation. J Clin Oncol 8:396–401, 1990.
McCracken JD, Janacki LM, Crowley JJ, et al: Concurrent chemotherapy/radiotherapy for limited small-cell carcinoma: A Southwest Oncology Group Study. J Clin Oncol 8: 892–898, 1990.
Seifter EJ, Ihde DC: Therapy of small cell lung cancer: A perspective on two decades of clinical research. Semin Oncol 15:278–299, 1988.

MALIGNANT MESOTHELIOMA

Mesothelioma is a tumor of serosal surfaces such as the pleura, peritoneum, and pericardium. The majority of patients with malignant mesothelioma give a history of occupational exposure to asbestos. The danger of asbestos to public health was not widely appreciated until about 1970, and even though measures are now being taken to reduce asbestos exposure, the incidence of the disease is expected to climb as patients exposed to asbestos in the past develop the disease. The latency period between exposure to asbestos and development of mesothelioma may be up to 40 years. Approximately 2000 cases of malignant mesothelioma are diagnosed in the United States annually; 80% arise in the pleura and 20% in the peritoneum, with rare cases arising in the pericardium or in the tunica vaginalis of the testis.

Malignant mesothelioma of the pleural space characteristically presents with chest pain and/or dyspnea associated with a pleural effusion. The pleural fluid is usually an exudate, often bloody. The visceral pleura is often encased by tumor, with disease extending into the interlobar fissures and occasionally into the lung parenchyma. Cytologic examination of pleural fluid or histologic examination of a Cope needle biopsy of the pleura rarely suffices to make a definitive diagnosis of mesothelioma, and open pleural biopsy is generally required. However, as long as non–small cell malignancy can be diagnosed with certainty from pleural fluid, distinguishing between pleural mesothelioma and metastatic adenocarcinoma is of academic interest only, since treatment is so poor for either condition.

Peritoneal mesotheliomas present with abdominal pain and increasing abdominal girth. The peritoneum may be studded with multiple plaques of tumor, but invasion into the gastrointestinal tract is rare.

All three major treatment modalities have been used to combat pleural malignant mesothelioma, but it is doubtful that any antineoplastic therapy meaningfully alters the dismal prognosis of this cancer. Radical removal of both pleura and lung (pleuropneumonectomy) is associated with an operative mortality as high as 30%, and 2-year survival is rare. Pleurectomy alone, often in conjunction with other modalities of cancer treatment, is a less morbid operation, but again, its effect on the ultimate course of the malignancy is uncertain. External beam radiation therapy is limited by the relative resistance of mesothelioma to tolerable doses of radiation. Some radiotherapists advocate complex treatment planning techniques or placement of implanted radiation sources in residual tumor at the time of thoracotomy. Radiotherapy can be used to palliate the severe pain that is characteristic of advanced stages of mesothelioma.

Adriamycin (doxorubicin), cisplatin, ifosfamide, and mitomycin C all have modest single-agent activity in mesothelioma (10 to 20% response rates), but to date, no meaningful impact has been demonstrated on survival with either single agents or drug combinations. Intrapleural chemotherapy for mesothelioma is an investigational approach. In short, given the mortality and morbidity associated with radical surgery for mesothelioma and the toxicity and lack of efficacy of nonsurgical therapy, one reasonable approach to this disease is withholding all anticancer therapy and treating patients with tube thoracostomy and sclerosis, analgesia, and similar palliative modalities.

REFERENCES

Alberts AS, Falkson G, Godehuls L, et al: Malignant pleural mesothelioma: a disease unaffected by current therapeutic modalities. J Clin Oncol 6:527–535, 1988.

Falkson G, Alberts AS, Falkson HC: Malignant pleural mesothelioma treatment: The current state of the art. Cancer Treat Rev 15:231–242, 1988.
Pisani RJ, Colby TV, Williams DE: Malignant mesothelioma of the pleura. Mayo Clin Proc 63:1234–1249, 1988.
Ruffie P, Feld R, Minkin S, et al: Diffuse malignant mesothelioma of the pleura in Ontario and Quebec: A retrospective study of 332 patients. J Clin Oncol 7:1157–1168, 1989.

MEDIASTINAL TUMORS

The majority of malignancies involving the mediastinum are metastatic, but primary mediastinal tumors do occur. The mediastinum is divided into anterior, middle, and posterior compartments. A primary tumor of the anterior mediastinum is usually a lymphoma, thymoma, or germ cell tumor, whereas neurogenic tumors are the most common posterior mediastinal tumors.

THYMOMA

Thymomas are rare tumors of the anterior mediastinum originating from epithelial elements of the thymus gland. They occur as an asymptomatic mass on a chest radiograph or present with local symptoms such as cough or dyspnea. Over half of patients with thymoma have associated autoimmune diseases, most commonly myasthenia gravis. Newly diagnosed myasthenic patients should have a chest radiograph and thoracic CT scan in order to detect thymoma. Resection of a thymoma in patients with myasthenia ameliorates the myasthenia in the great majority of cases. Other autoimmune syndromes in patients with thymoma include pure red cell aplasia and hypogammaglobulinemia.

Surgery is the treatment of choice for thymomas, and at the time of surgery, thymomas are classified as benign or malignant. About two-thirds of thymomas are noninvasive and well encapsulated at surgery, and these benign tumors have an excellent prognosis with 80 to 90% disease-free survival. About one-third of thymomas are invasive, and complete removal is frequently impossible. Radiotherapy is conventionally utilized to control these tumors. Nonetheless, invasive thymoma is associated with only 50% 10-year survival after surgery and/or radiotherapy. Malignant thymoma is a chemotherapy-responsive disease, and complete responses of metastatic lesions or recurrent intrathoracic disease have been observed with a variety of chemotherapy regimens. Investigational protocols are testing the use of chemotherapy earlier in the course of invasive thymoma.

REFERENCES

Fornassero A, Damel O, Ghiotto C, et al: Chemotherapy of invasive thymoma. J Clin Oncol 8:1419–1423, 1990.
Lewis JE, Wick MR, Scheithauer BW, et al: Thymoma: A clinicopathologic review. Cancer 60:2727–2743, 1987.
Suster S, Rosai J: Thymic carcinoma: A clinicopathologic study of 60 cases. Cancer 67:1025–1032, 1991.

14
GASTROINTESTINAL CANCERS

Susan Rosenthal

Despite the large and growing incidence of most cancers of the gastrointestinal tract and the increasing public awareness of these disorders, early diagnosis and adequate treatment of advanced disease remain unsolved problems. Although the epidemiology and natural history of these conditions are much better understood, relatively few major developments in therapy have occurred over the past several decades.

CANCER OF THE COLON AND RECTUM

INCIDENCE AND ETIOLOGY

According to National Cancer Institute estimates, 156,000 new cases of colorectal cancer will occur in the United States and 58,300 Americans will die of the disease in 1992. Fifteen percent of all cancers in Americans are of colorectal origin, and this disease is the second most common cause of cancer deaths (following lung cancer). The overall survival rate of 40 to 50% has not improved substantially over the past quarter century and probably will not improve until reliable methods for earlier detection are available. The incidence of colon cancer increases steadily with increasing age; 53% of cases occur in persons aged 55 to 74 and an additional 36% occur in persons over age 75. Males and females are approximately equally affected.

The etiology of colon cancer is unknown, but epidemiologic evidence implicates dietary factors. Within the United States, high incidence of colorectal cancer correlates with high socioeconomic status and high population density. Worldwide, the disease is more common in industrialized societies than in underdeveloped nations and may relate to high dietary fat and low dietary fiber intake. A variety of preexisting colonic conditions predispose to the development of cancer: familial colonic polyposis, Gardner's syndrome (colonic polyposis associated with osteomas, fibromas, and lipomas), ulcerative colitis and Crohn's colitis, villous adenomas, and Peutz-Jeghers syndrome. First-degree relatives of patients with colorectal cancer have three times the risk of colorectal cancer as the general population. The malignant potential of benign adenomatous polyps is controversial, but most authorities agree that at least some adenomatous polyps undergo malignant degeneration. Hyperplastic polyps, on the other hand, do not predispose to colonic malignancy. Characteristic genetic alterations are seen in colorectal cancers, and an accumulation of genetic changes accompanies the transition from adenomatous polyp to invasive carcinoma. These changes include mutation of the *ras* oncogene and deletions within chromosomes 5, 17, and 18 that may encode tumor suppressor genes (antioncogenes).

Cancer Prevention

The American Cancer Society suggests dietary modifications—increasing fiber intake and reducing fat intake—in an attempt to reduce the incidence of colon cancer. Confirmation of the benefit of such dietary changes requires complex, large-scale diet modification studies, which are currently being designed. A recent cancer prevention study of over 600,000 adults concluded that regular low-dose aspirin use may reduce the risk of fatal colon cancer. The authors theorize that the inhibition of prostaglandin synthesis by aspirin provides a protective effect, but this mechanism is speculative and further research is necessary.

PATHOLOGY

The vast majority of colorectal cancers are adenocarcinomas. Small numbers of carcinoid tumors, squamous cell carcinomas (especially near the anus), leiomyosarcomas, and lymphomas also occur. Multicentric invasive bowel cancers arise in 3% of patients, and

2% of patients develop a second bowel primary cancer at some time following initial diagnosis.

Carcinomas arise more frequently in the distal portion of the colon; over half of all colorectal cancers are within reach of the sigmoidoscope. Presenting symptoms vary with location and growth pattern. Cancers of the cecum and ascending colon tend to be large polypoid masses with little intramural invasion, whereas tumors of the descending and sigmoid colons are generally constricting, annular lesions. Rectal cancers may be bulky, friable, polypoid lesions or ulcerating and invasive.

STAGING

In 1932, Cuthbert E. Dukes observed that the prognosis of colon cancer depends on the degree of tumor penetration through the colonic wall, and this observation led to a pathologic staging system that bears his name. Table 14–1 gives a modified version of the Dukes system in widespread use. At the time of initial surgery, 40 to 70% of patients have regional lymph node metastases (Dukes C) and 15 to 25% have liver metastases (Dukes D).

DIAGNOSIS

Although large amounts of indirect evidence suggest a mortality benefit for screening large populations for colorectal cancer, no large-scale prospective controlled trials (such as the Health Insurance Plan [HIP] study and others in patients with breast cancer) demonstrate improved survival due to screening. Mass screening by fecal occult blood testing is currently under investigation in clinical trials. The American Cancer Society recommends an annual digital rectal exam and fecal occult blood testing for all asymptomatic patients over the age of 50, with proctoscopic exams every 3 to 5 years after two initial negative tests 1 year apart. Compliance with these recommendations is highly variable. Fecal occult blood testing, while imperfect, remains a worthwhile part of the general physical examination, and positive tests, even on an unrestricted diet, warrant further follow-up. Patients with symptoms suggestive of colorectal cancer obviously require further evaluation with colonoscopy and/or barium enema.

CLINICAL MANIFESTATIONS

Tumors in the cecum and ascending colon may remain clinically silent for long periods, since they rarely cause obstruction or obvious bleeding. Iron-deficiency anemia due to occult blood loss is often the initial manifestation of right-sided colon lesions. Cramping or colicky pain eventually occurs in the majority of patients. Weight loss is also common.

Cancers of the left colon, which tend to be annular and constricting, usually present with symptoms related to obstruction, pain, or change in bowel habit. Gross rectal bleeding is common, especially with rectal tumors, which may also cause tenesmus and pain. Physical examination of the colon cancer patient usually reveals either gross or occult gastrointestinal bleeding, an abdominal mass, or a rectal lesion on digital examination.

Table 14–1. **MODIFIED DUKES CLASSIFICATION OF COLON CANCER**

	DUKES STAGE	APPROXIMATE 5-YEAR SURVIVAL (%)
A	Confined to mucosa and submucosa	80
B_1	Penetration into muscularis	65
B_2	Extension through serosa	40–60
C_1	Positive lymph nodes; tumor within bowel wall	30–40
C_2	Positive lymph nodes; tumor extends through serosa	10–20
D	Involvement of adjacent organs or distant metastases	<5

Patients may also present with evidence of metastatic disease, usually hepatomegaly or supraclavicular adenopathy.

Figure 14–1 outlines the evaluation of the patient with signs or symptoms suggesting colorectal cancer. In one study, colonoscopy detected 12% more colorectal cancers than sigmoidoscopy and barium enema. The choice of diagnostic procedure may depend on the availability and quality of endoscopic and radiologic expertise.

TREATMENT

Surgery

Surgical excision is the only potentially curative treatment of colon cancer and should follow diagnosis as quickly as possible. Even in the presence of metastatic disease, surgery is often advisable to relieve or prevent obstruction, to reduce severe pain or bleeding, and to ameliorate disabling diarrhea and tenesmus. Modern surgical techniques now permit rectal sphincter preservation in all but the lowest lying rectal cancers, allowing colostomies to be avoided in the majority of cases.

Some authorities recommend surgical resection of solitary or multiple unilobar liver

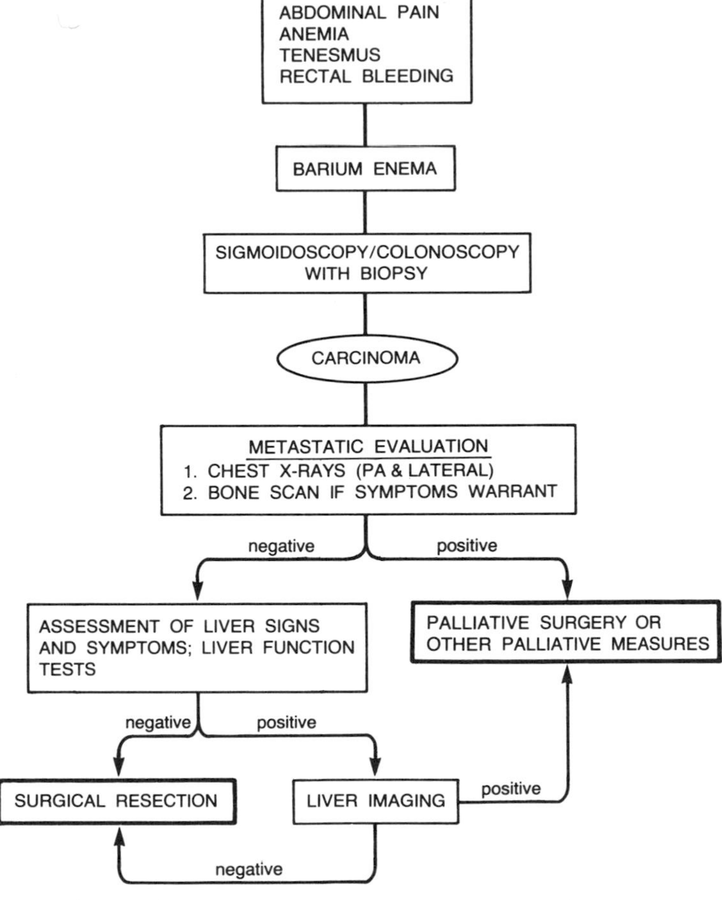

Figure 14–1. Flow diagram for evaluation of the patient with suspected colorectal cancer. (*From* Borg SA, Rosenthal S: Handbook of Cancer Diagnosis and Staging. A Clinical Atlas. New York, John Wiley & Sons, 1984.)

metastases in patients without evidence of extrahepatic metastases. Although no prospective trials comparing surgical to nonsurgical management in equivalent patients have been performed, survival following surgical resection of hepatic metastases in selected patients may extend to several years. Clearly surgery for liver metastases is not suitable for the vast majority of patients who have either extensive liver metastases, extrahepatic disease, or intercurrent illnesses that preclude partial hepatectomy.

Radiation Therapy

Rectal cancers arising below the peritoneal reflection tend to recur locally, causing serious morbidity that is difficult to palliate by either local or systemic measures. Preoperative radiotherapy for cancers of the rectum increases resectability and decreases local recurrence when compared with surgery alone. Most studies, however, fail to show any benefit in overall survival. Postoperative radiation for rectal and rectosigmoid lesions is also effective. However, postoperative combined modality therapy (see below) is currently the treatment of choice for high-risk rectal cancers. Highly selected patients with small rectal cancers may be treated with local excision and endocavitary irradiation as an alternative to abdominoperineal resection with permanent colostomy. Radiation therapy provides effective palliative treatment of locally recurrent tumor and painful bone metastases.

Adjuvant Chemotherapy

Because of the high relapse rate following surgery for Dukes C colorectal cancers, interest has focused on the potential for increasing the surgical cure rate by using chemotherapy in the postoperative period in patients presumed to have micrometastatic disease. Recently published results indicate some success with this approach, which is known as surgical adjuvant chemotherapy.

A large randomized trial recently demonstrated a substantial reduction in the risk of tumor recurrence and overall death rate in patients with Dukes C colon cancer treated with a combination of 5-fluorouracil (5-FU) and levamisole, an antihelminthic agent with immunomodulatory activity. At 3.5 years of follow-up, 37% of patients receiving adjuvant chemotherapy had disease recurrence and 29% died, versus a 53% recurrence rate and 45% death rate in the control group. Interestingly, levamisole alone in the adjuvant setting produces no benefit, and the combination of levamisole plus 5-fluorouracil in advanced disease is no more active than 5-fluorouracil alone. The National Institutes of Health (NIH) Consensus Conference advises that adjuvant therapy with levamisole plus 5-FU be offered to all patients with Dukes C colon cancer who are ineligible for clinical trials. Preliminary results from the Mayo Clinic suggest that patients with Dukes B_2 colon cancer may also benefit from adjuvant 5-FU plus levamisole. Research with flow cytometry and other methods continues to define high-risk subsets of patients for clinical trials with 5-FU plus levamisole and other adjuvant chemotherapy regimens.

Combined Modality Therapy

Postoperative chemotherapy and radiation therapy to the pelvis decrease the local recurrence rate and improve overall survival in patients with rectal cancer. However, controversy persists regarding the survival advantage conferred by radiotherapy (although most authorities agree that the local recurrence rate is definitely reduced) and the need for methyl-CCNU, a known leukemogen, used in these studies. A large trial with over 200 patients with stages B_2 and C rectal cancer compared postoperative radiotherapy with radiation treatment plus concurrent 5-fluorouracil as well as a course of 5-fluorouracil plus methyl-CCNU both preceding and following the radiation therapy. Local recurrences and distant metastases were significantly reduced in the combined modality group, and overall survival was prolonged. At 5 years, disease-free survival in the combined modality patients was 63%, compared with 42% in the patients treated with radiotherapy alone. The NIH Consensus Conference and subsequent Clinical Alert (March 1991) on this subject have recommended that all patients with rectal cancer receive postoperative local radiation therapy plus chemotherapy with 5-fluorouracil. Clinical trials now in progress are investigating whether 5-fluorouracil plus leukovorin and/or levamisole combined with radiation therapy will improve these results further.

Chemotherapy

Chemotherapy has a limited palliative role in the management of advanced colorectal carcinoma. Patients with rapidly advancing or symptomatic and measurable disease are the best candidates for a trial of chemotherapy. Those who are bedridden or deeply jaundiced are often better served by a regimen of supportive measures only. Debilitated patients with advanced colorectal cancer are unlikely to benefit from any form of chemotherapy.

Of the 40 cytotoxic drugs evaluated for efficacy in this disease, none is clearly superior to 5-fluorouracil. Although a wide range of response rates has been reported with 5-fluorouracil, an objective response rate of 15% is generally accepted for this drug used as a single agent in previously untreated patients. No single agent has been of any value following failure with 5-fluorouracil.

Attempts to increase the activity of 5-fluorouracil in this disease by alterations in dose, schedule, and route of administration have had limited success. Continuous intravenous infusion, portal vein infusion, and other approaches have produced improved response rates but no survival advantage compared with the conventional 5-fluorouracil regimen of 450 to 500 mg/m^2 IV daily for 5 days, repeated every 5 weeks.

Biochemical modulation of 5-fluorouracil with the use of leucovorin (folinic acid), however, has led to significant therapeutic advantages in response rate, quality of life, and survival in comparison with 5-fluorouracil alone. Many regimens are available, but a combination of 5-fluorouracil, 370 to 425 mg/m^2, and leucovorin, 20 mg/m^2, both given daily for 5 days and repeated every 4 to 5 weeks provides the advantages of superior activity with relatively mild side effects. Except in an investigational setting, 5-fluorouracil plus leucovorin represents the standard treatment for patients with advanced colorectal cancer. Treatment should continue in responding patients until disease progression, or for 2 to 3 months in the absence of response.

Combination Chemotherapy

Extensive experience with combination chemotherapy in advanced colorectal cancer has accumulated. No combination regimen has clear-cut superiority over 5-fluorouracil alone, and the combinations almost invariably cause greater toxicity. A recent study showed promising results with a combination of 5-fluorouracil plus recombinant alpha-2a-interferon. Further studies with this regimen (and others) are underway.

Hepatic Artery Infusion

Both 5-fluorouracil and 5-fluorodeoxyuridine have been administered intrahepatically to patients with liver metastases from colorectal cancer. Despite initial enthusiasm, this approach is clearly not a panacea for hepatic metastases. The complication and toxicity rates are high; the objective response rate is much lower than the 75% initially described; the requirement for laparotomy presents a problem for many patients; and importantly, the technique is inappropriate for the majority who have both hepatic and extrahepatic disease. Nevertheless, for selected patients with metastases confined to the liver, hepatic arterial infusion definitely produces higher response rates and greater response durations than systemic chemotherapy. Improvement in survival has not been convincingly demonstrated.

REFERENCES

Allison JE, Feldman R, Tekawa IS: Hemoccult screening in detecting colorectal neoplasm: Sensitivity, specificity, and predictive value. Ann Intern Med 112:328–333, 1990.

Bond JH: Screening for colorectal cancer: Need for controlled trials. Ann Intern Med 113:338–340, 1990.

Bruckner HW, Motwani BT: Chemotherapy of advanced cancer of the colon and rectum. Semin Oncol 18:443–461, 1991.
Cohen AM: Surgical considerations in patients with cancer of the colon and rectum. Semin Oncol 18:381–387, 1991.
Krook JE, Moertel CG, Gunderson LL, et al: Effective surgical adjuvant therapy for high-risk rectal carcinoma. N Engl J Med 324:709–715, 1991.
Moertel CG, Fleming TR, MacDonald JS, et al: Levamisole and fluorouracil for adjuvant therapy of resected colon carcinoma. N Engl J Med 322:352–358, 1990.
NIH Consensus Conference: Adjuvant therapy for patients with colon and rectal cancer. JAMA 264:1444–1450, 1990.
Poon MA, O'Connell MJ, Moertel CG, et al: Biochemical modulation of fluorouracil: Evidence of significant improvement of survival and quality of life in patients with advanced colorectal carcinoma. J Clin Oncol 7:1407–1418, 1989.
Ransohoff DF, Lang CA: Screening for colorectal cancer. N Engl J Med 325:37–41, 1991.
Thun MJ, Namboodiri BS, Heath CW: Aspirin use and reduced risk of fatal colon cancer. N Engl J Med 325:1593–1596, 1991.

CARCINOMA OF THE ESOPHAGUS

INCIDENCE AND ETIOLOGY

Malignant tumors of the esophagus are rare in the United States, comprising just over 1% of all forms of cancer and about 2% of cancer deaths. The National Cancer Institute estimates that 11,100 new cases and 10,000 deaths will occur in 1992. The disease arises more than twice as often in men as in women, and the incidence increases with age.

Worldwide, the incidence of esophageal cancer varies tremendously. Areas of high frequency include parts of Iran, Soviet Central Asia, Mongolia, northern China, India, several provinces in France, and parts of southern and eastern Africa. In the United States, the disease is much more common among blacks than among whites.

Etiologic factors contributing to the incidence of esophageal cancer include environmental carcinogens, nutritional deficiencies, chronic irritation, and mucosal damage. In North America and western Europe, excessive use of alcohol and tobacco are the major risk factors, accounting for 80 to 90% of cases. Other conditions that predispose to the development of esophageal cancer include esophageal stricture (especially due to lye ingestion), achalasia, gluten-sensitive enteropathy, Barrett's esophagus, and Plummer-Vinson syndrome. The highest association is with tylosis palmaris et plantaris, an inherited autosomal dominant condition characterized by epidermal thickening of the palms and soles. As many as 37% of affected persons develop esophageal cancer.

PATHOLOGY

More than 90% of upper- and middle-third esophageal cancers are squamous cell carcinomas, but an increasing proportion of carcinomas of the distal third are adenocarcinomas, probably arising in the gastric cardia and extending proximally. For unknown reasons, the incidence of adenocarcinomas of the distal esophagus and gastric cardia has risen extremely rapidly in recent years. Ten percent of esophageal cancers originate in the cervical esophagus, 40% in the upper half of the thoracic esophagus, and 50% in the lower half of the thoracic esophagus. These neoplasms spread via the lymphatic system, and since the esophagus lacks serosal layers, there is no effective barrier to early regional spread.

CLINICAL MANIFESTATIONS

Dysphagia is by far the most common presenting symptom of esophageal carcinoma. Dysphagia always requires investigation, and esophageal cancer is the presumptive diagnosis until proven otherwise. Weight loss, malaise, and anorexia also appear early. Vomiting, regurgitation, and pain in the epigastrium, chest or mid-back are frequent complaints. Vocal cord paralysis, nocturnal aspiration, and invasion of local organs occur with advancing disease. Physical signs other than evidence of weight loss are usually absent at the time of diagnosis.

Diagnosis is straightforward and depends on radiologic contrast examination (barium esophagram) followed by esophagoscopy with biopsy and brushings. Exfoliative cytology by esophageal lavage is also quite accurate but time consuming.

STAGING

Most patients have lymph node involvement and locally advanced disease at the time of diagnosis. Thorough examination prior to aggressive intervention should include bronchoscopy to detect any invasion of the tracheobronchial tree, chest x-ray, and computed tomography (CT) scan of the chest and upper abdomen to assess local involvement by direct extension of the primary tumor and to screen for adenopathy in the mediastinum and celiac axis. Metastases to lung, pleura, and liver can be detected by the same scan. Distant metastases, frequently asymptomatic, preclude major surgery, since these patients usually survive only 2 to 3 months.

Since the majority of patients with esophageal cancer also have significant nonmalignant disease, complete assessment of cardiopulmonary status is essential before considering surgery. Malnutrition among patients with esophageal cancer is common due both to the disease itself and often to preexisting alcoholism. Malnutrition adversely affects the outcome of therapy, but it is unclear whether nutritional intervention (enteral or intravenous hyperalimentation) will reverse the adverse effect. Nevertheless, nutritional assessment may contribute to therapeutic decision making.

The majority of patients have stage III disease at the time of diagnosis, explaining in large part the dismal 5-year survival rate of 5%. The survival of patients with esophageal cancer has not improved in the past 30 years.

TREATMENT

Despite advances in diagnosis and staging of esophageal cancer, the results of therapy remain unsatisfactory. No agreement exists on the best initial treatment of the disease; recommendations range from aggressive surgery to aggressive radiotherapy to symptomatic management alone. Many surgeons and radiation therapists are convinced that the disease is incurable and that their efforts should be directed toward palliative measures only. Others believe that therapy with curative intent is fully warranted, despite the substantial rate of major treatment complications.

Surgery

Because esophageal cancer is usually locally advanced at diagnosis, only a minority of patients are eligible for curative surgery. Major resections are often performed, nonetheless, for palliative purposes: to allow continued oral nutrition and to facilitate control of oral secretions. Radical esophagectomy with esophagogastrectomy is considered the procedure of choice. Ideal candidates for this procedure are patients whose tumors do not penetrate the esophageal wall, do not involve lymph nodes, and do not exceed 10 cm in length.

Surgical mortality is high (10 to 40%) and morbidity—including anastomotic leaks, strictures, respiratory failure, sepsis, and pulmonary embolism—considerable. Since only about 18% of patients survive even 1 year, radical surgery, with its substantial risk of postoperative death, serious complications, and prolonged and expensive hospitalization (often lasting for the remainder of the patient's life) represents a questionable choice for a terminally ill patient. Some authorities, including thoracic surgeons, question whether a procedure in which the operative mortality exceeds the cure rate by severalfold should continue to be recommended.

Palliative surgical procedures to improve dysphagia include endoscopic placement of an artificial tube, peroral esophageal dilatation, and gastric or colonic bypass without esophageal resection. Endoscopic laser therapy is also useful in some cases.

Radiation Therapy

Acute mortality following radiation therapy for esophageal carcinoma is uncommon, and treatment results are comparable to those of surgery. Therefore, many advocate radiation therapy rather than surgery for primary management of this disease. The best survival results with irradiation are achieved in patients with well-circumscribed tumors—the same group that does best with surgery. Unfortunately, no controlled prospective trial comparing surgery with irradiation for resectable tumors exists.

Several investigators claim that preoperative irradiation followed by esophagectomy confers a survival benefit over esophagectomy alone. However, two randomized trials refute this claim. Insufficient reported experience with postoperative irradiation precludes assessment of its value. The available data suggest that any benefit derived from combining surgery and irradiation is likely to be modest at best. Such combinations should not be used routinely.

Esophageal cancers that arise in the cervical esophagus are usually managed with primary irradiation. Surgical treatment results in major functional deficits and especially severe morbidity and high mortality. Primary irradiation results in comparable survival rates to those accomplished with surgery but avoids the complications.

Regardless of survival rates, however, radiation therapy offers significant palliation to 65 to 75% of patients with esophageal cancer. Radiotherapy is generally the initial palliative modality in patients ineligible for surgery. Average duration of improvement in dysphagia is approximately 6 months. Palliative surgical maneuvers may be necessary when dysphagia recurs following initial irradiation.

Contraindications to palliative radiotherapy include distant metastases (survival of these patients is extremely brief) and tracheoesophageal fistula.

Chemotherapy

Until recently chemotherapy results in esophageal carcinoma were extremely disappointing. Because of poor nutritional status, general debility, and lack of measurable disease to indicate response, patients with esophageal carcinoma are frequently poor candidates for chemotherapy. Table 14–2 summarizes the approximate response rates (from accumulated data) to single-agent chemotherapy. Most of the drugs listed have modest activity, with very rare complete responses and very brief (2 to 5 months) response durations.

Experience with several combination chemotherapy programs, most including cisplatin, has been more encouraging. Response rates range from 15 to 80%, with durations of 2 to 11 months. Toxicity is substantial, frequently leading to hospitalization for leukopenic sepsis. Clearly programs of this intensity are appropriate only for patients in relatively good general condition.

While combination chemotherapy for esophageal carcinoma appears beneficial, there are as yet no randomized trials comparing the effectiveness of combinations with that of single agents. Furthermore, it is not clear whether any chemotherapy improves survival in this disease. Until these questions have been answered, the role of chemotherapy in esophageal carcinoma should be considered investigational. Whenever possible, patients with esophageal carcinoma should be enrolled in controlled clinical trials.

Combined Modality Therapy

Combinations of surgery and radiotherapy have been discussed above. Recent evidence indicating activity of chemotherapy in this disease led to the study of various combinations

Table 14–2. **SINGLE AGENTS IN ESOPHAGEAL CANCER**

AGENT	RESPONSE RATE (%)
Methotrexate	12
Bleomycin	15
Mitomycin C	26
Adriamycin	15
5-Fluorouracil	15
CCNU	16
Methyl-GAG	17
Cisplatin	22
Vindesine	17
Etoposide	0

of local and systemic treatments. For patients with potentially operable disease, treatment programs combine preoperative chemotherapy or chemotherapy plus irradiation, often followed by a period of postoperative chemotherapy as well. Results of several such trials indicate that preoperative treatment can be delivered safely. Resectability rates are at least comparable to historical controls, and a 20 to 35% pathologically confirmed complete remission rate has been achieved in several studies following preoperative chemoradiotherapy.

Some investigators have questioned the need for surgery at all; patients with potentially operable tumors treated with high-dose radiation and concurrent chemotherapy have achieved palliation with median survivals of 1.5 to 2.0 years. A recent randomized study demonstrated a survival advantage for highly selected patients with good performance status treated with chemotherapy plus radiation compared with radiation alone. A second small study showed a survival advantage for patients receiving chemotherapy plus radiation prior to surgery compared with preoperative radiation alone. At present, the combined modality approach to the management of esophageal carcinoma appears very promising but should be offered only to selected patients capable of tolerating this rigorous course of therapy.

REFERENCES

Adelstein DJ, Forman WB, Beavers B: Esophageal carcinoma. Cancer 54:918–923, 1984.
Coia LR: Esophageal cancer: Is esophagectomy necessary? Oncology 3:101–110, 1989.
Hancock SL, Glatstein E: Radiation therapy of esophageal cancer. Semin Oncol 11:144–158, 1984.
Kelsen D: Chemotherapy of esophageal cancer. Semin Oncol 11:159–168, 1984.
Kelsen DP: Multimodality therapy of esophageal carcinoma: still an experimental approach. J Clin Oncol 5:530–531, 1987.
Kelsen DP, Minsky B, Smith M, et al: Preoperative therapy for esophageal cancer: A randomized comparison of chemotherapy versus radiation therapy. J Clin Oncol 8:1352–1361, 1990.
Leichman L, Berry BT: Experience with cisplatin in treatment regimens for esophageal cancer. Semin Oncol 18:64–72, 1991.

GASTRIC CARCINOMA

INCIDENCE AND ETIOLOGY

Gastric carcinoma is one of the leading causes of cancer deaths worldwide and a major public health problem in Japan, where more than 50% of all malignancies in males arise in the stomach. In the United States, carcinoma of the stomach accounts for about 2% of cancer deaths; the National Cancer Institute expects 24,400 new cases and 13,300 deaths in 1992. The incidence of gastric cancer rises with age, and the median age at diagnosis is 70. The male to female ratio is 1.5 to 1.0.

For unknown reasons, the incidence of gastric cancer in the United States has declined steadily over the past half century. In 1930, the age-adjusted death rate for gastric cancer was 28.9 per 100,000 population, and by 1967, it had fallen to 9.7 per 100,000. A similar decline has taken place in Australia, Canada, and England.

The incidence of gastric cancer in Japan, the highest in the world, is about eight times that in the United States. Other areas of high incidence include Central Europe, Finland, Iceland, parts of Latin America, and parts of the former Soviet Union. Native Americans, blacks, and native Hawaiians are also high-risk groups. Migrants from Japan to the United States continue to have a gastric cancer rate similar to that of Japan but their American-born children have a low rate. This observation suggests that the risk of gastric cancer is determined by environmental factors operating during the first several decades of life and is not substantially changed by migration to a low-risk area.

Epidemiologic evidence suggests that dietary substances play an important role in the causation of gastric cancer. No single food item can be implicated, but the following dietary pattern characterizes high-risk groups: low intake of animal fat and protein, high intake of complex carbohydrates, high salt and nitrate intake, and low intake of fresh fruits and vegetables. Nitrates and nitrites (formerly widely used as meat preservatives), converted during food preparation to carcinogenic nitrosamines, may be responsible for causing gastric cancer in many cases.

Several benign gastric conditions are thought to predispose to gastric cancer: chronic atrophic gastritis and gastric adenomas may be risk factors, and diffuse gastric polyposis is definitely premalignant. Patients with pernicious anemia were thought to be at high risk but recent data challenge this long-held view. Infection with *Helicobacter pylori,* associated with chronic atrophic gastritis, also increases the risk of gastric adenocarcinoma.

PATHOLOGY AND STAGING

Adenocarcinomas account for the majority of gastric malignancies; lymphomas comprise most of the rest. Leiomyosarcomas, other carcinomas, and carcinoids occur rarely. Gastric adenocarcinomas occur as ulcerating lesions, polypoid lesions, and diffusely (linitis plastica or scirrhous carcinoma). Prognosis correlates with the extent of disease. Survival decreases with increasing depth of tumor penetration through the gastric wall, with lymph node involvement, and with distant metastases (median survival 4 months). Tumor grade or degree of anaplasia also correlates with prognosis.

Preoperative staging should include upper abdominal computed tomography to assess liver involvement, spread to adjacent organs, and regional node involvement. Evidence obtained by CT scanning is reliable and obviates exploratory surgery in cases where the scan indicates unresectability.

CLINICAL MANIFESTATIONS AND DIAGNOSIS

Weight loss and abdominal pain are the most common complaints among patients with gastric cancer. Patients with tumor located in the pyloric region and adjacent antrum are likely to have anorexia, weight loss, early satiety, and eventually gastric outlet obstruction; those with tumors involving the cardia and distal esophagus complain of dysphagia. Symptoms related to anemia due to occult blood loss occur commonly; hematemesis is unusual and suggests peptic ulcer disease. Direct extension of gastric cancer to the transverse colon may produce symptoms of lower abdominal discomfort, constipation, and diarrhea. Intraperitoneal dissemination may result in ascites, small bowel obstruction, and pelvic masses (Krukenberg tumors). Hematogenous spread to liver, bones, adrenals, and lungs produces characteristic signs and symptoms.

Physical examination may reveal epigastric tenderness or a mass. Acanthosis nigricans, dermatomyositis, and left supraclavicular or left axillary adenopathy may be clues to underlying gastric cancer. Laboratory findings are generally nonspecific and rarely helpful in diagnosis, which depends on radiologic examination of the stomach, gastroscopy, and biopsy.

Barium upper gastrointestinal series is usually the initial diagnostic procedure in a patient with suspected gastric cancer. An accuracy of 90% can be expected if the examination is performed carefully and the patient cooperates fully . Radiologic findings of gastric cancer include ulceration, an obstructing lesion, enlarged gastric folds, or lack of distensibility. Benign gastric ulcers cannot be distinguished radiologically from malignant ulcers with total reliability; even the occurrence of healing, previously considered an infallible sign of benignity, is not reliable. Over 3% of radiologically benign gastric ulcers prove malignant, and about 1% of ulcers that heal radiologically are actually gastric cancers. For these reasons, gastroscopy with biopsy should be performed in all patients with gastric ulcer. A combination of multiple biopsies and brushings enhances the yield of the procedure.

TREATMENT

Surgery

Surgery is the only curative approach to gastric cancer, but the disease rarely presents in its early, curable stages. The lack of specific, readily recognized symptoms encourages diagnostic delay, which averages many months from onset of symptoms. At presentation about 25% of patients have inoperable lesions and are not explored. Of those explored, some have unresectable tumors, and others can be only incompletely resected. Overall, about one-third of patients with gastric cancer undergo curative resections, and the 5-year survival of this group averages less than 25%.

Table 14–3. **SINGLE AGENTS IN ADVANCED GASTRIC CARCINOMA**

AGENT	RESPONSE RATE (%)
5-Fluorouracil	21
Mitomycin C	24
BCNU	18
Methyl-CCNU	8
Adriamycin	25
Cisplatin	22

Depending on tumor location, size, and presence and extent of lymph node involvement, either a subtotal gastrectomy or total gastrectomy, with or without splenectomy, omentectomy, lymph node dissection, and partial pancreatectomy, may be performed. Subtotal gastrectomy is preferred to avoid the higher surgical mortality, metabolic consequences, and dumping syndrome associated with total gastrectomy. Tumors of the proximal stomach or gastroesophageal junction require a gastroesophagectomy, usually via a thoracoabdominal approach. Palliative surgery may be useful for patients with obstruction, bleeding, or perforation due to gastric cancer. The procedure employed depends on individual circumstances, but, in general, removal of the primary tumor, if possible, is advisable.

Radiation Therapy

Radiotherapy plays little part in the management of gastric cancer, other than in combined modality programs. Surrounding tissues and organs are unable to tolerate the high doses of radiation necessary to affect the tumor. Occasionally, local irradiation may control bleeding in patients with unresectable disease. Of course, radiotherapy is always useful in the treatment of brain metastases and painful bone metastases.

Chemotherapy

Chemotherapy has a palliative role in the treatment of gastric cancer. Its main use is in the management of patients with symptomatic metastatic disease. Although some have advocated the use of chemotherapy in patients with residual disease following surgery or in patients with asymptomatic metastases, there is no clear evidence that early treatment prevents or delays disease progression.

Treatment of Advanced Disease

Gastric carcinoma is the most responsive of the gastrointestinal adenocarcinomas. Table 14–3 summarizes the activity of the five most active single agents. Single-agent responses are usually brief, and no drug improves survival. Combination chemotherapy for advanced gastric cancer has been extensively explored. Table 14–4 summarizes recent results that require confirmation in multi-institutional randomized trials. The median survival of patients treated with these combinations is no better than that of patients treated with 5-fluorouracil alone and averages about 6 months.

A three-arm randomized study prospectively compared 5-fluorouracil alone with 5-fluorouracil plus Adriamycin (doxorubicin) and with the FAM (5-fluorouracil, Adriamycin

Table 14–4. **COMBINATION CHEMOTHERAPY IN GASTRIC CARCINOMA**

COMBINATION	RESPONSE RATE (%)
5-FU plus BCNU	42
5-FU, Adriamyin plus mitomycin C (FAM)	30–42
5-FU, Adriamyin plus cisplatin (FAP)	33–36
5-FU, Adriamycin plus methotrexate (FAMx)	0–58
Etoposide, Adriamycin plus cisplatin (EAP)	20–72
Etoposide, leucovorin plus 5-FU (ELF)	52

and mitomycin C) combination. No differences in response rate, survival (Fig. 14–2), or palliative effects were observed, but the combination regimens were far more toxic and expensive. More recent studies attempted to improve results by adding cisplatin, etoposide, or biomodulation with leucovorin or methotrexate. Response rates vary considerably (see Table 14–4), with most institutions being unable to duplicate the extremely high response rates initially reported. Significant morbidity and mortality also discourage widespread acceptance of the EAP (etoposide, Adriamycin, cisplatin) regimen. The FAMx (5-fluorouracil, Adriamycin, methotrexate) and ELF (etoposide, leucovorin, 5-fluorouracil) regimens result in apparently equivalent response rates and less toxicity. However, in the absence of large-scale, randomized studies, no combination is clearly superior to 5-fluorouracil alone, and patients should be entered on well-designed clinical trials whenever possible.

Treatment of Locally Unresectable Disease

A number of studies have explored the effectiveness of chemotherapy plus radiation therapy in the management of locally unresectable or recurrent gastric carcinoma. Despite early trials demonstrating clear-cut superiority for a combination of 5-fluorouracil and radiation over radiation alone, subsequent trials have led only to increased confusion.

A British randomized study of 5-fluorouracil plus radiation versus no further therapy failed to detect any difference in survival or in time to progression. The Gastrointestinal Tumor Study Group (GTSG) randomly assigned patients with locally advanced gastric cancer to a combination of 5-fluorouracil plus methyl-CCNU or to local radiation plus the same chemotherapy program. The median survival results favored the chemotherapy-alone arm (17 months versus 9 months) because of an excess of early deaths in the combined modality arm. However, during the second through fourth year of follow-up, the combined modality arm had a lower death rate, resulting in a superior 4-year survival for this arm.

A subsequent GTSG study, designed to avoid the high early death rate of the previous trial, compared chemotherapy alone (5-fluorouracil, Adriamycin, and methyl-CCNU) with chemotherapy plus radiation. Results from this trial failed to show any advantage in long-term (3-year) survival for the combined modality group. Similarly, the Eastern Cooperative Oncology Group (ECOG) performed a randomized comparison of 5-fluorouracil alone with 5-fluorouracil plus radiation for locally unresectable gastric cancer. There was no detectable difference in overall survival (median survival 9.3 months versus 8.2 months) or time to progression. The combined modality arm caused greater toxicity.

In summary, current information does not support the selection of any form of therapy as standard for locally unresectable disease. Further study of this problem by randomized controlled clinical trials will be necessary. Introduction of new chemotherapeutic agents

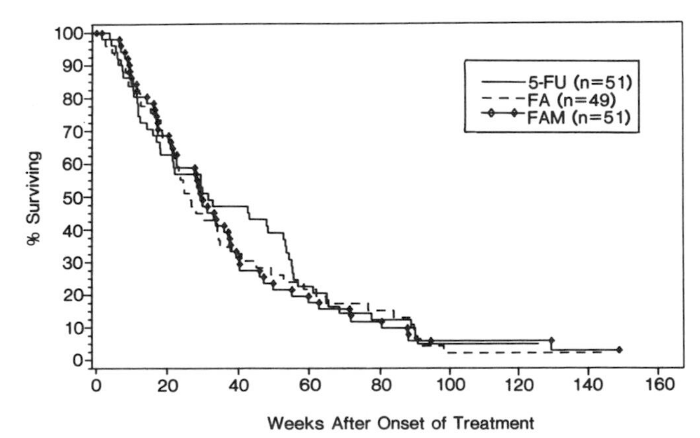

Figure 14–2. Gastric carcinoma. Survival from onset of treatment according to treatment regimen. (*From* Cullinan SA et al: A comparison of three chemotherapeutic regimens in the treatment of advanced pancreatic and gastric carcinoma. JAMA 253:2061–2067, 1985. Copyright 1985. American Medical Association.)

or combinations, innovative forms of radiation therapy, and other modalities may improve results.

Adjuvant Chemotherapy

Because of the extremely poor 5-year survival rate in gastric carcinoma, even among resected patients, interest has turned to adjuvant chemotherapy. Three studies have compared 5-fluorouracil plus methyl-CCNU to no further treatment following curative resection for gastric cancer. Both the Veterans Administration (VA) and the ECOG studies found no improvement in survival or disease-free survival associated with the treatment regimen, which was highly toxic. The GTSG noted a small improvement in favor of the treatment arm, at the expense of substantial toxicity, primarily hematologic.

A large international trial compared observation alone with FAM chemotherapy following surgery for operable gastric cancer. The FAM therapy conferred no improvement in either disease-free survival or overall survival in comparison with the no treatment control. At present, adjuvant chemotherapy for resected gastric carcinoma must be considered experimental. More active chemotherapy regimens will be required before improvement in results will occur.

REFERENCES

Coombes RC, Schein PS, Chilvers CE, et al: A randomized trial comparing adjuvant fluorouracil, doxorubicin, and mitomycin with no treatment in operable gastric cancer. J Clin Oncol 8:1362–1369, 1990.

Cullinan, SA, Moertel CG, Fleming TR, et al: A comparison of three chemotherapeutic regimens in the treatment of advanced pancreatic and gastric carcinoma. JAMA 253:2061–2067, 1985.

Gastrointestinal Tumor Study Group: The concept of locally advanced gastric cancer. Cancer 66:2324–2330, 1990.

Kelsen D, Atiq OT: Therapy of upper gastrointestinal tract cancers. Curr Probl Cancer 15:239–294, 1991.

Klaassen DJ, MacIntyre JM, Catton GE, et al: Treatment of locally unresectable cancer of the stomach and pancreas: Randomized comparison of 5-fluorouracil alone with radiation plus concurrent and maintenance 5-fluorouracil: An Eastern Cooperative Oncology Group study. J Clin Oncol 3:373–378, 1985.

Lawrence W: Gastric cancer. CA 36:216–236, 1986.

Macdonald JS: Chemotherapy of advanced gastric cancer: Present status, future prospects. Semin Oncol 15:42–49, 1988.

Preusser P, Wilke H, Achterrath W, et al: Phase II study with the combination etoposide, doxorubicin, and cisplatin in advanced measurable gastric cancer. J Clin Oncol 7:1310–1317, 1989.

Wilke H, Preusser P, Fink U, et al: New developments in the treatment of gastric carcinoma. Semin Oncol 17(suppl 2):61–70, 1990.

MALIGNANT TUMORS OF THE SMALL INTESTINE

Primary malignant tumors of the small intestine are uncommon. Accumulated series collected over many decades from large institutions rarely exceed 100 cases. The average annual incidence is 0.7 and 0.6 per 100,000 population for males and females, respectively. The National Cancer Institute estimates that 3400 new cases of small bowel cancers will occur in 1992, representing slightly more than 1% of all new gastrointestinal cancers.

Adenocarcinomas and malignant carcinoid tumors are the most common primary small bowel cancers. Small bowel adenocarcinomas arise more frequently in patients with Gardner's syndrome, Peutz-Jeghers syndrome, familial colonic polyposis, and regional enteritis than in the normal population. The majority of adenocarcinomas arise in the duodenum or jejunum within 20 cm of the ligament of Treitz. Carcinoids, on the other hand, increase in frequency with descent along the small bowel, occurring most often in the distal ileum. Lymphomas, leiomyosarcomas, and various other sarcomas comprise the remaining types of small bowel cancers; these tumors are uncommon in the duodenum. Metastatic tumors from other primary sites (gastric, ovarian, lung, and malignant melanoma) also occur in the small bowel either as multiple or solitary lesions.

Patients with small bowel malignancies generally present with nonspecific abdominal complaints; consequently, diagnosis is often delayed. Cramping, intermittent abdominal pain, nausea, vomiting, sporadic gastrointestinal bleeding, and weight loss are frequent. In many patients, symptoms precede the diagnosis by 6 months or more. In those patients who present with small bowel obstruction, however, surgery usually results in a prompt diagnosis.

For suspected small bowel cancer, fiberoptic endoscopy and barium examination of the stomach and small bowel are the most useful tests. Surgical resection provides both diagnosis and treatment. Prognosis depends on the depth of invasion, presence of lymph node involvement or distant metastatic spread, and histologic type. Five-year survival rates vary from 25 to 43%.

Several series of patients with small bowel carcinoids and adenocarcinomas report a high incidence of second (and third) primaries. Nearly 20% of patients develop either synchronous or metachronous second malignancies of both gastrointestinal and extraintestinal origin.

REFERENCES

Ashley SW, Wells SA: Tumors of the small intestine. Semin Oncol 15:116–128, 1988.
Barclay TH, Schapira DV: Malignant tumors of the small intestine. Cancer 51:878–881, 1983.
Johnson AM, Harman PK, Hanks JB: Primary small bowel malignancies. Am Surgeon 51:31–35, 1985.

LIVER, GALLBLADDER, AND BILE DUCT CARCINOMAS

Primary cancers of the liver and biliary passages are rare, comprising 1.5% of all cancers and 2.3% of cancer deaths. In 1992, the National Cancer Institute expects 15,400 new cases of cancer of the liver and biliary passages and 12,300 deaths. Hepatoma is more common than gallbladder cancer, which occurs more frequently than extrahepatic bile duct cancer. All three are rare before the age of 40 and increase in frequency with advancing age.

EPIDEMIOLOGY AND ETIOLOGY

The incidence of hepatoma varies widely worldwide. In parts of Africa and Asia, it is the most common malignancy in males, but it is rare in the United States and western Europe. Among Caucasians, hepatoma arises most often between the ages of 55 and 80, whereas among Africans and Asians, the disease is most common in the third and fourth decades. Males are two or three times more likely to develop hepatoma than females.

Sixty to 80% of patients with hepatoma have underlying cirrhosis, and about 4% of cirrhotics will develop hepatoma. Postnecrotic cirrhosis and cirrhosis associated with hemochromatosis have a relatively high risk of subsequent hepatoma. Chronic infection with hepatitis B or hepatitis C viruses and dietary exposure to aflatoxin (derived from moldy peanuts) also represent risk factors for hepatoma. Occupational exposure to vinyl chloride predisposes to the extremely rare hepatic angiosarcoma.

The pathogenesis of bile duct cancer involves chronic biliary inflammation and the excretion of carcinogens into the bile. Worldwide, infestation with the liver fluke *Clonorchis sinensis* in the Orient is the most common antecedent for bile duct carcinoma. Patients with ulcerative colitis have a 10 times greater risk of bile duct carcinoma than the general population and develop the disease several decades earlier. Neither the course nor the severity of the ulcerative colitis appears to affect the likelihood of subsequent bile duct cancer. Bile duct cancer is also strongly associated with the presence of congenital biliary tract cysts. In epidemiologic surveys, rubber workers and automotive workers share a greater risk for this disease.

The vast majority of patients with carcinoma of the gallbladder (65 to 90%) have cholelithiasis. In populations in which gallstones are infrequent, such as the Bantu, gallbladder cancer is extremely rare. Among groups in which the incidence of gallstones is high, such as the American Indians, carcinoma of the gallbladder is very common, accounting for 8.5 to 25% of all malignancies. The risk factors for gallstones—female sex, age over 55, parity, estrogen therapy, obesity, abnormalities of bile and lipoprotein metabolism— are therefore the risk factors for gallbladder cancer. Porcelain gallbladder and colonic polyposis also predispose to gallbladder cancer.

PATHOLOGY

Nearly all malignant tumors of the liver, gallbladder, and biliary tract are adenocarcinomas. In the liver, two major types occur: hepatocellular carcinoma and cholangiocarcinoma, with a 9:1 ratio. Rarely, hemangioendothelioma, sarcoma, and hepatoblastoma (especially in children) are encountered. Hepatomas may be single or multiple or may involve the liver diffusely. Vascular invasion is common, and extension of tumor into the portal vein, hepatic veins, and inferior vena cava leads to many of the characteristic thrombotic and embolic phenomena that distinguish this tumor. Metastases frequently involve the lung, pleura, bone, lymph nodes, and adrenals. Death results from hepatic failure or from hemorrhage due to esophageal varices. Spontaneous rupture of tumor with intra-abdominal hemorrhage is a dramatic and characteristic terminal event.

CLINICAL MANIFESTATIONS

Hepatomegaly, right upper quadrant pain, weakness, ascites, and weight loss are the most common findings of hepatoma. Upper gastrointestinal bleeding, respiratory failure due to pulmonary metastases, and acute abdominal crisis due to intraperitoneal hemorrhage occur less often. Paraneoplastic phenomena (Table 14–5) are described with varying frequency. Metastatic disease is identified at the time of initial diagnosis in about one quarter of cases.

The recognition of hepatoma in a patient with underlying hepatic cirrhosis may be difficult. The sudden development or worsening of jaundice, ascites, cachexia, fever, abdominal pain, or rapidly increasing hepatic size in a patient with cirrhosis suggests the possibility of hepatoma. The clinical course in patients with hepatoma consists of rapidly progressive deterioration. Liver function declines; portal hypertension often progresses with variceal bleeding and worsening ascites, and metastatic involvement proceeds. Tumor may extend into the hepatic veins and inferior vena cava; pulmonary emboli often result. Death follows diagnosis by only a few weeks or months.

Carcinoma of the gallbladder typically develops after years of symptomatic cholelithiasis. Symptoms of gallbladder cancer include right upper quadrant pain, anorexia, nausea, and jaundice. Unfortunately, these signs and symptoms mimic those of benign gallbladder disease, explaining why a preoperative diagnosis of gallbladder cancer is made in less than 10% of cases.

Most carcinomas of the bile ducts arise between the bifurcation of the common duct and the ampulla of Vater; consequently, jaundice, usually painless, is the most common finding. Tumors arising in the cystic duct may mimic acute cholecystitis, whereas those arising in one of the hepatic ducts may cause only pain, fever, and weight loss without jaundice. This last presentation is unusual, however.

Carcinomas of the ampulla of Vater deserve special mention, since their prognosis is far better than that of the other biliary tract cancers, probably due to early symptoms. These tumors present a similar clinical picture to those of common duct cancers and carcinomas of the head of the pancreas; i.e., obstructive jaundice, pain, weight loss, and nausea.

DIAGNOSIS

Various imaging techniques, including ultrasound, CT, and magnetic resonance imaging (MRI), demonstrate the presence of hepatic tumors, but biopsy is required for diagnosis.

Table 14–5. **PARANEOPLASTIC SYNDROMES ASSOCIATED WITH HEPATOMAS**

Hypercalcemia	Vitamin B_{12}–binding protein
Hypoglycemia	Variant alkaline phosphatase
Erythrocytosis	Alpha-fetoprotein
Hyperlipidemia	Feminization
Dysfibrinogenemia	Porphyria cutanea tarda
Abnormal prothrombin	

Despite the vascular nature of these tumors, ultrasound- or CT-guided percutaneous liver biopsy carries negligible risk and provides diagnostic material in over 85% of cases. Levels of alpha-fetoprotein are elevated in most patients with hepatoma; however, elevated levels also occur in patients with germ cell malignancies, other gastrointestinal cancers, and rarely with nonmalignant liver disease.

Most cases of gallbladder and biliary carcinomas are diagnosed at surgery. If a tumor of the bile ducts is suspected preoperatively, percutaneous transhepatic cholangiography usually demonstrates the lesion. Endoscopic retrograde cholangiopancreatography (ERCP) may be helpful in selected cases (Fig. 14–3).

TREATMENT

Surgery

With each of these tumor types, surgical resection offers the only hope of cure. Although most patients with hepatocellular carcinoma have diffuse or multicentric lesions, solitary tumors occur occasionally and may be amenable to curative resection. Preoperative angiography is usually recommended to determine whether the lesion is truly solitary. Only 7 to 30% of patients have resectable hepatomas, and the 5-year survival even in these selected patients is a disappointing 10%.

Curative surgery is rarely possible in patients with gallbladder carcinoma unless the tumor is discovered incidentally at surgery in a patient thought to have uncomplicated benign gallbladder disease. In most cases, the tumor has spread to lymph nodes and adjacent liver tissue by the time of diagnosis. Less than 5% of patients survive 5 years, and less than 15% survive 1 year following diagnosis.

Curative resections of bile duct cancers are rarely successful, since tumor usually extends into the liver, vessels, pancreas, or duodenum. For localized tumors, pancreatico-duodenectomy is usually the procedure of choice and produces a 5-year survival rate of 20% in selected patients. Surgical drainage of the obstructed biliary system into a jejunal

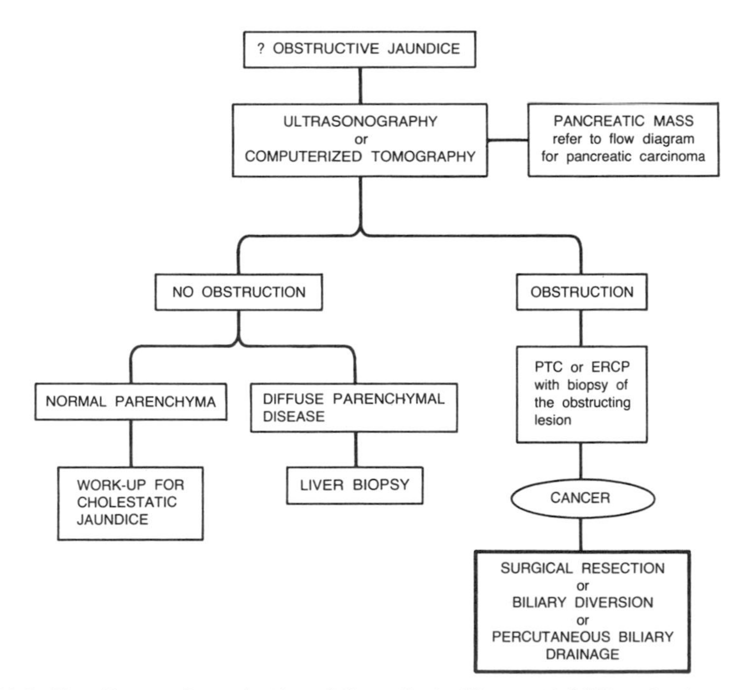

Figure 14–3. Flow diagram for evaluation of the patient with suspected biliary tract cancer. (*From* Borg SA, Rosenthal S: Handbook of Cancer Diagnosis and Staging. A Clinical Atlas. New York, John Wiley & Sons, 1984.)

loop (choledochojejunostomy) or percutaneous transhepatic biliary drainage under radiologic guidance provides useful palliation in the majority of unresectable cases.

Carcinomas of the ampulla of Vater usually are low grade and produce symptoms early while the tumor remains small and localized; they therefore have a far better prognosis with surgical resection than other biliary tract tumors. Pancreaticoduodenectomy is the surgical procedure of choice with cure rates of 30 to 35%.

Radiation Therapy

Conventional radiation therapy is ineffective in hepatocellular carcinoma. It provides neither palliation nor survival prolongation. The role of radiation therapy in the management of gallbladder and bile duct cancers is controversial; some authorities report significant palliation, whereas others find no benefit. Since some patients improve with radiation, although the effect on survival is negligible, palliative radiotherapy is an option for patients with unresectable gallbladder and bile duct cancers. Bile duct carcinomas may respond better to radiation than gallbladder carcinomas.

Experimental radiation therapy techniques show some promise in the treatment of these tumors. Trials employing radiolabeled antibody for hepatoma demonstrate responses. Interstitial radiation therapy using surgically or percutaneously implanted iridium wires produces relief of biliary obstruction in some cases of cholangiocarcinoma, with a possible effect on survival. These modalities are currently undergoing further investigation.

Chemotherapy

Chemotherapy has a very limited role in the treatment of hepatocellular carcinoma. Adriamycin, 5-fluorouracil, and the nitrosoureas are active agents. Response rates in small series vary but are generally under 20%. In 348 patients treated by the Eastern Cooperative Oncology Group with a variety of single-agent and combination regimens, the overall response rate was less than 10% and the median survival only 17 weeks. The best regimen achieved a 19% response rate but no improvement in median survival and was accompanied by an unacceptably high incidence (63%) of severe toxic side effects. At present, no chemotherapeutic program is standard treatment for advanced hepatoma; whenever possible patients with this disease should enter clinical trials.

Better results have been claimed for hepatic arterial infusion of cytotoxic agents in patients with hepatoma confined to the liver. However, these reports include only small numbers of highly selected patients without comparison to systemic chemotherapy in similar patient cohorts. Lack of uniform definition of response, variation in method of drug administration, and exclusion of patients with early deaths from the analysis make precise evaluation of this modality very difficult.

Experience with chemotherapy in advanced bile duct and gallbladder cancers is limited. The largest trial, reported by ECOG, randomized 53 patients with advanced gallbladder cancer and 34 with bile duct cancer to 5-fluorouracil alone, 5-fluorouracil plus streptozocin, and 5-fluorouracil plus methyl-CCNU. There was no significant difference among treatments for either tumor type with respect to response or survival. The overall response rate was less than 10%. The addition of streptozocin or methyl-CCNU to 5-fluorouracil resulted in additional toxicity without any improvement in outcome.

A recent study of 14 patients with bile duct carcinoma treated with the FAM combination (see section on Gastric Cancer) reported a 31% partial response. This encouraging trial requires confirmation.

REFERENCES

DiBisceglie AM, moderator. Hepatocellular carcinoma. Ann Intern Med 108:390–401, 1988.

Flickinger JC, Epstein AH, Iwatsuki S, et al: Radiation therapy for primary carcinoma of the extrahepatic biliary system. Cancer 68:289–294, 1991.

Ihde DC, Matthews MJ, Makuch RW, et al: Prognostic factors in patients with hepatocellular carcinoma receiving systemic chemotherapy. Am J Med 78:399–406, 1985.

Nagorney DM, McPherson GAD: Carcinoma of the gallbladder and extrahepatic bile ducts. Semin Oncol 15:106–115, 1988.

Norton RA, Foster EA: Bile duct cancer. CA 40:225–233, 1990.

Shieh CJ, Dunn E, Standard JE: Primary carcinoma of the gallbladder. Cancer 47:996–1004, 1981.
Wands JR, Blum HE: Primary hepatocellular carcinoma. N Engl J Med 325:729–731, 1991.

PANCREATIC CARCINOMA

INCIDENCE AND ETIOLOGY

Pancreatic carcinoma is now more common than gastric cancer in the United States; over the past 40 years the incidence of this disease has tripled from 3 per 100,000 to more than 10 per 100,000. Pancreatic cancer, comprising approximately 3% of all cancers and 5% of cancer deaths, is the second most frequent gastrointestinal malignancy and the fifth most frequent cause of cancer deaths in the United States. Most cases occur between the ages of 35 and 70, with peak incidence in the 55- to 74-year age group. The National Cancer Institute expects 28,300 new cases of pancreatic cancer and 25,000 deaths in 1992. Despite the rapidly increasing incidence, treatment remains unsuccessful, and the 5-year survival rate (0.4%) is among the lowest of all cancers. About 90% of patients with pancreatic cancer die within 1 year of diagnosis.

Although the etiology of pancreatic carcinoma is unknown, several risk factors have been identified in epidemiologic studies. Cigarette smoking is clearly associated with pancreatic carcinoma and may be responsible for almost half the cases among American males. Certain chemical carcinogens and particular occupations (chemists, petroleum industry workers, coke and metal workers, and gas plant employees) have been implicated. Alcoholism, diabetes, industrial pollution, and high fat diets also may play an etiologic role.

PATHOLOGY AND STAGING

Approximately 75% of pancreatic cancers are adenocarcinomas arising from duct epithelium. Other histologies are uncommon and include giant cell, adenosquamous, mucinous, and anaplastic carcinomas. Sixty-one percent of pancreatic cancers arise in the head of the pancreas; 20% in the body and tail. The remainder involve the pancreas diffusely. At the time of diagnosis 14% of tumors are limited to the pancreas (stages I and II), 21% have lymph node involvement (stage III), and 65% have distant spread (stage IV).

CLINICAL MANIFESTATIONS

Abdominal pain, weight loss, and obstructive jaundice are the most common presenting symptoms of pancreatic carcinoma and develop eventually in almost all patients. Tumors of the pancreatic head cause obstruction of the common bile duct in 75 to 90% of patients, and the resulting jaundice is unrelentingly progressive. Painless jaundice, long thought characteristic of carcinoma of the head of the pancreas, is in fact uncommon; in most patients, pain precedes the first evidence of jaundice. (Painless jaundice is more suggestive of carcinoma of the ampulla of Vater or biliary tract.) Pain usually centers in the epigastrium and frequently radiates to the back. Weight loss is often dramatic and may exceed 10% of ideal body weight. Anorexia, malabsorption, and diabetes mellitus all contribute to the weight loss. Acute pancreatitis is an unusual presenting manifestation of pancreatic cancer, but pancreatitis without apparent cause should suggest the possibility of this diagnosis.

Carcinomas involving the body and tail of the pancreas generally produce severe pain with radiation to the back. By the time of diagnosis, these tumors are often bulky and locally invasive. Jaundice is uncommon unless extensive liver metastases have occurred. Gastrointestinal bleeding may result from tumor erosion into colon or small bowel or from esophageal varices due to portal hypertension. Nausea, vomiting, weight loss, and anorexia also occur in most patients. Tables 14–6 and 14–7 describe presenting signs and symptoms of pancreatic cancer.

DIAGNOSIS

When carcinoma of the pancreas is suspected on clinical grounds, abdominal CT and ultrasonography are the most useful imaging techniques. Endoscopic retrograde cholan-

Table 14–6. **PRESENTING SYMPTOMS IN 100 CASES OF PANCREATIC CANCER**

SYMPTOM	NUMBER OF PATIENTS
Weight loss	75
Abdominal pain	72
Anorexia	47
Vomiting	33
Acholic stools	34
Constipation	34
Dark urine	32
Jaundice	24
Nausea	22
Diarrhea	12

From Gudjonsson B, Livistone EM, Spiro HM: Cancer of the pancreas. Diagnostic accuracy and survival statistics. Cancer 42:2494–2506, 1978.

giopancreatography (ERCP) and percutaneous transhepatic cholangiography (PTC) provide useful information in selected cases (Fig. 14–4). Tissue confirmation of a characteristic radiologic or ultrasound picture is mandatory. If CT or ultrasound clearly demonstrates a pancreatic mass, percutaneous fine needle aspiration biopsy is safe and reliable and may obviate exploratory surgery. Other cases require exploratory laparotomy to obtain a tissue diagnosis.

In the past, surgeons were reluctant to biopsy pancreatic masses for fear of complications including hemorrhage, acute pancreatitis, and pancreatic fistula formation. However, since 85% of cases have lymph node and/or liver involvement at diagnosis, biopsy of the pancreas itself is usually unnecessary. In those cases without local or regional spread, a large pancreatic mass more than 3 cm in diameter can be safely biopsied directly. A smaller pancreatic tumor can be sampled with a fine needle, just as would be done percutaneously, or with a larger needle via the transduodenal route. Pancreatic resection should never be performed without tissue confirmation of the diagnosis, and exploratory laparotomy for suspected pancreatic cancer should rarely fail to provide a tissue diagnosis.

Because of the dismal prognosis of advanced disease, investigators have attempted to identify serum markers for pancreatic cancer allowing early diagnosis. A number of enzymes, isoenzymes, hormones, and fetal antigens have been evaluated, but as yet none has proved clinically useful. Unless the disease can be prevented, earlier diagnosis remains the best hope for improving the outlook for patients with pancreatic cancer.

TREATMENT

The treatment of pancreatic carcinoma is far from satisfactory, as reflected in the appalling 5-year survival rate. In an aggregate of 37,000 patients drawn from 144 clinical studies reviewed by Gudjonsson, the overall 5-year survival rate was 0.4% (Fig. 14–5). No improvement in survival was seen in the more recent reports.

Surgery

Potentially curative resections are possible in only about 10% of patients with carcinoma of the head of the pancreas, and the morbidity and mortality (16% in series published

Table 14–7. **PHYSICAL FINDINGS IN 100 CASES OF PANCREATIC CANCER**

FINDING	NUMBER OF PATIENTS
Hepatomegaly	54
Jaundice	39
Blood in stool	27
Abdominal mass	16
Ascites	12

From Gudjonsson B, Livistone EM, Spiro HM: Cancer of the pancreas. Diagnostic accuracy and survival statistics. Cancer 42:2494–2506, 1978.

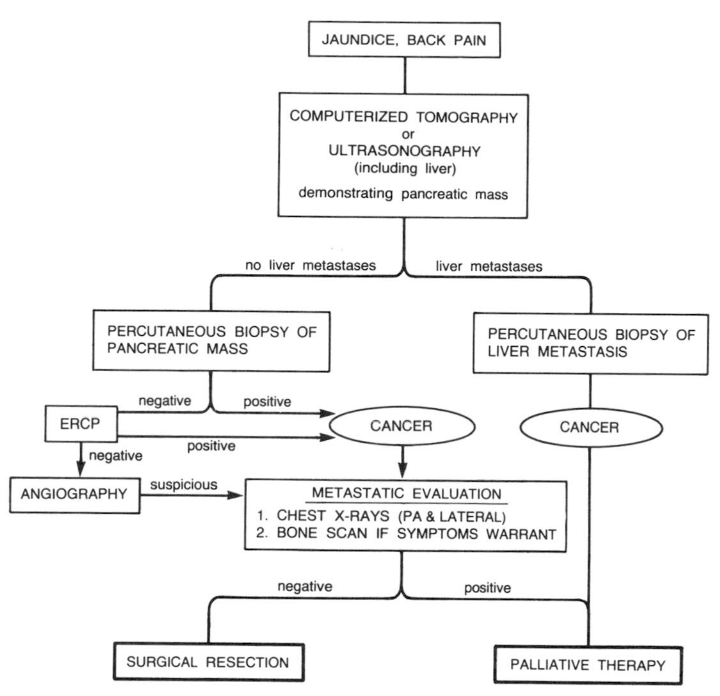

Figure 14–4. Flow diagram for evaluation of the patient with suspected pancreatic carcinoma. (*From* Borg SA, Rosenthal S: Handbook of Cancer Diagnosis and Staging. A Clinical Atlas. New York, John Wiley & Sons, 1984.)

since 1980) of the most commonly performed operation, pancreaticoduodenectomy (Whipple procedure), are substantial. Some surgeons favor a total pancreatectomy to ensure adequate margins and address the problem of tumor multifocality, but the advantages of this procedure have not been demonstrated. Moreover, total pancreatectomy guarantees both

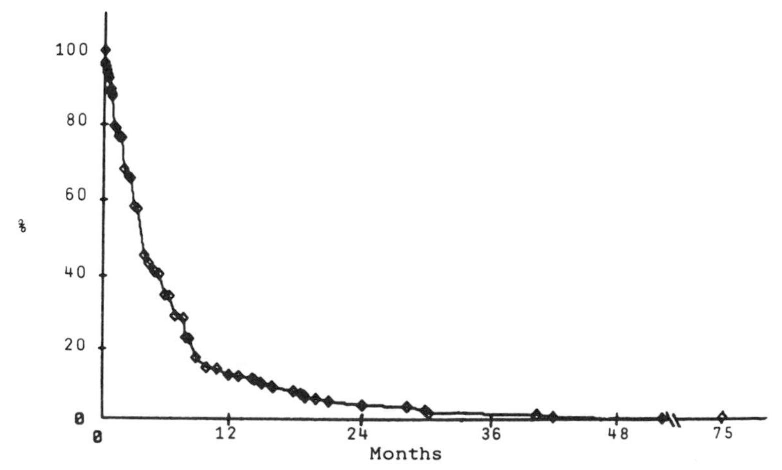

Figure 14–5. Survival of patients with pancreatic carcinoma. (*From* Gudjonsson B: Cancer of the pancreas: 50 years of surgery. Cancer 60:2284–2303, 1987.)

diabetes mellitus and pancreatic exocrine insufficiency. Other surgeons believe that the complications of pancreatic resection outweigh the benefits and prefer to perform only palliative bypass procedures. Resection with curative intent requires surgical expertise in this area, and only carefully selected patients with small (2 to 3 cm) tumors and good general health are candidates for the procedure.

Carcinomas of the body and tail of the pancreas are rarely, if ever, recognized early enough to permit surgical treatment with curative intent. These patients are usually diagnosed and treated with nonsurgical methods.

Although surgical cure is rarely possible, many patients benefit from surgical palliation of jaundice by means of biliary diversion. Even in the absence of jaundice, a choledochojejunostomy should be performed, since the majority of patients with carcinoma of the head of the pancreas will develop jaundice at some point in the course of their disease. In some instances, gastroenterostomy is necessary as well to relieve or prevent duodenal obstruction from local spread of tumor.

Percutaneous internal drainage of malignant obstructive jaundice is safe and effective in many cases. This procedure involves introducing a catheter into the obstructed biliary system and passing it through the obstructed area under radiologic guidance. Side holes in the catheter above and below the point of obstruction allow passage of bile into the duodenum. With this method jaundice can be relieved without surgery.

Radiation Therapy

External beam radiotherapy offers no significant palliation or improvement in survival for patients with locally unresectable pancreatic carcinoma. External radiation plus 5-fluorouracil, however, improves both symptomatic response and survival when compared with radiation alone in patients with unresectable disease. In a study reported by the Gastrointestinal Tumor Study Group, the median survival for patients treated with 5-fluorouracil–containing programs was almost twice as great (10 months versus 5.5 months) as that of patients receiving radiotherapy alone. At 1 year, 40% of the group treated with the combined modality programs were alive compared to 10% of patients treated with radiotherapy alone. These differences were statistically significant. Nevertheless, only 10% of patients treated with the combined modality programs were alive at 2 years.

Interestingly, patients who received the combined modality treatment had no fewer distant recurrences than patients who received only local therapy. This observation suggests that the 5-fluorouracil enhanced the local effect of the radiation therapy, serving as a radiation sensitizer rather than as a systemic agent.

Although the combination of 5-fluorouracil plus radiation is superior to radiation alone in the management of patients with locally unresectable (nonmetastatic) disease, it is not clear whether the combination is superior to chemotherapy alone. The ECOG reported the results of a randomized comparison of 5-fluorouracil alone with 5-fluorouracil plus radiation. Surprisingly, 5-fluorouracil alone was equivalent to the combined modality program in terms of time to disease progression and median survival (8.2 versus 8.3 months). Toxicity was substantially greater in the group receiving the combined modality program. However, a subsequent study comparing SMF (streptozocin, mitomycin, 5-fluorouracil) alone with SMF plus radiation demonstrated a significantly superior 1-year survival (41% versus 19%) for the combined modality approach.

Experimental radiation techniques, including implantation of radioisotopes in the pancreas, intraoperative radiation, hyperthermia, radiation sensitizers, and particle beam

Table 14–8. **SINGLE-AGENT ACTIVITY IN PANCREATIC CANCER**

AGENT	RESPONSE RATE (%)
5-Fluorouracil	17
Mitomycin C	23
Streptozocin	17
CCNU	16
Adriamycin	8
Methotrexate	4
Actinomycin D	4
Melphalan	2

Table 14–9. **COMBINATION CHEMOTHERAPY IN PANCREATIC CARCINOMA**

COMBINATION	RESPONSE RATE (%)
5-FU plus BCNU	26
5-FU, streptozocin, plus mitomycin C (SMF)	28
5-FU, Adriamycin, plus mitomycin C (FAM)	28

irradiation, provide hope for future improvements in the radiotherapeutic management of this tumor.

Chemotherapy

At present, no chemotherapeutic agent or combination offers the hope of long-term remission or cure for patients with pancreatic cancer. This assessment is especially disturbing since 85 to 90% of pancreatic cancers extend beyond the pancreas at the time of diagnosis and could potentially benefit from effective systemic therapy.

The single-agent experience with this tumor is adequate for only a handful of drugs (Table 14–8). 5-Fluorouracil, mitomycin C, and streptozocin are the most effective, with roughly a 20% response rate for each agent. Responses to single-agent therapy are partial and very brief, and have no impact on survival. Reported experience with combination chemotherapy is only slightly more encouraging. Several combinations appear to have higher objective response rates than any of the single agents (Table 14–9) and responses are occasionally durable (more than 6 months). Toxicity has generally not been severe.

However, the value of combination chemotherapy in advanced pancreatic carcinoma is not clear. High response rates in small numbers of patients are of interest but may result from patient selection factors rather than therapeutic benefit. The North Central Cancer Treatment Group and the Mayo Clinic conducted a prospective randomized comparison of 5-fluorouracil alone, 5-fluorouracil plus Adriamycin, and FAM in patients with advanced pancreatic carcinoma. Neither of the combinations achieved superiority in response rate, palliative effects, or survival compared to 5-fluorouracil alone. Toxicity and cost were substantially greater with the combinations. In view of the lack of therapeutic advantage, as measured by either survival prolongation or palliation of symptoms, and the increased cost in both dollars and side effects, combination chemotherapy with either of these regimens cannot be recommended. Whenever possible, patients with advanced pancreatic cancer should enter clinical trials attempting to identify new agents and combinations with activity in this disease.

Patients with poor performance status or extensive liver metastases rarely respond to chemotherapy of any sort and benefit most from comfort measures and supportive care.

REFERENCES

Beazley RM: Update on pancreatic cancer. CA 38:310–317, 1988.

Cullinan SA, Moertel CG, Fleming TR, et al: A comparison of three chemotherapeutic regimens in the treatment of advanced pancreatic and gastric carcinoma. JAMA 253:2061–2067, 1985.

Gudjonsson B: Cancer of the pancreas: 50 years of surgery. Cancer 60:2284–2303, 1987.

Haller DG: Chemotherapy in gastrointestinal malignancies. Semin Oncol 15:50–64, 1988.

Harter KW, Dritschilo A: Cancer of the pancreas: Are chemotherapy and radiation appropriate? Oncology 3:27–37, 1989.

Kalser MH, Barkin J, MacIntyre JM: Pancreatic cancer: Assessment of prognosis by clinical presentation. Cancer 56:397–402, 1985.

O'Connell MJ: Current status of chemotherapy for advanced pancreatic and gastric cancer. Semin Oncol 3:1032–1039, 1985.

Warshaw AL, Swanson RS: Pancreatic cancer in 1988. Ann Surg 208:541–553,1988.

15
GENITOURINARY MALIGNANCIES

Martin Brower

RENAL CELL CARCINOMA

INCIDENCE AND ETIOLOGY

The National Cancer Institute expects 26,500 new cases of renal cell carcinoma in the United States in 1992, with 10,700 deaths during the same period. Renal cell carcinoma accounts for about 2% of all malignancies diagnosed in this country. Males are affected approximately twice as often as females, and the disease is uncommon before age 40. The incidence has been increasing steadily in the United States for unknown reasons. Worldwide, the highest incidence is found in northern Europe and North America, and the lowest incidence is in Africa, Asia, and South America.

The etiology of renal cell carcinoma is unknown. In hamsters, the disease can be induced by estrogens. In these animals, diethylstilbestrol produces an elevated progesterone receptor level in the kidney; this is the earliest consistent premalignant change. However, similar elevated hormone receptor levels have not been demonstrated in human renal cell carcinoma. Tobacco use (cigarette, cigar, and pipe smoking and chewing tobacco) is the only environmental factor consistently associated with increased incidence. Genetic factors rarely play a role except in the case of von Hippel-Lindau syndrome (cerebelloretinal hemangioblastomatosis), an autosomal dominant disorder that has up to a 25% incidence of renal cell carcinoma.

PATHOLOGY

The majority of renal cancers are adenocarcinomas. The terms *renal cell carcinoma, clear cell carcinoma,* and *hypernephroma* are all used interchangeably in the literature to refer to renal adenocarcinoma. These tumors may occur at any location within the kidney; there is no predilection for any intrarenal site. Renal cell carcinomas are bilateral in 2 to 5% of cases.

Renal cell carcinomas may be composed of clear, granular, spindle-shaped, or sarcomatoid cells or a mixture of these patterns. Compared to other carcinomas, renal cell carcinomas tend to be well differentiated with little nuclear pleomorphism and relatively few mitoses. The tumor may be solid, cystic, papillary, or tubular, but none of these forms has been clearly shown to correlate with prognosis.

Transitional cell carcinoma of the renal pelvis is the second most common renal malignancy. Primary renal sarcomas and lymphomas are rare, as is Wilms' tumor in the adult.

CLINICAL MANIFESTATIONS

The most common presenting feature of renal cell carcinoma is hematuria, present in 50% of patients at the time of diagnosis. Flank pain and abdominal mass are two other common presenting complaints. The classic triad of hematuria, flank pain, and palpable mass occurs in only about 10 to 15% of patients. In 10 to 25% of patients, the presenting symptoms represent metastatic disease involving liver, lung, bone, or brain. In some patients, the disease is asymptomatic and detected during routine physical examination or through the evaluation of microscopic hematuria.

Renal cell carcinoma has long been known as the internist's tumor because of its association with many paraneoplastic syndromes. Fever, weight loss, anemia, erythrocytosis, hypercalcemia, hepatic dysfunction unrelated to metastases, amyloidosis, and neuromyopathy may all be manifestations of an occult renal malignancy.

DIAGNOSIS AND STAGING

Excretory urography (IVP), performed to evaluate hematuria or other suggestive symptoms, usually demonstrates a renal mass, enlargement of the kidney, or distortion of the renal outline and caliceal pattern. Since the vast majority of renal masses are benign cysts, however, further evaluation with either computed tomography (CT) or ultrasonography is necessary.

Radiologic diagnosis of renal cell carcinoma on the basis of characteristic CT findings is highly accurate, but tissue confirmation is almost invariably recommended. This is usually obtained at surgery, but if the patient has metastatic disease or is otherwise not a surgical candidate, fine needle aspiration biopsy under CT guidance is a simple, safe, and reliable method to obtain tissue.

The Robson (Table 15–1) staging system for renal cell carcinoma is in general use. Preoperative staging requires an abdominal CT scan to assess local tumor extent, liver metastases, and renal vein and inferior vena caval involvement. Magnetic resonance imaging (MRI) may also be useful, particularly for assessing renal vein and inferior vena caval invasion. Chest x-ray is performed routinely, but additional studies to detect metastatic disease (i.e., bone scan, head CT) should not be obtained unless clinical indications suggest abnormalities. Renal angiography and inferior vena cavography are sometimes required by the urologist to assist in planning surgery.

NATURAL HISTORY

Survival in renal cell carcinoma correlates with stage. About one-third of patients present with tumor confined to the kidney; with radical nephrectomy this group can expect a 65 to 70% 5-year survival. About one-third have more advanced nonmetastatic disease. Those with involvement of perirenal fat and/or invasion of the renal vein or inferior vena cava have a 5-year survival rate of about 45 to 65%. Those with lymph node involvement have a considerably worse prognosis, particularly if there is macroscopic lymph node involvement at surgery; 5-year survival is 20% or less in most series.

Approximately 25 to 33% of patients have metastatic disease at the time of presentation. Patients with metastatic disease have a median survival of 6 months, but some have a remarkably indolent course, and as many as 10% may be alive 5 years after the detection of metastases. The most common metastatic sites are lymph nodes, lung, bone, adrenal, liver, opposite kidney, and brain. Renal cell carcinoma has a predilection for unusual metastatic sites; it may spread to the paranasal sinuses, eye and orbit, vagina, larynx, and various other unusual locations.

Late recurrences, more than 10 years after surgical resection, occur in about 10% of patients with renal carcinoma—much more commonly than with other carcinomas. Such late recurrences imply either an extremely long tumor doubling time or the presence of host defense mechanisms that are able to control the disease for long periods.

The literature contains about a hundred well-documented case reports of regression of renal cell carcinoma without treatment and additional reports of regression of metastatic lesions after resection of the primary cancer. The mechanism is not understood. Although these spontaneous regressions are intriguing, in the vast majority of cases once metastases have occurred, relentless progression of disease in spite of active therapeutic intervention is the rule.

TREATMENT

Surgery

Surgical excision of localized renal cell carcinoma is the only form of curative therapy. Most urologists believe that radical nephrectomy (including excision of the involved

Table 15–1. **THE ROBSON STAGING CLASSIFICATION OF RENAL CELL CARCINOMA**

STAGE	DESCRIPTION
I	Tumor confined to the kidney
II	Extension into perinephric fat
III	Involvement of renal vein, inferior vena cava, or regional nodes
IV	Involvement of adjacent organs or distant metastases

kidney, adrenal, surrounding fat, Gerota's fascia, and regional lymph nodes) achieves better results than simple nephrectomy. Operative mortality ranges from 2 to 6% for this procedure. Recently, experience with partial nephrectomy and tumor enucleation has accumulated in patients with renal cell carcinoma in a solitary kidney. Survival of these patients appears equivalent to that of patients undergoing radical nephrectomy.

Nephrectomy may be justified in the presence of metastatic disease in order to control disabling symptoms of pain and hematuria. Nephrectomy in a patient with an asymptomatic primary tumor and multiple metastases or poor performance status in the hope of causing regression of distant metastases is unacceptable; the operative mortality far exceeds the likelihood of regression. However, occasional long-term survival is achieved after nephrectomy and excision of *solitary* metastases in patients with good performance status, minimal weight loss, and low-grade tumors. Solitary recurrences many years following nephrectomy should also be excised; such aggressive surgical therapy may prolong survival.

In patients with multiple metastases and uncontrollable pain or bleeding from a primary tumor, renal artery occlusion by means of transcatheter arterial embolization of various materials (e.g., autologous clot, plastic spheres, gelatin sponge) may achieve palliation with less morbidity than nephrectomy, especially in patients who are poor surgical risks.

Radiation Therapy

Neither preoperative nor postoperative radiotherapy appears to enhance the survival rate of patients with resectable renal cell carcinoma. Nevertheless, radiotherapy has an important role in the palliation of this disease. Painful bone metastases, brain metastases, and recurrences in the renal bed can be radiated with relief of symptoms, although the doses required may be high.

Hormonal Treatment

Renal cancers in several rodent species are clearly hormone dependent and often regress with various forms of hormonal therapy. During the 1960s and early 1970s several investigators reported response rates of 7 to 33% in patients with metastatic renal cell carcinoma treated with progestins or androgens. More recent studies using modern criteria for defining objective response report response rates of 5% or less for progestins in this disease. Combinations of hormonal agents or of hormones with chemotherapy also have shown no benefit.

Chemotherapy

Experience with chemotherapy in renal cell carcinoma has been uniformly discouraging. All agents tested achieved less than a 10% response rate, with the exception of vinblastine and infusions of fluorodeoxyuridine. Those responses that have occurred have been brief and incomplete. Without effective single agents, combination chemotherapy is unlikely to succeed, a fact confirmed by a large number of trials. Transitional cell carcinoma of the renal pelvis, however, appears to be sensitive to the same chemotherapeutic regimens used in bladder carcinoma (see below).

Immunotherapy

Certain features of the natural history renal cell carcinoma—spontaneous regressions, delayed recurrences—have long suggested that host immune mechanisms influence the course of the disease and that immunotherapy could play a role in treatment. Occasional responses have been reported with immune ribonucleic acid (RNA), autologous tumor cell vaccines, transfer factor, thymosin, and bacille Calmette-Guérin (BCG). In one study, transcatheter renal arterial occlusion, producing infarction of the tumor and postulated release of tumor antigens, followed by nephrectomy and then by progesterone therapy produced a 24% response rate, perhaps by stimulating an immune response in the host.

Interleukin-2 (IL-2)–based therapies cause tumor regressions in a substantial minority of patients with renal cell carcinoma. At the National Cancer Institute (NCI) over 200 patients with metastatic renal cell carcinoma have been treated with IL-2–based regimens. Thirty percent of these patients responded to treatment; 10% had complete remissions; and some complete remissions have lasted over 3 years. Unfortunately, at tertiary referral centers outside the NCI overall response rates have been substantially lower, with about 15% of patients having partial responses. Because IL-2–based therapies can be extraordinarily toxic, commonly requiring intensive care unit hospitalization for hypotension, massive fluid retention, and respiratory insufficiency, such treatment is an option only for very fit patients. Ongoing research is attempting to improve the efficacy of IL-2–based therapy in renal cell carcinoma and to decrease the toxicity.

High doses of alpha interferon also have antitumor efficacy in renal cell carcinoma. As with IL-2 therapy, response rates vary with patient selection. Patients with small volumes of pulmonary metastases may have response rates as high as 30%. Interferon also has multiple toxicities. A national randomized trial is testing the use of alpha interferon as a surgical adjuvant after resection of high-risk localized renal cell carcinomas.

In summary, there is no standard therapy for patients with metastatic renal cell carcinoma. Entry of appropriate patients on research protocols must be encouraged.

REFERENCES

Fisher RI, Coltman CA, Doroshow JH, et al: Metastatic renal cell cancer treated with interleukin-2 and lymphocyte activated killer cells: A phase II clinical trial. Ann Intern Med 108:518–523, 1988.

Harris DT, Maguire HC (eds): Renal cell carcinoma. Semin Oncol 10:365–436, 1983.

Neves RJ, Zincke H, Taylor WF: Metastatic renal cell cancer and radical nephrectomy: Identification of prognostic factors and patient survival. J Urol 139:1173–1176, 1988.

Pritchett TR, Lieskovsky G, Skinner DG: Clinical manifestations and treatment of renal parenchymal tumors. *In* Skinner DG, Lieskovsky G (eds): Diagnosis and Management of Genitourinary Cancer. Philadelphia, WB Saunders, 1988, pp 337–361.

Quesada JR: Biologic response modifiers in the therapy of metastatic renal cell carcinoma. Semin Oncol 15:396–407, 1988.

Rosenberg SA, Lotze MT, Yang JC, et al: Experience with the use of high-dose interleukin-2 in the treatment of 652 cancer patients. Ann Surg 210:474–485, 1989.

BLADDER CANCER

INCIDENCE AND ETIOLOGY

The National Cancer Institute expects 51,600 new cases of bladder cancer in the United States in 1992, with 9500 deaths due to this disease. The male:female ratio for bladder cancer is 2.8 to 1 with the majority of patients in the 50 to 70 age range. Smokers have two to three times the incidence of bladder cancer as nonsmokers. Other risk factors include industrial exposure to chemicals such as benzidine and naphthylamine (used in rubber manufacturing) and aniline dyes (used in paint and in the textile industry). Data conflict on the possible role of coffee and artificial sweeteners in the etiology of bladder cancer. Heavy users of phenacetin-containing analgesics are at increased risk, and infection with *Schistosoma haematobium* leads to an increased risk of bladder cancer in endemic areas (especially Egypt).

PATHOLOGY

Ninety percent of bladder cancers are transitional cell carcinomas; 8% are squamous cell and 2% are adenocarcinomas. The overwhelming majority of tumors are superficial, and most arise near the ureteral orifices. Multicentric tumors occur frequently. Tumor grade, growth pattern, depth of invasion, and multifocality all influence prognosis and treatment selection.

Histologic grade has an important bearing on prognosis. The grade depends on the number of mitoses present and on the degree of nuclear and cytoplasmic atypia. Grade I tumors are well differentiated, grade II moderately differentiated, grade III poorly differentiated, and grade IV anaplastic.

CLINICAL MANIFESTATIONS

Most patients present with symptoms similar to those of urinary tract infection: dysuria, frequency, urgency, and hematuria. For this reason, diagnosis is often delayed, sometimes by as much as 1 to 3 years. Less common symptoms indicating advanced disease include urethral or ureteral obstruction, edema of the lower extremities, pelvic pain, bowel obstruction, and symptoms due to bone or lung metastases.

DIAGNOSIS AND STAGING

When bladder cancer is suspected, cystoscopy with multiple endoscopic biopsies usually yields a tissue diagnosis. The biopsies must be sufficiently deep to allow assessment of muscle invasion. Any visualized lesion should be resected or fulgurated. Random biopsies in multiple other areas also should be obtained because of the propensity of bladder cancer to produce widespread occult disease. Bimanual examination under anesthesia helps to define the local extent of disease and detect the presence of fixation. Excretory urography may demonstrate intraluminal filling defects. The Jewett-Strong-Marshall (Table 15–2, Fig. 15–1) staging system is commonly used. Stage 0 and stage A cancers are considered superficial, whereas stage B and C cancers are considered invasive.

If invasive cancer is diagnosed, pelvic CT scanning is indicated to detect perivesical fat infiltration, extension to the pelvic wall, and lymph node and seminal vesicle involvement. Patients with invasive bladder cancer should have a chest x-ray and blood chemistries. Bone scan and liver imaging are obtained if clinically indicated by abnormalities in the history, physical examination, or laboratory testing.

MANAGEMENT OF SUPERFICIAL BLADDER CANCER

Bladder cancer represents a wide spectrum of biologic-pathologic entities with a corresponding variety of clinical behaviors. The majority (75 to 85%) present as superficial tumors; most can be treated successfully with transurethral resection and/or fulguration. Many will develop additional superficial recurrences requiring either further transurethral resections, intravesical chemotherapy, or both.

Perhaps 25% of patients who present with superficial bladder tumors eventually develop invasive disease; the challenge for the urologist is to determine, in advance, which patients are in this group. Features of superficial bladder cancers indicating a high risk of subsequent invasion are high grade, high stage, tumor multicentricity in space or time, the presence of in situ carcinoma in close proximity to a superficial bladder cancer, and in situ disease with diffuse involvement and/or severe symptoms of bladder irritability. Biopsy or cytologic evidence of disease persisting 6 to 12 months after intravesical chemotherapy also suggests high risk. Aneuploid tumors identified by flow cytometry have a worse prognosis than diploid tumors. Whether patients with these poor prognostic

Table 15–2. **JEWETT-STRONG-MARSHALL AND ABBREVIATED TNM STAGING FOR BLADDER CANCER**

JEWETT-STRONG-MARSHALL STAGE	TNM EQUIVALENT STAGE	DEFINITION
0	T1s	Confined to mucosa (carcinoma in situ)
0	T1a	Confined to mucosa (papillary)
A	T1	Confined to submucosa (no invasion beyond lamina propria)
B1	T2	Superficial muscle involvement (up to 50% full thickness)
B2	T3a	Deep muscle involvement
C	T3b	Invasion of perivesical fat
D1	T4a	Involvement of adjacent organs such as prostate, uterus, or vagina
D1	T4b	Tumor fixed to pelvic or abdominal wall
D1	N1–3	Regional lymph node involvement
D2	M1	Distant metastases

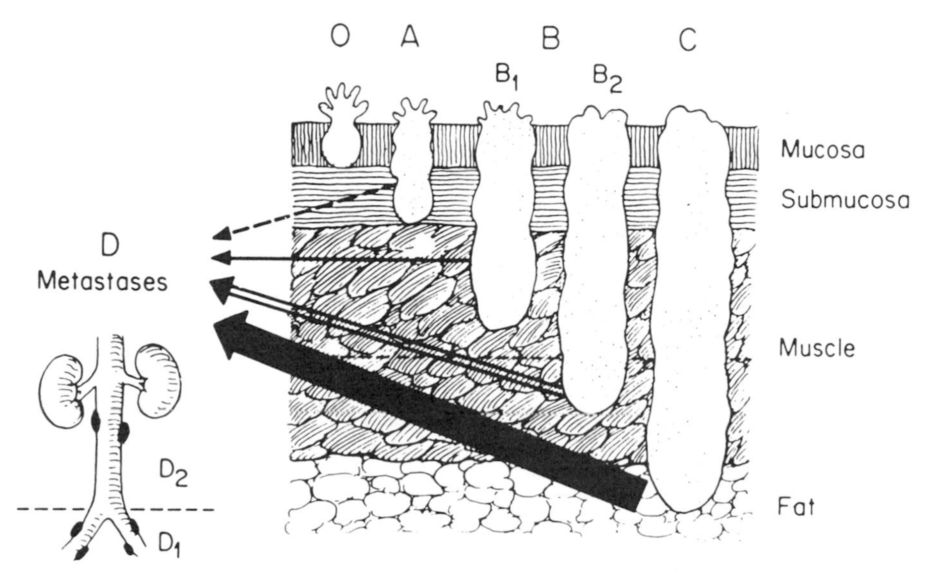

Figure 15–1. Jewett-Strong-Marshall staging classification for bladder cancer. (*From* Skinner DG: Current state of classification and staging of bladder cancer. Cancer Res 37:2840, 1977. © 1977, The Williams & Wilkins Company, Baltimore.)

variables should be offered immediate radical cystectomy, prior to development of invasive disease, depends on individual factors and the philosophy of the urologist.

Superficial transitional cell carcinomas (stages 0 and A) are treated by transurethral resection (TUR) and/or fulguration. Forty to 85% recur within 1 year. Recurrence rate is proportional to tumor grade, stage, size, and number of lesions.

Topical (intravesical) chemotherapy is used to decrease the likelihood of further recurrence and to treat multifocal disease and carcinoma in situ. Thiotepa, Adriamycin (doxorubicin), mitomycin C, and BCG are most frequently used. The three chemotherapeutic drugs are approximately equally effective in preventing recurrence of papillary tumors, but BCG is superior in treating carcinoma in situ. Thiotepa is by far the least expensive of the chemotherapy drugs, but systemic absorption of thiotepa can lead to myelosuppression. Adriamycin can cause substantial bladder irritation. BCG can cause bladder irritation, fever, chills, and rarely disseminated mycobacterial disease.

Several studies have demonstrated a significant reduction in the number of recurrences and/or a delay in time to recurrence with the use of intravesical chemotherapy compared to historical controls. Two large randomized controlled studies have confirmed the efficacy of intravesical chemotherapy in delaying and reducing recurrences. Most authorities agree that intravesical chemotherapy is indicated for both prophylactic and definitive treatment of superficial bladder cancers. Urine cytology and cystoscopy every 3 months provide adequate follow-up of treated superficial bladder cancer. Flow cytometric analysis of the urine may be more sensitive in detecting recurrences, but whether this improves the ultimate clinical outcome is unknown.

New therapies under evaluation for superficial bladder cancer include photodynamic therapy using hematoporphyrin derivative and intravesicular interferon.

MANAGEMENT OF INVASIVE BLADDER CANCER

Surgery

Standard treatment for invasive disease and superficial tumors at high risk of recurrence is radical cystectomy. Nevertheless, the majority of patients develop distant metastases within 2 years after surgery and ultimately succumb to the disease. Only 35 to 50% of patients undergoing cystectomy survive 5 years. Radical cystectomy in men includes prostatectomy, removal of seminal vesicles, and urethrectomy in cases of diffuse disease or urethral involvement. Impotence was formerly universal, although newer surgical techniques reduce the incidence of this complication. In women, the procedure includes removal of the ovaries, fallopian tubes, uterus, urethra, and vaginal cuff in addition to the bladder. Pelvic lymph node dissection offers prognostic information but does not appear to alter the survival rate. Pelvic lymph node involvement is present in 10 to 50% of patients at the time of cystectomy and serves as the harbinger of distant metastatic disease. The 5-year survival for patients with positive regional lymph nodes is less than 20%; the survivors are limited to patients without macroscopic lymph node involvement and with three or fewer involved nodes. Segmental resection or partial cystectomy alone as treatment for invasive bladder cancer is rarely indicated owing to the multifocal nature of the disease and the frequency of involvement in the region of the urethra and ureteral orifices—circumstances that require total cystectomy.

Radiotherapy

Preoperative radiotherapy prior to radical cystectomy was popular in the past on the basis of uncontrolled studies, but randomized data indicate no survival benefit, and in most centers this procedure has been abandoned.

Radiation therapy alone has long been used to treat invasive bladder cancer in patients unfit for radical surgery or who refuse cystectomy. Radical cystectomy and definitive radiation therapy have never been directly compared, but it is likely that surgical treatment provides a survival advantage over radiotherapy. Nonetheless, in very elderly patients or in those unlikely to be cured with surgery (i.e., those with nodal involvement), radiotherapy offers a much less toxic form of treatment than surgery or chemotherapy.

Experience in treating invasive bladder cancer with combined radiotherapy and chemotherapy is accumulating. If a complete response to this therapy is documented, the bladder is preserved. Patients with less than a complete response or who relapse in the bladder undergo salvage cystectomy. Bladder preservation is accomplished in over 50% of patients treated on such protocols, but whether long-term survival is equivalent to that following radical cystectomy is not yet known; such treatment must still be considered experimental in patients who are able to undergo cystectomy.

Chemotherapy

Because distant dissemination kills the majority of patients with invasive bladder cancer despite surgery or radiotherapy, researchers have advocated preoperative (neoadjuvant) or postoperative (adjuvant) chemotherapy for these patients. It is clear that preoperative chemotherapy can cause marked tumor regression in over 50% of patients, including occasional complete pathologic response. Preliminary results with adjuvant chemotherapy following radical cystectomy demonstrate that such treatent is feasible. Whether neoadjuvant or adjuvant chemotherapy will yield meaningful long-term survival benefits for patients with invasive bladder cancer is unknown. A major national study is testing neoadjuvant chemotherapy plus cystectomy versus cystectomy alone in invasive bladder cancer, and a large European trial is testing neoadjuvant chemotherapy plus either cystectomy or radiotherapy versus local treatment only. The only prospective randomized trial of postoperative adjuvant chemotherapy in invasive bladder cancer published to date (1991) demonstrated a prolongation in median survival from 2.3 to 4.2 years, but the long-term (5-year) survival advantage in the chemotherapy-treated group was minimal. Adjuvant chemotherapy in bladder cancer remains experimental and should be given only in the context of a controlled clinical trial. Participation in such studies should be encouraged, however, since results with surgery and/or radiotherapy are unlikely to improve.

TREATMENT OF METASTATIC DISEASE

Several cytotoxic agents are active in metastatic carcinoma of the bladder. Cisplatin is the most active agent; carboplatin, methotrexate, vinblastine, and Adriamycin are also active.

Two combination chemotherapy regimens have consistently demonstrated high response rates and occasional complete responses in metastatic bladder cancer: M-VAC (methotrex-

Table 15–3. **COMBINATION CHEMOTHERAPY FOR BLADDER CANCER**

REGIMEN	DRUGS	DOSE (IV)	SCHEDULE
M-VAC	Methotrexate	30 mg/m^2, days 1, 15, 22	Cycle repeats every 28 days
	Vinblastine	3 mg/m^2, days 2, 15, 22	
	Adriamycin	30 mg/m^2, day 2	
	Cisplatin	70 mg/m^2, day 2	
CMV	Cisplatin	100 mg/m^2, day 2	Cycle repeats every 21 days
	Methotrexate	30 mg/m^2, days 1, 8	
	Vinblastine	4 mg/m^2, days 1, 8	

ate, vinblastine, Adriamycin, and cisplatin) and CMV (cisplatin, methotrexate, and vinblastine [Velban]) (Table 15–3). In single institutions, response rates to these regimens approach 70%, with 20 to 30% complete responses. M-VAC has been directly compared to cisplatin as a single agent in a cooperative group trial. Response rate was only 35% but there was a clear survival advantage to the combination, with median survival increasing from 7 to 12 months. CMV or M-VAC can be considered standard therapy for patients with metastatic bladder cancer who are able to tolerate aggressive combination chemotherapy. Researchers are attempting to improve the effectiveness of these regimens by using colony-stimulating factors to permit dose escalations.

REFERENCES

Lum BL, Torti FM: Adjuvant intravesicular pharmacotherapy for superficial bladder cancer. J Natl Cancer Inst 83:682–694, 1991.

Raghavan D, Shipley WU, Garnick MB, et al: Biology and management of bladder cancer. N Engl J Med 322:1129–1138, 1990.

Scher HI, Splinter TAW: Neoadjuvant treatment of invasive bladder cancer. Semin Oncol 17:515–640, 1990.

Shipley WU, Prout GR, Kaufman DS: Bladder cancer: Advances in laboratory innovations and clinical management, with emphasis on innovations allowing bladder-sparing approaches for patients with invasive tumors. Cancer 65:675–683, 1990.

Skinner DG, Daniels JR, Russell CA, et al: The role of adjuvant chemotherapy following cystectomy for invasive bladder cancer: A prospective comparative trial. J Urol 145:459–467, 1991.

Sternberg CN, Yagoda A, Scher HI, et al: Methotrexate, vinblastine, doxorubicin, and cisplatin for advanced transitional carcinoma of the urothelium. Cancer 64:2448–2458, 1989.

CANCER OF THE PROSTATE

INCIDENCE

According to NCI statistics, cancer of the prostate is the most common malignancy in men, with 132,000 new cases expected in 1992. The incidence rises rapidly with advancing age. Eighty percent of clinical cases are in men over age 65, and microscopic prostatic carcinoma has been found at autopsy in 15 to 20% of men in the sixth decade and in as many as 60% in the ninth decade. Relatively few of these cases are clinically apparent before death, but even so, prostate cancer is the third leading cause of cancer deaths in men, with 34,000 deaths annually. The etiology is not clear, but prolonged stimulation of prostatic tissue by testosterone seems the most likely cause. Prostate cancer does not develop in men castrated at any early age. For unknown reasons, the disease is twice as common in American blacks than in whites, whereas Americans of Asian descent have half the incidence rate of white Americans.

PATHOLOGY

Most adenocarcinomas of the prostate arise either from the peripheral zone of the gland (70%) and present as nodules detectable on rectal examination or in the transitional zone (20%) removed during transurethral resection of the prostate (TUR). Serial sections of the prostate frequently demonstrate multifocal cancers. Histologic grade of the tumor correlates closely with prognosis. Pathologists commonly use Gleason's scoring system to grade prostate cancer. In this system, the average pattern of the tumor and the most undifferentiated pattern of the tumor are each given a rating from 1 to 5. Adding these two ratings yields a score from 2 to 10. Tumors with scores of 2 to 4 are low grade, 5 to 7 intermediate, and 8 to 10 high grade. Prognosis worsens markedly as tumor grade increases. Recently, it has also been shown that aneuploid prostate cancers have a much worse prognosis than diploid cancers of identical stage and histologic grade.

Immunohistochemistry for prostate-specific antigen can be invaluable in determining the nature of a metastatic lesion of apparently unknown primary origin.

Transitional cell carcinoma and small cell carcinoma are unusual variants of prostate cancer with poor prognosis.

SCREENING, DIAGNOSIS, AND STAGING

Few topics in oncology are more controversial than how best to screen healthy men for occult prostate cancer. The American Cancer Society currently recommends a digital rectal examination as part of the annual physical examination for men over age 50. It is clear that far more men will be diagnosed with prostate cancer if screening tests more sensitive than physical examination are used; i.e., serum prostate-specific antigen (PSA) levels and prostatic ultrasound. Unfortunately, these tests are not specific. Many men have elevated serum PSA levels or positive ultrasounds in the absence of carcinoma.

The major problem with aggressive screening for prostate cancer is that many older men have small foci of occult cancer, and the natural history of localized prostate cancer can be extremely indolent. If screening does not differentiate between aggressive carcinomas that are likely to kill the host within his lifetime and indolent carcinomas that are not likely ever to become symptomatic, then thousands of men will undergo morbid procedures such as radical prostatectomy without benefit. Conceivably, the surgical mortality from aggressive treatment of small prostate cancers detected by screening could outweigh any reduction in mortality from cancer. A national randomized study is planned to determine whether reduction in cancer mortality can actually be achieved with intense PSA and/or ultrasound screening.

When prostate cancer is suspected, needle biopsy of the prostate usually establishes the diagnosis, but transurethral or suprapubic biopsies are required under some circumstances. The presence of characteristic blastic bone metastases and an elevated serum PSA provide strong evidence of prostatic carcinoma; even if needle biopsy of the prostate is negative in such a patient, a presumptive diagnosis of metastatic prostate cancer can be made and a therapeutic trial of endocrine therapy given.

PSA determinations have replaced acid phosphatase determinations in the management of prostate cancer. More patients with advanced prostate cancer have elevations of PSA than of acid phosphatase, and abnormal serum PSA values in the absence of a diseased prostate are extraordinarily rare. Unfortunately, PSA alone cannot distinguish between benign prostatic hypertrophy and prostate cancer, though PSA levels tend to be higher in malignancy.

When prostate cancer is diagnosed, a thorough history and physical examination are required, along with a complete blood count, intravenous pyelography (IVP), abdominal computed tomography (CT) scan to assess local tumor extent, PSA level, chest x-ray, liver function tests, and bone scan. In some centers, lymphangiography is employed to detect involvement of the pelvic lymph nodes. Needle aspiration of abnormal pelvic lymph nodes or staging lymphadenectomy is often useful and appropriate; the detection of lymph node involvement (i.e., stage D1) indicates incurable disease and the futility of radical surgery or radical radiation therapy.

The American Urological System for staging prostate cancer (Fig. 15–2) possesses the advantages of simplicity and familiarity and is used almost exclusively in the United States.

CLINICAL FEATURES

Because most prostate cancers arise in the posterior portion of the gland, urinary symptoms tend to occur late in the course of the disease, and the diagnosis is often made by palpation of a hard nodule on routine rectal examination. Local symptoms, when present, usually relate to bladder obstruction.

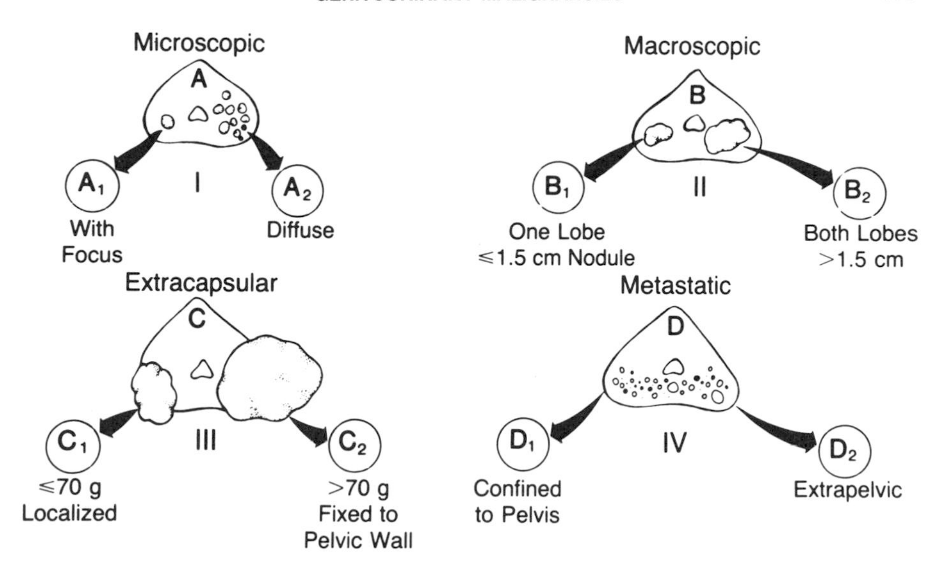

Figure 15–2. Staging of prostate cancer. (*From* Gittes RF: Carcinoma of the prostate. N Engl J Med 324:240, 1991.)

Stage A accounts for 20% of newly diagnosed prostatic carcinomas. By definition, this stage is clinically inapparent; it is discovered on pathologic examination following resection for (presumed) benign prostatic hypertrophy. In autopsy series, stage A prostate cancer increases markedly with age: in men between the ages of 50 and 59, an incidence of 5% is encountered; from 60 to 69, 18%; from 70 to 79, 41%; from 80–89, 54%; and 90 and over, 83%. Patients with stage A1 disease have the same survival as age-matched controls. Stage A2 disease with diffuse involvement and poor differentiation behaves more aggressively.

Stage B lesions account for one-third of cases. The finding of a prostatic nodule on rectal examination leads to their detection. Clinical behavior in this stage correlates with nodule size and grade. As many as 25 to 45% of clinical stage B lesions are upstaged to stage C or D1 disease at time of surgery and lymph node dissection.

Twenty percent of cases present with stage C lesions, defined as local extension beyond the prostatic capsule. These patients may complain of obstructive symptoms. Up to 70% have lymph node involvement when staged with lymphadenectomy, upstaging this group to stage D1. Tumor size and histologic grade correlate with nodal involvement.

Twenty to 30% of patients present with stage D disease. Bone metastases usually dominate the clinical picture, and bone pain is often accompanied by anemia and weight loss. Lung, liver, distant lymph nodes, brain, and soft tissue sites may also harbor metastases from prostate cancer.

TREATMENT

Few topics in medicine are as controversial as the treatment of prostate cancer. Multiple treatment options exist for each stage of the disease (Table 15–4), and choice of therapy

Table 15–4. **TREATMENT OPTIONS IN PROSTATE CANCER BY STAGE**

STAGE	OBSERVATION	SURGERY	RADIATION	HORMONAL Rx
A1	Standard	Rarely	Rarely	Never
A2	In selected cases	Standard	Standard	Never
B	In selected cases	Standard	Standard	Never
C	In selected cases	Occasionally	Standard	Occasionally
D1	Often	Rarely	Often	Standard
D2	Often	Never	For palliation	Standard

must be based on careful deliberation by patient and physician, with full explanation of treatment options.

Localized Disease (Stages A,B,C)

The three major treatment options for patients with localized prostate cancer are observation, surgery (radical prostatectomy), and radiotherapy.

Patients with stage A1 prostate cancer (small foci of well-differentiated carcinoma as an incidental finding on a TUR specimen) have long been managed with observation. Some urologists advocate immediate surgery for younger patients (e.g., less than age 60) with A1 cancer, but usually specific anticancer therapy is deferred until symptoms develop or rapid tumor growth or more aggressive histology become evident. Recent data suggest that such an approach may also be reasonable in selected patients with well-differentiated stage B lesions. Five-year progression-free survival in a group of Swedish patients followed expectantly after the diagnosis of stage A or B prostate cancer was 83% in those with highly differentiated tumors but only 27% with poorly differentiated tumors. Five-year survival after correcting for nonprostate cancer–related deaths was 93%; more than 80% of deaths in this cohort were due to causes other than prostate cancer. Median time before specific treatment was required was over 10 years, and median survival was in excess of 15 years in another series of 75 patients with stage B prostate cancer followed expectantly.

The standard surgical approach to localized prostate cancer is radical prostatectomy, which in the past uniformly led to impotence and caused urinary incontinence in perhaps 10% of patients. The incidence of these complications is reduced, although not eliminated, using newer nerve-sparing prostatectomy techniques. Surgical mortality from radical prostatectomy is approximately 1%. Most authorities believe that lymph node sampling should be performed at the time of surgery, and most but not all urologists agree that radical prostatectomy should not be performed on patients with positive lymph nodes.

Long-term survival rates after radical prostatectomy depend on the stage and especially on the grade of the cancer, as well as on the number of deaths from unrelated conditions in this elderly population. Typically, 10-year survival is about 75% and 15-year survival about 50%, with most deaths from causes other than prostate cancer; only 15 to 20% of patients have recurrences of their malignancy.

Radiotherapy is very commonly used as an alternative to radical prostatectomy for localized prostate cancer. Radiotherapists can deliver 6600 cGy to a small prostate field using external beam treatment, and higher doses can be delivered using interstitial radiotherapy (brachytherapy) techniques. Radiotherapy to pelvic lymph nodes is often administered to patients with high-stage or high-grade lesions. Complications of radiotherapy include proctitis, cystitis, and impotence, but overall radiotherapy produces less morbidity than surgery. The largest experience with radiotherapy for prostate cancer is at Stanford University, where survival of patients treated for stage A prostate cancer matches that of age-matched California men without cancer, and survival of patients with stage B disease (45% at 15 years) is only slightly less than that of the age-matched cohort. Disease-specific survival depends greatly on tumor grade: the disease-specific death rate is 20% at 15 years for low-grade tumors versus 80% at 15 years for high-grade tumors. Radiotherapy may be particularly suited for managing patients with clinically evident stage C disease who have a poor long-term survival and in whom palliation rather than cure is the realistic goal. The 15-year survival rate for stage C prostate cancer treated with radiotherapy is about 20%.

Available data do not permit definite determination of superiority among the three treatment options for localized prostate cancer. Comparison of surgical series with radiotherapy and observation series is hampered by the exclusion from surgical series of most frail or very elderly patients and patients with clinically occult lymph nodes found to be involved with cancer at staging lymphadenectomy. Only one small randomized trial has directly compared radical prostatectomy with radiotherapy for stages A2 and B disease. In the initial follow-up, only 4 of 41 patients assigned to surgery had failed, compared to 17 of 56 patients assigned to radiotherapy. However, stratification based on tumor grade was not employed. Moreover, survival differences have yet to emerge from this study. A large intergroup study is underway, randomizing surgically staged A2 and B patients to radical prostatectomy or radiotherapy. It is hoped that this study will provide definitive data on this controversial issue.

Hormonal therapy is rarely appropriate for localized prostate cancer. It certainly should not be employed in the ordinary patient with stage A or B disease. Randomized studies of the VA Cooperative Urologic Research Group (VACURG) showed increased mortality with supplemental estrogen after radical prostatectomy in such patients. In stage C disease, randomized studies to date have demonstrated a prolonged disease-free interval with immediate adjunctive hormonal therapy after definitive local therapy, but no survival benefit. Research is underway to determine whether survival benefit can be achieved with adjuvant use of some of the newer hormonal therapies in stage C disease. Hormonal therapy alone may be appropriate in selected symptomatic frail elderly patients with locally advanced cancer in whom surgery or even radiotherapy is deemed inappropriate.

Hormonal Therapy of Stage D Prostate Cancer

Metastatic prostate cancer has a variable natural history. Although most men live 1 to 2 years after the diagnosis of metastatic disease, about 20% survive 5 years or longer. An early study by the VACURG compared immediate treatment with delay of treatment until the onset of symptoms and demonstrated no survival benefit to immediate treatment, although interpretation of this study remains controversial. Most medical oncologists recommend therapy for stage D prostate cancer only to relieve symptoms or for rapidly progressing disease.

Hormonal manipulations in symptomatic stage D prostate cancer decrease androgenic stimulation of the carcinoma by interfering with androgen production or blocking androgen action on the target tissue. Methods of accomplishing this include:

- Bilateral orchiectomy
- Estrogen therapy
- Luteinizing hormone–releasing hormone analogue therapy (leuprolide, goserelin)
- Antiandrogen therapy (flutamide, megestrol acetate)
- Antiadrenal therapy (aminoglutethimide, prednisone, ketoconazole)

Bilateral orchiectomy reduces the serum testosterone level by 95% and effectively relieves symptoms in the vast majority of men with metastatic prostate cancer, but many men refuse this procedure for psychological reasons.

Exogenous estrogen binds to a receptor in the hypothalamus, inhibiting release of luteinizing hormone–releasing hormone (LHRH) and eventually LH and testosterone; estrogen probably has a direct antitumor effect on prostate cancer cells as well. Estrogen causes gynecomastia, which can be prevented by pretreatment breast irradiation. High doses of estrogen (5 mg daily of diethylstilbestrol [DES] or equivalent) clearly increase mortality from cardiovascular disease. One milligram of DES daily has much less thrombogenic potential, and many physicians combine this low dose of DES with a low dose of aspirin to try to reduce the cardiovascular risk (although no proof of the success of this strategy exists). One milligram of DES daily does not suppress plasma testosterone levels to castrate levels, but most patients respond to this lower dose of the drug; the dose can be increased to 3 mg daily for patients progressing on the lower dose. The advantages of DES are low cost and oral administration.

The LHRH analogues initially stimulate LH and testosterone release, but after the initial flare, they cause long-term reduction of LH and testosterone levels. Leuprolide and goserelin, which are the commercially available LHRH analogues at this time, cost approximately $300 monthly and must be administered monthly parenterally for life; however, they avoid the psychologic trauma of orchiectomy and the cardiovascular problems of estrogens.

Antiandrogens inhibit uptake and/or binding of testosterone to the target cell nuclear receptor in a manner analogous to the action of antiestrogens like tamoxifen. They have not been extensively evaluated as single agents in initial treatment of advanced prostate cancer, although they clearly are active in this setting. These drugs are most commonly either combined with LHRH analogues in initial therapy or used as salvage treatment after failure of initial hormonal treatment. Antiandrogens are very expensive: the wholesale cost of flutamide is over $200 monthly. Flutamide when used as a single agent in prostate cancer does allow retention of potency in many men. The activity of progestational drugs such as megestrol acetate in prostate cancer probably is related to their weak antiandrogenic effects.

The major nontesticular source of testosterone in men is the adrenal gland, and adrenal suppression reduces adrenal testosterone production in men with worsening prostate cancer. Aminoglutethimide, low doses of exogenous corticosteroids, or ketoconazole can be used.

Several major randomized trials have addressed the issue of optimal initial therapy for symptomatic stage D prostate cancer. Leuprolide was compared to DES, 3 mg daily, and found to be equally effective (85% favorable responses lasting a median of 14 months). Leuprolide caused more hot flashes, but DES caused more gynecomastia, nausea, and edema, and 7% of patients had thrombosis, phlebitis, or pulmonary emboli. It is not known whether DES, 1 mg, could have achieved similar results with less toxicity.

It has been hypothesized that "total androgen blockade" would be more effective in treating prostate cancer than any single hormonal therapy. Spectacular results (median duration of favorable responses over 2 years) were obtained in uncontrolled pilot series using the combination of leuprolide and flutamide. Controlled clinical trials have tested this hypothesis. A large American trial demonstrated a slight benefit to the combination of leuprolide and flutamide (16.5- versus 13.9-month progression-free interval) compared to leuprolide alone. Differences were most marked in patients with minimal metastatic disease. However, European and Canadian trials testing combined androgenic blockade have not proved confirmatory. Many experts think the benefit to combined therapy in the U.S. trial occurred because flutamide blocked the "flare" in testosterone levels and in tumor growth seen when LHRH therapy is first initiated. A major U.S. trial testing flutamide versus placebo in patients treated with orchiectomy (who do not have tumor flare) will help determine whether flutamide confers any benefit other than blocking the initial flare seen with LHRH analogues.

In short, selection of initial therapy for patients with symptomatic or rapidly progressive stage D prostate cancer should be individualized. Options include low-dose DES, flutamide alone, orchiectomy, an LHRH analogue, or the combination of orchiectomy and flutamide or an LHRH analogue and flutamide.

Once prostate cancer becomes resistant to the initial hormonal manipulation, responses to secondary hormonal manipulations are uncommon; no more than one-third of these patients have stabilization or shrinkage of tumor with secondary treatments. Patients treated initially with estrogens can undergo orchiectomy, and those treated with orchiectomy can receive DES, antiandrogen, or antiadrenal therapy. There are anecdotal reports of accelerated progression of cancer when estrogen therapy is suddenly stopped in patients with slowly worsening prostate cancer and intact testicles; maintaining testosterone suppression for life should be considered even in hormone-refractory patients.

Chemotherapy of Stage D Prostate Cancer

Oncologists rarely use cytotoxic chemotherapy in prostate cancer. Many patients have painful bone metastases that are best treated with radiotherapy, and many patients are of such advanced age and poor performance status that they are poor candidates for chemotherapy. Nevertheless, several agents appear to have activity in this disease. Adriamycin (doxorubicin), cisplatin, and cyclophosphamide each produce brief responses in up to 30% of patients. Adriamycin in a low-dose weekly schedule can be given with acceptable toxicity. Although combination chemotherapy may increase the response rate, it has no effect on survival and produces substantial morbidity.

Recently several authors have analyzed the overall experience with chemotherapy in advanced prostate cancer and have reached several conclusions:

- Quality of survival and survival duration have been all but ignored in chemotherapy trials in favor of response rate, a parameter that has little value to the patient.
- Response criteria in chemotherapy trials have been insufficiently rigorous. So-called partial responses and stable disease categories may reflect the natural history of the disease in certain patients rather than the effect of chemotherapy.
- No chemotherapeutic agent has convincingly demonstrated a meaningful prolongation of survival in this disease.
- Chemotherapy produces significant toxicity; the impact of chemotherapy on the quality of life in prostate cancer has not been carefully examined.
- Future trials should randomly assign eligible patients either to a chemotherapy regimen or supportive care only so that the overall effect of chemotherapy in this disease can be adequately assessed.

Regardless of which form of systemic therapy for advanced prostate cancer is used, palliative measures play an important role in producing and maintaining patient comfort. The majority of patients require palliative radiotherapy for painful bone metastases or spinal cord compression. Blood transfusions may control symptoms of anemia caused by bone marrow invasion. Nutritional support and physical therapy are important considerations in many patients. Virtually all patients need high doses of narcotic analgesics in the end stages of this disease.

REFERENCES

Andrioli GL, Catalona WT (eds): Advanced prostate carcinoma. Urol Clin North Am 18:1–159, 1991.
Badalamant RA, Drago JR: Prostate cancer. Disease-A-Month 37:199–268, 1991.
Crawford ED, Eisenberger MA, Mcleod DG, et al: A controlled trial of leuprolide with and without flutamide in prostatic carcinoma. N Engl J Med 321:419–424, 1989.
Gittes RF: Carcinoma of the prostate. N Engl J Med 324:236–245, 1991.
Hanks GE: Radical prostatectomy or radiation therapy for early prostate cancer: two roads to the same end. Cancer 61:2153–2160, 1988.
Hinman F: Screening for prostatic carcinoma. J Urol 145:126–130, 1991.
Johansson J-E, Adami H-O, Andersson S-O, et al: Natural history of localised prostatic carcinoma: A population based study in 223 untreated patients. Lancet 1:799–803, 1989.
Lyss AP: Systemic treatment for prostate cancer. Am J Med 83:1120–1128, 1987.
Smith JA (ed): Early detection and treatment of localized carcinoma of the prostate. Urol Clin North Am 17:689–891, 1990.
Tannock IF: Is there evidence that chemotherapy is of benefit to patients with carcinoma of the prostate? J Clin Oncol 3:1013–1021, 1985.
Whitmore WF, Warner JA, Thompson IM: Expectant management of localized prostate cancer. Cancer 67:1091–1096, 1991.

TESTICULAR CARCINOMA

INCIDENCE AND ETIOLOGY

Testicular carcinoma accounts for only 1% of cancers in males (6300 new cases in 1992; 350 deaths), but it represents the most common carcinoma in the 15 to 35 age group, and its incidence is increasing. The social and economic impact of testicular carcinoma is out of proportion to its incidence, since the patient is often the father and breadwinner of a young family. For reasons unknown, testicular cancers are much less common in blacks, Asians, and Africans than in whites.

The etiology of testicular carcinoma is unknown. Risk factors include cryptorchidism (undescended testis), which is associated with a 20- to 40-fold increase in incidence that is not altered by orchipexy after age 6. Polythelia (supernumerary nipples) is associated with a 4.5-fold increase in risk. A history of trauma or infection frequently precedes the diagnosis of testicular cancer, but this association is probably fortuitous.

PATHOLOGY

Testicular carcinomas arise from the germinal epithelium and are characterized as either seminomatous or nonseminomatous (Table 15–5). Seminomas account for 40% of all

Table 15–5. **HISTOLOGIC CLASSIFICATION OF TESTICULAR GERM CELL TUMORS**

Tumors of a single histologic type
Seminoma
Nonseminomatous
Embryonal carcinoma
Teratocarcinoma
Choriocarcinoma
Yolk sac tumor (endodermal sinus tumor)
Mixed tumors

germ cell cancers; embryonal cell carcinomas, 20%; teratocarcinomas, 30%; and choriocarcinomas, 0.3%. Yolk sac tumors are rare. Since tumors of mixed cell types are common, multiple sections from each specimen are required in order to identify all cell types present for proper histologic classification, prognosis, and treatment selection.

Totipotential germ cells may be present in testicular tumors and may metastasize. When in a new environment, they may differentiate into a different histologic type. For example, up to 30% of seminomas may metastasize as embryonal carcinoma, teratocarcinoma, or choriocarcinoma. Therefore, when orchiectomy reveals seminoma but serum markers (see below) suggest a nonseminomatous tumor, metastatic lesions should be biopsied to identify other histologic types.

DIAGNOSIS AND STAGING

Approximately 90% of germ cell cancers present as an asymptomatic testicular mass; the remaining 10% produce some symptoms. If after a relatively brief period of observation the mass persists, biopsy by means of a high inguinal orchiectomy should be performed. Transscrotal biopsy is inappropriate, since it increases the risk of local recurrence and lymphatic dissemination.

The clinical staging system in common use for testicular carcinoma is shown in Table 15–6. The staging evaluation consists of a thorough history and physical examination, chest x-ray, liver function tests, and abdominal CT scan for assessment of the retroperitoneal nodes. The abdominal CT scan is highly accurate when positive, but false-negative scans are common (30 to 40%).

All patients should have determinations of serum levels of alpha-fetoprotein (AFP) and the beta subunit of human chorionic gonadotropin (β-HCG). These tumor markers are extremely useful in diagnosis, in assessing response to treatment, and in detecting recurrence. At least one of these markers is elevated in 87 to 91% of patients with nonseminomatous germ cell cancers. Persistent elevation of the markers following orchiectomy and lymphadenectomy indicates residual disease.

In adults, AFP is normally absent, but it is detectable in 70% of patients with nonseminomatous germ cell tumors. It is also elevated in 70% of patients with hepatoma and is minimally increased in some patients with ataxia-telangiectasia and gastrointestinal malignancies. The serum half-life of AFP is 5 days.

The beta subunit of HCG is elevated in 50% of patients with nonseminomatous germ cell cancers and is a product of syncytiotrophoblastic elements in the tumor. The half-life of HCG is 16 to 30 hours. About 10% of men with seminoma have slightly increased levels of β-HCG (usually <100 units). These patients are not treated differently than men with marker-negative seminoma, but the pathologist must take great care to exclude the possibility of a mixed tumor that would require a different therapeutic approach.

Serum marker levels and radiologic examinations are highly accurate when positive, but all have a high false-negative rate. When all methods for detecting retroperitoneal lymph node disease are grouped together, the false-negative rate as a whole is still 20 to 30%. This observation provides one of the strongest arguments for surgical lymphadenectomy after orchiectomy in patients without clinical evidence of metastases (see below).

TREATMENT

Seminomas

Because of differences in clinical behavior and natural history, the treatment of pure seminoma differs considerably from that of the other histologic types. Pure seminoma

Table 15–6. **CLINICAL STAGING SYSTEM FOR TESTICULAR CARCINOMA**

STAGE	DESCRIPTION
I	Disease limited to the testes
IIA	Microscopic positive retroperitoneal lymph nodes at lymphadenectomy
IIB	Macroscopic positive retroperitoneal lymph nodes (e.g., >2 cm)
IIC	Huge (palpable) retroperitoneal lymphadenopathy
III	Supradiaphragmatic or visceral involvement

metastasizes in an orderly fashion, first to common iliac and paraaortic nodes with subsequent spread to the mediastinum and supraclavicular nodes. Parenchymal metastases to such sites as lungs, liver, brain, and bone occur only late in the course of the disease.

Seminomas are extremely radiosensitive. Dosages in the range of 2000 to 3000 cGy almost invariably eradicate this disease. Patients with stages I and IIA disease receive radiation therapy to paraaortic and ipsilateral iliac lymph nodes (hockey stick field). Retroperitoneal lymphadenectomy is not indicated because of the extreme radiosensitivity of this disease. Approximately 90 to 95% of patients are cured. The addition of prophylactic mediastinal radiation confers no survival benefit.

Stage IIB seminomas are treated in the same way. Approximately 10% relapse in the mediastinum or supraclavicular area but most of these can be salvaged with chemotherapy. Initial inclusion of the mediastinum in the radiation field in a prophylactic manner provides no survival benefit and compromises the subsequent administration of chemotherapy to the minority of patients who relapse.

The management of bulky retroperitoneal disease (stage IIC) is more difficult. About 60 to 75% of patients with an abdominal mass greater than 5 cm in diameter can be cured with radiotherapy. The proper extent of radiation therapy is controversial: some radiotherapists treat the mediastinum and supraclavicular areas, some limit treatment to subdiaphragmatic nodes, and others advocate whole abdominal radiotherapy. More recently, many authorities have treated stage IIC seminoma with primary chemotherapy followed by surgical resection of residual masses.

Patients with seminoma who present with disease above the diaphragm and those with early-stage disease who relapse following radiation therapy should receive combination chemotherapy as described below for nonseminomatous germ cell cancers. The cure rate for these patients is about 90%. Patients who have had radiation therapy to the lungs should receive a chemotherapy regimen that does not contain bleomycin to avoid the 10% incidence of pulmonary fibrosis encountered when these two agents are combined.

Nonseminomatous Germ Cell Tumors

The treatment of nonseminomatous germ cell tumors of the testis has been revolutionized in the past 2 decades with the advent of highly effective systemic chemotherapy for advanced disease. This development has altered the role of surgery and led to the abandonment of radiation therapy for this disease in the United States. Nevertheless, controversies remain over several issues in management.

Traditionally, patients with clinical stage I disease have undergone elective retroperitoneal lymphadenectomy (RPLND) for accurate staging and therapy. Half of those with positive lymph nodes are cured by RPLND alone and are spared the toxicity of chemotherapy. Patients who undergo elective RPLND and who subsequently relapse almost invariably recur with nonbulky pulmonary disease (where recognition requires only a chest x-ray and serum marker levels) rather than in the retroperitoneum. Early detection and subsequent chemotherapy result in cure in almost 100% of this group.

Recently, many experts have advocated orchiectomy alone without RPLND for these men. Twenty to 25% of patients with clinical stage I disease who do undergo RPLND have microscopic involvement of retroperitoneal nodes and would relapse if the procedure were omitted, but advocates of observation without RPLND point out that the vast majority of these men can be cured with chemotherapy at the time of relapse. Certain features (vascular or lymphatic invasion, involvement of the epididymis or spermatic cord, or predominance of embryonal cell carcinoma) define a population at particularly high risk for occult retroperitoneal lymph node involvement. Fewer than 10% of stage I patients with no adverse prognostic features have positive lymph nodes compared with up to two-thirds of patients with multiple poor prognostic features. Close follow-up of patients who omit RPLND requires cooperation; if the patient fails to comply with scheduled examinations, recurrence may be bulky when first recognized and therefore less likely to be cured with chemotherapy. Recurrence in the retroperitoneum is more likely in patients who have not had RPLND; detection in this area is more difficult and requires frequent abdominal CT scans.

The argument for observation alone for patients with clinical stage I disease relies on two issues. First, 75 to 80% of these patients will have negative retroperitoneal nodes and therefore will derive no benefit from the surgery. Second, while the surgical mortality is low (<0.5%) in experienced hands, morbidity in the form of infertility due to ejaculatory dysfunction is high. At present, this question is unresolved. The appropriate standard of care is probably elective RPLND outside the context of a clinical trial, but observation can be offered to highly motivated and reliable men with low-risk stage I disease.

Patients who have surgically documented retroperitoneal lymph node involvement need close follow-up with monthly serum markers and chest x-rays for the first year and bimonthly examinations for the second year. This surveillance allows detection of relapse at a sufficiently early stage so that a 100% cure rate with chemotherapy can be expected. Adjuvant chemotherapy can be administered immediately after RPLND, but equivalent high cure rates are achieved if chemotherapy is delayed until clinical relapse if strict surveillance is maintained. About half of these stage II patients will be cured with RPLND alone but half will eventually relapse. In a patient who will comply with a stringent schedule of monthly visits, adjuvant chemotherapy should not be necessary, but a less reliable individual might be better served by immediate treatment.

Patients with a palpable abdominal mass, a mass that appears unresectable by CT, distant metastases, and those whose serum markers remain elevated following RPLND require chemotherapy. Five drugs have significant single-agent activity in testicular cancer: cisplatin, vinblastine, etoposide, bleomycin, and ifosfamide. Because bleomycin and cisplatin are relatively nonmyelosuppressive, they can be combined with myelosuppressive drugs such as vinblastine and etoposide without compromising dose. The Einhorn regimen (Table 15–7) consisting of cisplatin, vinblastine, and bleomycin (PVB), first given in the mid 1970s, achieved a 70% complete and a 30% partial remission rate in advanced testicular carcinoma. About one-third of the partial responses were converted to complete responses after surgical resection of residual disease.

More recently, even better survival with less morbidity has been achieved by substituting etoposide for vinblastine. Four cycles of cisplatin, bleomycin, and etoposide over 12 weeks is now standard therapy for advanced testicular cancer. Overall, about 70 to 80% of patients with advanced testicular carcinoma will be cured: over 90% of patients with marker-only disease or small bulk but only 50 to 65% of patients with very bulky disease (e.g., > 10 cm tumor masses).

Residual tumor remaining following chemotherapy either in the retroperitoneum, lungs, liver, mediastinum, or elsewhere should be surgically resected if at all possible, as long as serum marker levels have returned to normal. Approximately 40% of such residual masses contain only fibrous tissue or necrotic, nonviable tumor; about 40% contain benign teratoma; and the remainder contain persistent viable carcinoma. Patients in the first two categories require no additional therapy and have a high likelihood of cure. Two additional courses of chemotherapy are administered to those patients with persistent tumor, and many will also be cured.

All patients who enter complete remission with chemotherapy alone or chemotherapy plus surgery require close follow-up. Monthly physical examinations, chest x-rays, and serum marker levels should be obtained during the first year posttherapy and bimonthly during the second year. Recurrences after 2 years are rare, so that follow-up after this point may take place at longer intervals.

Patients whose marker levels do not normalize following induction chemotherapy should not undergo postchemotherapy surgical resection. This group, and those with normal markers but unresectable residual viable tumor, require salvage chemotherapy. Patients whose tumor was still shrinking with cisplatin, bleomycin, and etoposide but who did not

Table 15–7. **CHEMOTHERAPY REGIMENS FOR TESTICULAR CANCER**

REGIMEN	DRUGS	DOSES	SCHEDULE
PVB	Cisplatin	20 mg/m^2, days 1–5	Repeat cycle every 21 days
	Vinblastine	0.15 mg/kg, days 1–2	
	Bleomycin	30 U, days 1, 8, 15	
BEP	Bleomycin	30 U, days 1, 8, 15	Repeat cycle every 21 days
	Etoposide	100 mg/m^2, days 1–5	
	Cisplatin	20 mg/m^2, days 1–5	
VIP	Etoposide	75 mg/m^2, days 1 5 or	Repeat cycle every 21 days
	Vinblastine	0.11 mg/kg, days 1, 2	
	Ifosfamide	1.2 g/m^2, days 1–5 with mesna uroprotection	
	Cisplatin	20 mg/m^2, days 1–5	

achieve complete response after four cycles can be treated with cisplatin, ifosfamide, and vinblastine once there is unequivocable evidence of active residual tumor. Patients with tumor that grows during treatment with a cisplatin-based regimen have a very poor prognosis. Very high-dose chemotherapy with autologous marrow rescue may salvage some patients with refractory testicular cancer.

EXTRAGONADAL GERM CELL TUMORS

Extragonadal germ cell tumors include teratocarcinomas, embryonal cell carcinomas, choriocarcinomas, endodermal sinus tumors, and benign teratomas. The most common site for these tumors is the mediastinum. Serum marker levels (AFP, β-HCG) may be elevated in some cases.

Treatment of malignant extragonadal germ cell tumors consists of the same cisplatin-based combination chemotherapy regimens used to treat testicular carcinomas. The prognosis of this group is somewhat worse than that of patients with testicular cancers, probably due to the large size that the mediastinal tumors often attain prior to diagnosis.

Young patients who present with poorly differentiated adenocarcinoma, undifferentiated carcinoma, or similar pathologic diagnoses with pulmonary or mediastinal metastases and without an evident primary tumor may actually have occult extragonadal germ cell cancers. Serum marker levels should be obtained, and, if possible, immunohistochemical studies should be performed on their tumor tissue in an attempt to detect AFP and β-HCG in the tumor cells. Such patients frequently respond to cisplatin-based combination chemotherapy even in the absence of a firm histologic diagnosis of germ cell tumor.

REFERENCES

Einhorn LA: Treatment of testicular cancer: A new and improved model. J Clin Oncol 8:1777–1781, 1990.

Fung CY, Garnick MB: Clinical stage I carcinoma of the testis: A review. J Clin Oncol 6:734–750, 1988.

Greco FA, Hainsworth JD (eds): Germ cell neoplasms. Hematol/Oncol Clin North Am 5:1095–1322, 1991.

Motzer RJ, Bosl GJ, Geller NL, et al: Advanced seminoma: The role of chemotherapy and adjunctive surgery. Ann Intern Med 108:513–518, 1988.

Williams SD, Birch R, Einhorn LH, et al: Treatment of disseminated germ-cell tumors with cisplatin, bleomycin, and either vinblastine or etoposide. N Engl J Med 316:1435–1440, 1987.

Williams SD, Stablein DM, Einhorn LH, et al: Immediate adjuvant chemotherapy versus observation with treatment at relapse in pathological stage II testicular cancer. N Engl J Med 317:1433–1438, 1987.

16
GYNECOLOGIC ONCOLOGY

Joanne R. Carignan

The female genital organs contain tissues that undergo dramatic structural and functional changes throughout life. Maturation, menstruation, pregnancy, and hormone production make these organs among the most susceptible to neoplastic transformation in the body. The symptoms and signs of gynecologic neoplasia range from the subtle to the overwhelming and life threatening. Detailed histories and careful physical examinations are essential to the evaluation of these patients. Diagnostic studies include Papanicolaou (Pap) smears, endometrial tissue biopsies, needle aspirations and biopsies, and serum tumor markers. Ultrasonography can reliably detect ascites, adnexal masses, uterine enlargement, and some omental masses. Computed tomography (CT) scanning, while sometimes disappointing in evaluating the extent of cervical and ovarian cancers, can be helpful in assessing lymph nodes, detecting ascites, and examining liver parenchyma and the urinary system. Magnetic resonance (MR) scanning shows diagnostic promise for staging cervical and possibly ovarian cancers. Monoclonal antibody tumor imaging is under active investigation.

Surgery is usually necessary for the diagnosis, staging, and treatment of gynecologic malignancies. Because the initial surgical procedure frequently both establishes the tissue diagnosis and accomplishes the primary oncologic treatment, meticulous planning and state of the art surgical techniques are mandatory for optimal results. Severely ill patients or those with an uncommon or aggressive gynecologic cancer should be considered for referral to a specialized gynecologic oncology unit. These centers provide specialized surgery, research protocols, and the multidisciplinary support that may be required for complex oncologic problems.

OVARIAN CARCINOMA

The National Cancer Institute (NCI) estimates that 21,000 new cases of ovarian cancer and 13,000 deaths from this disease will occur in 1992. Ovarian cancer accounts for 4% of cancer diagnoses and 5% of cancer deaths in American women. One in 70 American women will develop ovarian cancer (compared with one in nine who will develop breast cancer). The incidence of ovarian cancer has increased slightly, whereas survival has not changed over the past 30 years.

The etiology of ovarian cancer is unknown, but epidemiologic evidence reveals an association between duration of uninterrupted ovulation and risk of ovarian carcinoma. Pregnancy, hysterectomy, tubal ligation, and oral contraceptive use reduce risk. Infertility and late menopause appear to increase risk. Theoretically, pregnancy and oral contraceptive use provide rest periods for the ovarian surface mesothelium, which is disrupted with each ovulation and potentially more susceptible to tumor promoters as a consequence. Tubal ligation may protect against ovarian cancer by limiting the exposure of the peritoneal surface to carcinogens like talc. Women with breast cancer have twice the baseline risk of ovarian cancer, and women with ovarian cancer have three to four times the baseline risk of a subsequent breast cancer.

PATHOLOGY

Primary malignant tumors of the ovary are classified according to the tissue of origin: epithelium, gonadal stroma, and germ cells. Table 16–1 is a simplified classification based on the World Health Organization (WHO) schema. Eighty-five to 95% of ovarian cancers arise from the epithelium. Epithelial ovarian cancers include tumors of low malignant potential as well as the much more common higher-grade invasive adenocarcinomas, subclassified as serous, mucinous, endometrioid, clear cell, and undifferentiated. Gonadal stromal tumors make up about 4% of ovarian cancers and germ cell tumors only 2 to 3%.

Table 16–1. **PATHOLOGY OF OVARIAN CANCER**

EPITHELIAL ORIGIN	GERM CELL ORIGIN
Serous	Dysgerminoma
Mucinous	Endodermal sinus tumor
Endometrioid	Embryonal carcinoma
Clear cell	Polyembryoma
Brenner	Choriocarcinoma
Mixed	Teratoma
Undifferentiated	Mixed tumors
GONADAL STROMAL ORIGIN	
Granulosa-stromal tumors	
Granulosa cell tumor	
Theca-fibroma tumor	
Androblastomas; Sertoli-Leydig cell tumors	
Gynandroblastomas	
Unclassified	

DIAGNOSIS

Most cases of ovarian cancer (about 65%) occur in women between the ages of 40 and 65. Early symptoms are unusual, and most cases are discovered on routine pelvic examination or after a period of vague abdominal or pelvic discomfort. About three-quarters of all patients with ovarian carcinoma present with extensive disease that has spread beyond the pelvis, manifested by ascites and widespread intra-abdominal seeding along peritoneal surfaces. Pleural effusions account for most metastatic involvement outside the abdomen. Epithelial ovarian cancer uncommonly metastasizes to the lung or liver parenchyma, bone, or brain.

An ovarian mass in a woman younger than age 45 has only a 7% likelihood of malignancy, whereas in women older than age 45, the risk of malignancy increases to 33%. In peri- or postmenopausal women, ovarian masses must be considered malignant until proven otherwise. In the premenopausal patient, cystic adnexal masses under 5 cm may sometimes be observed, whereas those over 5 cm should be promptly evaluated. Ultrasound or CT scan evaluation is seldom sufficient, however, since definition of a cystic mass does not prove benignity. Operative biopsy remains the standard method of evaluation for adnexal masses. In some cases, fiberoptic laparoscopy with biopsy and washings can be very useful. Nevertheless, if uncertainty exists following the procedure, patients should undergo operative biopsy (and surgical staging if necessary).

The development of a monoclonal antibody–based serum assay for an ovarian cancer antigen, CA-125 (positive >35 U/mL), provides an additional diagnostic tool. CA-125 levels are elevated in over 80% of patients with ovarian carcinoma, and the presence of an elevated CA-125 in a postmenopausal patient with a pelvic mass or ascites is highly suggestive of malignancy; however, nonovarian cancers (pancreas, lung, breast, endometrium, colon, and others) are also associated with elevated levels. Premenopausal women with endometriosis and other benign gynecologic conditions may have elevated CA-125 levels, decreasing the value of this marker for diagnosis of ovarian cancer in this age group. Eventually further work with CA-125 and other ovarian cancer antigens may lead to useful screening tests, particularly for patients at high risk on the basis of a positive family history.

STAGING

As in other gynecologic malignancies, the International Federation of Gynecology and Obstetrics (FIGO) staging classification is used for ovarian cancer. A simplified version is shown in Table 16–2. Meticulous surgical assessment of the abdominal contents and diaphragmatic surfaces and complete examination of the pelvic structures are central to appropriate oncologic management. Incomplete operative staging results in inadequate treatment in a significant number of patients. Surgical debulking (cytoreductive surgery) is usually undertaken along with the staging procedure. Although no prospective randomized trial has ever critically evaluated the role of cytoreductive surgery, it is clear that patients who have minimal disease volume after surgery have a much better response

Table 16–2. **FIGO* STAGING FOR CARCINOMA OF THE OVARY**

Stage I	Growth limited to the ovaries.
Stage IA	Growth limited to one ovary; no ascites. No tumor on the external surface; capsule intact.
Stage IB	Growth limited to both ovaries; no ascites. No tumor on the external surfaces; capsules intact.
Stage IC	Tumor either stage IA or IB but with tumor on the ovarian surface, or with capsule ruptured, or with cytology-positive peritoneal fluid.
Stage II	Growth involving one or both of the ovaries with pelvic extension.
Stage IIA	Extension and/or metastases to the uterus and/or tubes.
Stage IIB	Extension to other pelvic tissues.
Stage IIC	Tumor either stage IIA or IIB but with tumor on the ovarian surface, or with capsule ruptured, or with cytology-positive peritoneal fluid.
Stage III	Tumor involving one or both ovaries with peritoneal implants outside the pelvis and/or positive retroperitoneal or inguinal nodes and/or superficial liver metastases.
Stage IIIA	Tumor grossly limited to the true pelvis with negative nodes but with microscopic seeding of the abdominal peritoneal surfaces.
Stage IIIB	Tumor implants of the abdominal peritoneal surfaces smaller than 2 cm. Nodes negative.
Stage IIIC	Abdominal implants larger than 2 cm and/or positive retroperitoneal or inguinal nodes.
Stage IV	Ovarian cancer with distant metastases (includes cytology-positive pleural fluid and parenchymal hepatic metastases).

*International Federation of Gynecology and Obstetrics (1987).

rate and survival following subsequent chemotherapy. Whether the poor prognosis associated with bulky residual disease is due to the increased tumor burden per se or to greater intrinsic virulence of such tumors remains unresolved. Nevertheless, most gynecologic oncologists recommend aggressive surgical debulking whenever technically feasible.

The survival of patients with epithelial ovarian cancer depends on the clinical stage, the histologic grade of the tumor, and the postsurgical tumor burden (measured as the diameter of the largest residual tumor nodule). Tumor stage is the single most important factor, and within each stage, tumors with higher histologic grades have a poorer prognosis than those of lower grade. Preliminary studies with flow cytometry indicate that diploid stage III tumors have a better prognosis than aneuploid tumors. More aggressive ovarian cancers tend to have more frequent genetic abnormalities such as amplification of the HER-2/*neu* oncogene, which is associated with increased tumor invasiveness and greater antineoplastic drug resistance.

TREATMENT OF EPITHELIAL OVARIAN CANCER

Limited Disease

About 20 to 30% of patients with ovarian cancer present with limited (stages I and II) disease. Clinical trials have indicated that these patients can be divided into a low-risk and a high-risk group. Low-risk tumors are characterized by disease limited to the ovary, an intact capsule, low tumor grade, and the absence of ascites or malignant cells in peritoneal washings. These patients have a 5-year survival greater than 90% when treated by total abdominal hysterectomy, bilateral salpingo-oophorectomy, and omentectomy. Adjuvant treatment with either chemotherapy or irradiation does not appear to be helpful.

Patients with stage II and less favorable stage I (positive fluid cytology or higher tumor grade) disease are treated with a similar surgical approach. However, in these patients, postsurgical adjuvant therapy may be indicated. In a recent randomized study, the 5-year survival rate for such patients treated with either intraperitoneal ^{32}P (chromic phosphate) or 10 courses of systemic adjuvant melphalan was about 80% for both treatments. However, owing to the lack of an untreated control arm, the true value of adjuvant chemotherapy in this group remains uncertain. Previous studies have suggested that abdominopelvic radiation therapy may also be useful in locoregional ovarian cancer, and this modality requires further study in comparison with both systemic chemotherapy and intraperitoneal ^{32}P. Because of the higher response rate of advanced ovarian carcinoma to cisplatin-based chemotherapy, the Gynecologic Oncology Group is currently conducting a randomized trial comparing three cycles of cyclophosphamide plus cisplatin with intraperitoneal ^{32}P in patients with stages I and II disease. The results of this and similar studies will have a major impact on the management of early stage ovarian cancer.

Advanced Disease

Cisplatin-based combination chemotherapy is the mainstay of treatment for stages III and IV ovarian cancer following cytoreductive surgery. The outcome is largely dependent on the residual tumor volume. Data from M.D. Anderson Cancer Center show that patients with minimal residual disease have a 4-year survival of 51% compared to 19% for those with residual masses greater than 2 cm in diameter.

The optimal chemotherapy regimen for advanced ovarian cancer remains a subject of intense investigation. Combination chemotherapy with cyclophosphamide plus cisplatin is more effective than single-agent alkylating chemotherapy (i.e., melphalan) and as effective but less toxic than combinations that also include Adriamycin (doxorubicin) or hexamethylmelamine. With cyclophosphamide plus cisplatin, the Gynecologic Oncology Group achieved a negative second-look laparotomy (pathologic complete remission) rate of 30% and an overall response rate of 70%.

The toxicity of cisplatin-containing regimens is appreciable, with significant nausea, vomiting, alopecia, renal impairment, and bone marrow suppression. Substituting carboplatin for cisplatin reduces gastrointestinal, neurologic, and renal toxicity with therapeutic equivalency demonstrated in two recent studies. Bone marrow toxicity increases with the carboplatin regimen. The treatment regimen consists of six cycles of carboplatin (300 mg/m^2) and cyclophosphamide (600 mg/m^2) administered intravenously every 4 weeks. Very ill or elderly patients, who are unlikely to tolerate cisplatin or carboplatin, can be treated with melphalan, 0.1 to 0.2 mg/kg/day for 5 days every 4 to 6 weeks. Response rates are approximately 50% with this approach, which produces very little toxicity other than myelosuppression.

After six cycles of chemotherapy, if no disease is clinically apparent on physical examination and pelvic ultrasound or CT scan, a second-look laparotomy is sometimes recommended. CA-125 levels can predict laparotomy findings: persistently elevated levels ($>$35 U/mL) usually indicate residual active disease; levels below 35 U/mL after three cycles of chemotherapy were associated with a 75% clinical remission rate and 66% negative second-look laparotomy rate. However, the value of the second-look laparotomy remains controversial. Prognostic information is definitely obtained; in one series at 3 years survival was 81% with negative findings at second-look laparotomy, 49% with less than 2 cm residual disease, and 30% with gross residual disease. But the value of additional debulking and of the early detection of residual disease following completion of chemotherapy is questionable in the absence of highly effective salvage chemotherapy. Therefore, second-look laparotomies are best reserved for those patients who would be considered for investigational protocols following second-look surgery.

Unfortunately, even patients with negative second-look laparotomies have a substantial relapse rate estimated at about 33% within 2 years of the procedure. Only the minority of patients with well-differentiated tumors and minimal residual disease following initial surgery are likely to have long-term survival. An NCI follow-up study of patients with advanced ovarian cancer treated with cisplatin combination chemotherapy found an overall 4-year survival of 15%. Patients who fail to respond to initial chemotherapy, those who achieve only a partial remission, and those who relapse following an initial response develop progressive disease rapidly. Standard approaches to treatment with second-line chemotherapeutic agents (alkylating agents, antimetabolites, hormones) achieve minimal response rates, and survival is measurable in months. Such patients should be considered for experimental clinical trials.

Intensive efforts to improve the efficacy of ovarian cancer treatment continue. Current research directions include intraperitoneal chemotherapy with cisplatin (and other chemotherapeutic agents) for first-line therapy of minimal residual disease and for minimal residual disease at second-look laparotomy. High dose intensity chemotherapy with a colony-stimulating factor (CSF) (granulocyte-CSF or granulocyte-macrophage-CSF) or autologous bone marrow transplant support is an option for young and otherwise healthy patients able to tolerate such treatments. New agents such as taxol and ifosfamide show promise and are under active investigation. The role of biological response modifiers (interferons, interleukins) is also being defined.

GONADAL STROMAL TUMORS

Gonadal stromal tumors represent fewer than 5% of ovarian malignancies. These tumors are associated with the secretion of androgens or estrogens in the majority of cases, although the hormone secreted does not always correlate with the cell type. The granulosa cell tumor is the most common in this group. It arises most frequently during the fifth to seventh decades. In postmenopausal patients, it is associated with endometrial cancer in 15% of cases. Granulosa cell tumors are almost always unilateral and localized. Standard therapy is total abdominal hysterectomy and bilateral salpingo-oophorectomy. Young patients are sometimes treated with unilateral salpingo-oophorectomy to preserve fertility. Recurrences may occur many years following initial diagnosis and eventually cause death. These tumors are not very radiosensitive, although radiation has been used for incompletely resected primary tumors. Chemotherapy experience is anecdotal, but recent interest has centered on cisplatin, vinblastine, and bleomycin.

GERM CELL TUMORS

Germ cell tumors comprise 2 to 3% of ovarian cancers. They are usually seen in women under the age of 30. Dysgerminomas are the most common type and are sometimes associated with pregnancy. They are frequently unilateral and confined to the ovary. Dysgerminomas may be treated with unilateral salpingo-oophorectomy as long as careful operative staging confirms the absence of extraovarian spread. When the tumor consists of pure dysgerminoma confined to the ovary, the cure rate exceeds 80%.

Germ cell tumors may produce human chorionic gonadotropin (HCG), which can be used to monitor disease recurrence or the results of treatment, analogous to the management of testicular nonseminomatous germ cell carcinomas in males. Less common types of germ cell tumors include endodermal sinus tumors, teratomas, and mixed germ cell tumors; in these cases, surgical cures are much less likely. An M.D. Anderson study of 26 patients with dysgerminomas and nondysgerminomas who were treated with a combination of cisplatin, etoposide, and bleomycin achieved a 96% sustained remission rate.

REFERENCES

Friedman JB, Weiss NS: Second thoughts about second-look laparotomy in advanced ovarian cancer. N Engl J Med 322:1079–1082, 1990.
Gershenson DM, Morris M, Cangir A, et al: Treatment of malignant germ cell tumors of the ovary with bleomycin, etoposide, and cisplatin. J Clin Oncol 8:715–720, 1990.
McClay EF, Howell SB: A review: Intraperitoneal cisplatin in the management of patients with ovarian cancer. Gynecol Oncol 36:1–6, 1990.
Niloff JM: The role of the CA-125 assay in the management of ovarian cancer. Oncology 2:67–76, 1988.
Ozols RF (ed): Ovarian cancer. Semin Oncol 18:177–313, 1991.
Young RC, Walton LA, Ellenberg SS, et al: Adjuvant therapy in stage I and stage II epithelial ovarian cancer. N Engl J Med 322:1021–1027, 1990.

ENDOMETRIAL CARCINOMA

The National Cancer Institute estimates that in 1992 there will be 32,000 new cases of endometrial cancer and 5,600 deaths due to the disease. Endometrial cancer is a disease of middle-aged women, with the peak incidence occurring between 50 and 64 years of age. Predisposing factors include obesity, diabetes, hypertension, and a history of infertility, menstrual irregularity, late menopause, or exogenous estrogen use. One woman per 1000 will develop endometrial cancer each year. The overall cure rate worldwide approximates 75%, although in selected early cases the cure rate with surgery alone approaches 95 to 100%.

An underlying derangement in endogenous estrogen metabolism is presumed to play a role in the development of these tumors. Unopposed estrogenic stimulation as seen in the

Stein-Leventhal syndrome, granulosa-theca cell tumors, obesity, and anovulatory menstrual cycles increases the risk of endometrial cancer. Unopposed exogenous estrogen supplementation also markedly enhances the incidence of endometrial cancer; this risk diminishes if progesterone accompanies the estrogen therapy.

PATHOLOGY

About 90% of cancers arising in the uterine corpus are adenocarcinomas of the endometrium. Like cervical cancer, endometrial carcinoma appears to develop from atypia through a continuum of changes to frank carcinoma. Cystic endometrial hyperplasia and adenomatous hyperplasia frequently regress after a course of progestin therapy; only a minority of cases evolve over many years to carcinoma in situ or invasive carcinoma.

Pathologic studies show that a significant percentage of endometrial carcinomas contain elements of squamous tissue, either benign (adenoacanthoma) or malignant (adenosquamous carcinoma). Adenoacanthomas are no more virulent than adenocarcinomas. Adenosquamous, clear cell, and papillary serous endometrial cancers behave more aggressively, with a greater risk for dissemination and lower survival rates.

DIAGNOSIS

Postmenopausal bleeding is the hallmark of endometrial cancer. Diagnosis requires histologic examination of endometrial tissue; routine Pap tests are only 50 to 65% accurate, and curettage is usually necessary to obtain adequate histologic material. The fractional curettage under general anesthesia represents the standard for endometrial evaluation. Aspiration curettage, frequently without local anesthesia, can be performed on an outpatient basis with very good diagnostic yield. It may provide an acceptable method for outpatient screening of high-risk patients.

The staging classification for endometrial carcinoma is shown in Table 16–3. Examination under anesthesia provides valuable preoperative staging information. An intravenous pyelogram, chest x-ray, and cystoscopy and proctoscopy, if indicated, provide additional preoperative staging. Research studies indicate that ultrasonography (transabdominal and transvaginal) and MRI scans may provide helpful noninvasive information regarding depth of myometrial invasion and lymph node or pelvic wall involvement. Operative staging, including lymph node biopsy, helps in planning radiation therapy and in determining prognosis. More than three-quarters of all cases of endometrial carcinoma are diagnosed while still confined to the uterus, accounting for the relatively low death rate from this disease.

Prognosis and survival vary according to the determinants outlined in Table 16–4. Positive hormone receptor status, especially a positive progesterone receptor, is associated with improved survival. Aneuploidy predicts a greater risk of distant metastases. Most patients with endometrial cancer are cured but 25 to 30% have recurrences and require further therapy.

Table 16–3. **FIGO* STAGING OF ENDOMETRIAL CANCER**

Stage 0	Carcinoma in situ.
Stage I	The carcinoma is confined to the corpus.
Stage Ia	The length of the uterine cavity is 8 cm or less.
Stage Ib	The length of the uterine cavity is more than 8 cm.
Stage II	The carcinoma involves the corpus and the cervix.
Stage III	The carcinoma extends outside the uterus but not outside the true pelvis.
Stage IV	The carcinoma extends outside the true pelvis or involves the bladder or rectum.
Stage IVa	Spread to adjacent organs.
Stage IVb	Spread to distant organs.

*International Federation of Gynecology and Obstetrics (1987).

Table 16–4. **FOUR-YEAR PROGRESSION-FREE SURVIVAL OF PATIENTS WITH ENDOMETRIAL CANCER STRATIFIED BY PROGNOSTIC DETERMINANTS**

PROGNOSTIC VARIABLE	SURVIVAL (%)
DNA ploidy	
Diploid	88
Nondiploid	57
Surgical stage	
1 and 2	87
3 and 4	48
Grade (Broders')	
1 and 2	88
3 and 4	54
Myometrial invasion	
Inner two-thirds	86
≥Two-thirds	62

Modified with permission from Britton LC, et al: DNA ploidy in endometrial carcinoma: Major objective prognostic factor. Mayo Clin Proc 65:643–650, 1990.

TREATMENT

Premalignant Disease

Progesterone (Depo-Provera, 1000 mg intramuscularly, monthly; or Megace, 40 mg orally, three times daily) will eliminate many cases of mild or moderate adenomatous hyperplasia. Clomiphene or ovarian wedge resection can reestablish an ovulatory pattern that will reverse hyperplasia in premenopausal women. Endometrial biopsies must be repeated after 3 months of treatment. If hyperplasia persists or atypia is present, hysterectomy may be required.

Stage I Disease

The treatment of stage I endometrial carcinoma consists of total abdominal hysterectomy and bilateral salpingo-oophorectomy with peritoneal cytologic washings. For well-differentiated lesions (grade 1) and for those without deep myometrial invasion (grades 1 and 2), the surgical results are so good (5 to 15% recurrence rate) that no further treatment is indicated. Stage I cancers with poorly differentiated histology or deep myometrial invasion have a less favorable survival rate; recurrence rates vary from 10 to 45% (see Table 16–4). Most centers advocate external pelvic irradiation following surgery for these patients.

Stage II Disease

Extension of endometrial cancer to the cervix decreases survival rates and increases the risk of vaginal, parametrial, and regional lymph node involvement. Treatment approaches vary widely, but combined radiation therapy plus surgery is most common. Radiation therapy aims to sterilize the lymph node metastases that occur in 30% of stage II cancers, and surgery removes bulk disease in the uterus. Considerable controversy surrounds the issue of the most appropriate sequence and details of treatment. Microscopic cervical involvement often is treated with preoperative therapy followed by surgery.

The role of adjuvant chemotherapy and hormonal therapy for high-risk early-stage endometrial cancer is a subject of current research.

Stage III Disease

Stage III disease with vaginal and/or parametrial involvement accounts for only 3 to 13% of endometrial cancers. If the only extrauterine disease involves the ovaries or fallopian tubes, the outlook is much better than if other pelvic involvement is present (20% relapse rate versus 73%). These more favorable patients are usually treated with surgery followed by radiation therapy.

Bulky stage III disease may be treated with radiation therapy alone. Radiation doses are increased and no surgery is planned. While survival may be better for those patients who receive surgery and radiation therapy, this probably reflects patient selection on the basis of tumor extent rather than a significant treatment superiority. Treatment for patients with stage III endometrial carcinoma is best decided by close cooperation between gynecologist and radiation oncologist on an individual case basis. Because of the high risk of disease recurrence, current clinical trials are investigating the role of adjuvant chemotherapy with cyclophosphamide, Adriamycin, and cisplatin. Randomized trials of adjuvant chemotherapy are needed.

Stage IV and Recurrent Disease

Patients with stage IV or recurrent disease are treated with palliative intent. Radiation therapy can sometimes provide prolonged disease-free survival and symptomatic relief for those with extensive pelvic disease. Patients with symptomatic distant metastases are best treated with progesterone (Megace, 160 to 320 mg daily; or Depo-Provera, 1 to 3 g weekly), and 30% will demonstrate objective response. For patients who fail to respond or who progress after response, single-agent Adriamycin with a response rate of 36% can provide some palliative benefit. Cyclophosphamide and cisplatin also have single-agent response rates between 20 and 30%, but while some trials of combination therapy exist, no advantage for combination chemotherapy over single-agent treatment has been demonstrated.

UTERINE SARCOMAS

Uterine sarcomas are rare tumors. Although they have been subclassified according to pathologic type, for each stage all sarcomas have a similar prognosis. Like endometrial carcinoma, the sarcomas commonly present with vaginal bleeding and are frequently associated with obesity and hypertension. Therapy consists of surgery or surgery plus radiation therapy. Adjuvant chemotherapy with Adriamycin offers no advantage over observation alone following local treatment. The disease recurs within 2 years in two-thirds of patients, and distant metastases are almost invariably present. The most frequent sites of distant failure are the upper abdomen and the lungs. Both Adriamycin and cisplatin have single-agent activity in the treatment of advanced uterine sarcomas. A recent unconfirmed study reported a 73% response rate when Adriamycin and cisplatin were combined in the treatment of measurable advanced disease. The number of patients treated was small, and larger, randomized studies of chemotherapy as an adjuvant and for advanced disease are needed.

REFERENCES

Boronow RC: Advances in diagnosis, staging, and management of cervical and endometrial cancer, stages I and II. Cancer 65:648–659, 1990.

Gusberg SB: Current concepts in the control of carcinoma of the endometrium. CA 36:245–253, 1986.

Moore TD, Phillips PH, Nerenstone SR, Cheson BD: Systemic treatment of advanced and recurrent endometrial carcinoma: Current status and future directions. J Clin Oncol 9:1071–1088, 1991.

Peters WA, Rivkin SE, Smith MR, Tesh DE: Cisplatin and Adriamycin combination chemotherapy for uterine stromal sarcomas and mixed mesodermal tumors. Gynecol Oncol 34:323–327, 1989.

Pliskow S, Penalver M, Averette HE: Stage III and IV endometrial carcinoma: A review of 41 cases. Gynecol Oncol 38:210–215, 1990.

Symonds DA: Prognostic value of pathologic features and DNA analysis in endometrial carcinoma. Gynecol Oncol 39:272–276, 1990.

GESTATIONAL TROPHOBLASTIC DISEASE

Trophoblastic tumors are products of conception and result from abnormal proliferation of the chorionic villi of the placenta. Pathologically these tumors are divided into three entities:

- Hydatidiform mole, usually benign with large hydropic villi and trophoblastic proliferation
- Chorioadenoma destruens, or invasive mole, a hydatidiform mole with myometrial invasion
- Choriocarcinoma, an anaplastic invasive tumor with syncytiotrophoblastic and cytotrophoblastic elements

About half of all gestational choriocarcinomas follow molar pregnancies; 40% follow normal pregnancies or abortions. The remainder arise from ectopic pregnancies. The incidence of molar pregnancies is 10 times higher in Asians and Mexicans than in Americans. Likewise, the incidence of choriocarcinoma is 1 in 1382 pregnancies in Manila but only 1 in 16,000 in Chicago. These differences are not due to genetic factors, since Asian immigrants in the United States have a low incidence.

Hydatidiform moles are considered either complete or partial based on pathology, morphology, and chromosome analysis. Complete moles lack fetal remnant tissue and are always diploid (46, XX), and 15 to 20% develop persistent trophoblastic tumor. The chromosomes of complete moles are both derived paternally (androgenesis). The mechanism requires either duplication of the paternal haploid genome or fertilization by two sperm (dispermy) within an ovum with inactive or absent maternal chromosomes. Partial moles usually have detectable fetal tissue and a triploid karyotype resulting from fertilization of a normal ovum by two sperm. After uterine evacuation of a partial mole, the risk of persistent trophoblastic tumor is 4 to 10%.

Gestational trophoblastic disease may produce certain serious medical complications. Hyperthyroidism, pulmonary tumor emboli, respiratory distress, preeclampsia-eclampsia, hemorrhage, and coagulation defects can be severe and life threatening.

DIAGNOSIS

An abnormally elevated β-HCG level in the clinical setting of current or recent pregnancy indicates possible gestational trophoblastic disease. The clinical presentation is variable. Common findings in pregnant patients include a uterus larger than expected for gestational age, absent fetal heart tones after 18 weeks of pregnancy, and bleeding associated with passage of villiform tissue.

Some patients present after induced abortion or ectopic pregnancy with abnormal uterine bleeding and a positive pregnancy test. Occasionally patients present with serious medical complications following a normal delivery. Recurrent pulmonary emboli despite heparinization, particularly during the postpartum period, may be due to tumor emboli from gestational trophoblastic disease.

CLINICAL ASSESSMENT

After evacuation of a molar pregnancy, the patient should have a complete history and physical examination as well as complete blood counts, β-HCG levels, and hepatic, renal, and thyroid function tests. Staging work-up consists of an abdominal and pelvic ultrasound, chest x-ray, and a head CT scan, which can detect asymptomatic brain metastases in patients with extensive tumor burden. Patients who do not have metastases are followed by weekly β-HCG determinations and monthly pelvic examinations and chest x-rays. In 85% of these cases, the β-HCG is undetectable by 8 weeks, and no further therapy is required. Patients are asked to avoid pregnancy for 1 year.

Patients initially without metastases who experience a rise in β-HCG titer, a plateau in β-HCG for 3 weeks, or subsequent evidence of metastases require systemic therapy. Occasionally patients with nonmetastatic trophoblastic disease hemorrhage from uterine perforation. These patients require both surgery (either hysterectomy or bilateral hypogastric artery ligation) and systemic chemotherapy. Indications for treatment of postmolar trophoblastic disease are summarized in Table 16–5.

The presence of invasive mole or choriocarcinoma on histologic examination or detection of distant metastases indicates the need for systemic therapy. Metastatic work-up (Table 16–6) includes the same tests as for those patients with molar disease, supplemented by CT scans of the chest, abdomen, and pelvis (some centers prefer MR scans of the abdomen and pelvis). Patients with metastases should have a lumbar puncture for cytology and

Table 16–5. **INDICATIONS FOR TREATMENT OF POSTMOLAR TROPHOBLASTIC DISEASE**

Abnormal HCG regression curve
- Plateau for 3 or more consecutive weeks
- Rise in titer over 2 consecutive weeks

Presence of metastases
Tissue diagnosis of choriocarcinoma
Uterine hemorrhage
Patient at high risk who cannot be followed

cerebrospinal fluid HCG. A ratio of plasma HCG to cerebrospinal fluid HCG of less than 60:1 suggests central nervous system involvement. Patients with metastases are then divided into low-risk and high-risk categories (Table 16–7), depending on the HCG level, duration of disease, and the presence of liver or brain metastases.

TREATMENT

Low-risk patients with nonmetastatic gestational trophoblastic disease and those with metastases confined to the lung and vagina have a cure rate of 68 to 90% with single-agent chemotherapy. Methotrexate, actinomycin D, and etoposide each have excellent single-agent response rates. The current regimen of choice is methotrexate, 1 mg/kg, intramuscularly every other day for four doses followed by leukovorin, 0.1 mg/kg, 24 hours after each methotrexate dose. Of patients achieving complete remission, 82% require only one course of this treatment.

A decrease of one log or greater in the β-HCG level over the succeeding 18 days allows cessation of treatment. Additional therapy is administered at least every 18 days for those patients with a lesser decrease, plateau, or increase in the β-HCG titer until the titer normalizes for 3 weeks. The rare patient who does not achieve lasting remission with this induction regimen will almost always achieve complete remission with combination chemotherapy. Toxicity with this methotrexate regimen is quite modest, with low rates of bone marrow suppression (<10%) and asymptomatic, transient, liver enzyme elevations (14%).

High-risk patients (see Table 16–7) should receive combination chemotherapy, supplemented by brain and/or hepatic irradiation as dictated by metastatic site. The most effective single agents, etoposide, methotrexate, and actinomycin D, are combined with cyclophosphamide and vincristine (Oncovin) in the EMA/CO regimen, which achieves survival rates of 91% in previously untreated, high-risk patients and 78% in those with resistant disease or disease that has progressed following previous chemotherapy. Although the EMA/CO regimen has not been compared with other multidrug regimens in randomized studies, its apparent superior response rates and decreased toxicity make it a reasonable choice for high-risk and resistant cases. Because high-risk gestational trophoblastic disease is a rare and potentially curable malignancy, referral of patients to specialized centers should be considered.

Table 16–6. **STAGING STUDIES FOR MALIGNANT GESTATIONAL TROPHOBLASTIC DISEASE**

Complete history and physical examination
Blood studies
- Serum HCG titer, CBC with differential and platelet count, prothrombin time, and partial thromboplastin time, electrolytes, renal functions, liver functions, thyroid panel, blood type and Rh type

Radiographic studies
- CT scans of the brain and abdomen, pelvic ultrasound

Electrocardiography
Indicated consultations
Optional studies
- CT scan of the lung, IVP, selective arteriography, lumbar puncture for cerebrospinal fluid HCG levels and electroencephalography

Table 16–7. **PROGNOSIS OF METASTATIC GESTATIONAL TROPHOBLASTIC DISEASE**

GOOD PROGNOSIS
Metastases present and:
1. Serum β-HCG less than 40,000 mIU/mL.
2. Symptoms of malignancy have been present for <4 months.
3. Brain and liver metastases are not present.
4. The patient has had no chemotherapy.

POOR PROGNOSIS
Metastases are present and:
1. Serum β-HCG greater than 40,000 mIU/mL.
2. Symptoms of malignancy have been present for >4 months.
3. Brain or liver metastasis.
4. Unsuccessful previous chemotherapy.
5. Antecedent term pregnancy.

REFERENCES

Berkowitz RS, Goldstein DP: Gestational trophoblastic diseases. Semin Oncol 16:410–416, 1989.

Bolis G, Bonazzi C, Landoni F, et al: EMA/CO regimen in high risk gestational trophoblastic tumor (GTT). Gynecol Oncol 31:439–444, 1988.

Hunter V, Raymond E, Christensen C, et al: Efficacy of the metastatic survey in the staging of gestational trophoblastic disease. Cancer 65:1647–1650, 1990.

Jones WB: Gestational trophoblastic disease: What have we learned in the past decade? Am J Obstet Gynecol 162:1286–1295, 1990.

Rustin GJS, Newlands ES, Begent RHJ, et al: Weekly alternating etoposide, methotrexate, and actinomycin, with vincristine and cyclophosphamide chemotherapy for the treatment of CNS metastases of choriocarcinoma. J Clin Oncol 7:900–903, 1989.

CANCER OF THE CERVIX

The National Cancer Institute estimates that in 1992 13,500 new cases of invasive cervical cancer and 4,400 deaths from this disease will occur. Over the past 30 years, mortality from cervical cancer has dropped 53% in the United States, although the decrease appears to be leveling out recently. While the decline is in part due to improved therapy, it is largely attributed to the Pap smear and the resulting early detection of invasive, in situ, and premalignant cervical lesions. Extensive epidemiologic surveys indicate that the incidence and mortality of invasive cervical cancer could be reduced by 90% with regular Pap smear screening. While some controversy still exists regarding the optimal timing of Pap tests, the National Cancer Institute recommends that young, sexually active women have three annual Pap tests followed by Pap tests every 3 years thereafter until age 65.

EPIDEMIOLOGY

The risk of cervical cancer increases with low socioeconomic status, early sexual intercourse, multiple sexual partners, and poor prenatal and postnatal care. Cervical cancer has been twice as common in blacks as in whites, although the difference is decreasing among the younger age groups. It is far less common among celibates and Jewish women whose partners are circumcised. Recent evidence suggests that squamous cell carcinoma of the cervix represents a venereal disease, primarily related to infection with human papilloma virus. Cigarette smoking, pelvic radiation, immunodeficiency, and other factors may also play a role. Oral contraceptives have been tentatively linked with increased incidence of cervical adenocarcinoma. Barrier contraceptives may decrease the risk of cervical cancer.

DIAGNOSIS

Postcoital bleeding is classically associated with cervical cancer; however, most cervical cancers are asymptomatic until locally advanced. The cervix may appear normal or quite abnormal with bleeding, friability, and visible tumor growth. Many patients have advanced disease at presentation with large bleeding masses that extend to the pelvic sidewalls. After local extension, disease spreads within the abdomen and to the lungs and the supraclavicular lymph nodes.

Tissue diagnosis requires cervical biopsy, sometimes assisted by colposcopy. Staging usually requires an examination under anesthesia as well as cystoscopy to evaluate the bladder. Additional studies should include a chest x-ray and either a pelvic CT or MRI to assess local extent and nodal involvement. (Recent studies indicate that MRI scans may be more accurate.) The staging classification of the International Federation of Gynecology and Obstetrics (FIGO) is used (Table 16–8).

TREATMENT

A variety of local techniques, including biopsy, hot and cold cautery, laser treatment, surgical excision, cone biopsy, and hysterectomy, can eradicate preinvasive cervical neoplasia. The treatment of invasive cancer depends on the stage. Very early, superficially invasive (microinvasive) cancers may be treated with cone biopsy, although hysterectomy is more commonly employed. Once cancer progresses beyond microinvasion, more extensive treatment is required. This may include radical hysterectomy with pelvic and paraaortic lymph node dissection or radiation therapy. Surgery is more commonly used in younger women for ovarian preservation and avoidance of long-term radiation changes in uninvolved structures (bone marrow, bladder, rectum, and intestines). Radiation therapy is as effective as surgery for early-stage and for locally advanced disease. CT or MR scanning of paraaortic lymph nodes can detect disease requiring alteration in surgical or radiation approaches. Occasionally ultraradical surgery (pelvic exenteration) with creation of an ileal bladder and colostomy may be required for radiation failures. A current study is investigating whether the addition of cisplatin to radiation therapy will improve disease control rates for locally advanced disease.

Patients with distant metastases and those with recurrent cervical cancer present major management problems and are generally treated in a palliative fashion. Chemotherapy responses are infrequent and of limited duration. Cisplatin given at a dose of 50 mg/m^2 every 3 weeks achieves a response rate of 21 to 44% and is the most commonly used agent. However, responses usually last only a few months. Cisplatin-based combination chemotherapy regimens have been extensively studied; while some have had promising results, no substantial survival benefits occur owing to the brevity of response durations. Current research focuses on dose-intensive chemotherapy regimens aided by colony-stimulating factors and/or autologous bone marrow transplants, and clinical trials with cisplatin analogues and combined modality therapy with radiation and chemotherapy.

SURVIVAL

Stage-for-stage survival figures are the same for radiation therapy and for surgery. Disease rarely recurs after 3 years so that 5-year survival approximates cure. All patients

Table 16–8. **FIGO* STAGING FOR PRIMARY CARCINOMA OF THE CERVIX**

Stage	Description
Stage 0	Carcinoma in situ.
Stage I	Carcinoma confined to the cervix.
Stage Ia	Microinvasive carcinoma.
Stage Ib	All other cases of stage I.
Stage II	Carcinoma extends beyond cervix but not to the pelvic wall or lower vagina.
Stage IIa	No obvious parametrial involvement.
Stage IIb	Obvious parametrial involvement.
Stage III	Carcinoma extends to the pelvic wall or lower vagina or causes ureteral obstruction.
Stage IIIa	Extension onto the pelvic wall.
Stage IIIb	Extension onto the pelvic wall and hydronephrosis or nonfunctioning kidney.
Stage IV	Carcinoma beyond the true pelvis or invading bladder or rectum.
Stage IVa	Spread to adjacent organs.
Stage IVb	Spread to distant organs.

*International Federation of Gynecology and Obstetrics (1987).

with stage 0 are cured; 85 to 90% of those with stage I; 70 to 75% of those with stage II; 30 to 35% of those with stage III; and less than 10% of patients with stage IV disease are cured.

REFERENCES

Alberts DS, Mason-Liddil N: The role of cisplatin in the management of advanced squamous cell cancer of the cervix. Semin Oncol 16(suppl 6):66–78, 1989.
Cobby M, Browning J, Jones A, et al: Magnetic resonance imaging, computed tomography and endosonography in the local staging of carcinoma of the cervix. Br J Radiol 63:673–679, 1990.
Devesa SS, Young JL, Brinton LA, Fraumeni JF: Recent trends in cervix uteri cancer. Cancer 64:2184–2190, 1989.
Eddy DM: Screening for cervical cancer. Ann Intern Med 113:214–226, 1990.
Rader JS, Haraf DJ, Halpern HJ, et al: Radiation therapy in the treatment of cervical cancer: The University of Chicago/Michael Reese Hospital experience. J Surg Oncol 44:157–165, 1990.

VAGINAL CARCINOMA

Primary vaginal carcinoma is rare, accounting for only 1 to 2% of gynecologic malignancies. Metastatic cancer to the vagina is more common than primary vaginal cancer. The most common sites of origin are (in order of frequency): endometrium, colon, sarcoma, and breast.

Over 90% of vaginal carcinomas are of the squamous cell type, sharing characteristics of etiology, detection, and diagnosis with squamous cell cancer of the cervix. However, vaginal carcinoma has its peak incidence in the sixth and seventh decades. Squamous cell carcinomas of the vagina may arise many years after radiation treatment for other gynecologic malignancies and may be radiation induced. Clear cell adenocarcinomas of the vagina (and cervix) occur in women with a history of in utero exposure to diethylstilbestrol (DES). As little as 1.5 mg of DES daily initiated before the eighteenth week of gestation has been associated with vaginal adenocarcinoma in female offspring.

DIAGNOSIS AND STAGING

Vaginal discharge and bleeding are the only common symptoms of vaginal cancer, and 10 to 15% of patients present with silent lesions detected on routine pelvic examination and Pap smear. Colposcopy is valuable in directing vaginal biopsies and detecting in situ or preinvasive disease. The DES progeny often have benign changes associated with their previous drug exposure.

The staging of vaginal carcinoma has been outlined by the International Federation of Obstetrics and Gynecology (not shown). Stage depends largely on the degree of local invasion. Because local invasion has already occurred in many patients, most treatments achieve only limited success.

TREATMENT

Carcinoma in situ of the vagina has been successfully treated with 5-fluorouracil (5-FU) cream, which causes full-thickness desquamation of the underlying epithelium. Other locally ablative techniques include laser therapy and hot or cold cautery.

Radical surgery for vaginal cancer is difficult because of the close proximity of the bladder, urethra, and rectum and because of the advanced age of many of the patients. Most patients with invasive disease are treated with radiation therapy. A combination of external and intracavitary radiation is used. Vaginal atresia is a common complication, unless estrogen supplementation, vaginal dilatation, and/or regular sexual relations are maintained. Cure rates for stages I and II vary between 94 and 43%. Survival for patients with stages III and IV disease is less likely, and survival rates range from 50 to 0%.

Currently, no effective treatment exists for recurrent or advanced vaginal cancer. Research interests include combined modality treatment with radiotherapy and chemotherapy and new or multiple-agent chemotherapy regimens.

CARCINOMA OF THE VULVA

Vulvar cancer is uncommon, accounting for only 4% of gynecologic malignancies. Risk factors include a history of cervical cancer and infections with herpes simplex virus type II and human papilloma viruses. Five percent of vulvar cancers develop apparently within vulvar condylomata. Early superficially invasive disease may present as a single, raised, discolored papule. In older women, a long history of pruritus is typical. Cancers arise in areas of both chronic hyperplasia and atrophy.

The clinical appearance of vulvar cancer varies. Lesions are usually elevated and of variable color from white to pink to brown and often confluent or multicentric. Because of the association with cervical cancer, a complete pelvic examination and Pap smear are required. The FIGO classification is used for staging vulvar cancer (not shown). It is based on an assessment of the primary tumor, regional lymph nodes, and distant metastases. Chest x-ray, abdominopelvic CT or MR scanning, and possibly cystoscopy and proctoscopy may be required for clinical evaluation.

The mainstay of treatment is surgery. Most patients undergo a radical vulvectomy and bilateral inguinal node dissection. Patients with small or superficially invasive disease have also been treated with wide and deep local excision and unilateral superficial inguinal lymphadenectomy, whereas those with advanced disease are treated with radical vulvectomy, bilateral inguinal node dissection, and pelvic exenteration. In one recent study, the 5-year survival rate was 85% without inguinal node involvement and 39% when the inguinal or femoral nodes did show tumor involvement. Radiation therapy (sometimes supplemented with 5-FU) may decrease the need for the more radical surgical approaches for patients with early disease, and it may increase survival when patients with positive inguinal nodes receive pelvic node irradiation.

Recurrences may be local or systemic. Results with chemotherapy resemble those for vaginal and cervical cancer. Radiation is generally not effective for recurrent disease.

REFERENCES

Cavanagh D, Fiorica JV, Hoffman MS, et al: Invasive carcinoma of the vulva: Changing trends in surgical management. Am J Obstet Gynecol 163:1007–1015, 1990.

Pao WM, Perez CA, Kuske RR, et al: Radiation therapy and conservation surgery for primary and recurrent carcinoma of the vulva: Report of 40 patients and a review of the literature. Int J Radiat Oncol Biol Phys 14:1123–1132, 1988.

Perez CA, Camel HM, Galakatos AE, et al: Definitive irradiation in carcinoma of the vagina: Long-term evaluation of results. Int J Radiat Oncol Biol Phys 15:1283–1290, 1988.

Spirtos NM, Doshi BP, Kapp DS, Teng N: Radiation therapy for primary squamous cell carcinoma of the vagina: Stanford University experience. Gynecol Oncol 35:20–26, 1989.

17
SARCOMAS OF SOFT TISSUE AND BONE

Deepak Sahasrabudhe

SOFT TISSUE SARCOMAS

Malignant tumors of the primitive mesoderm are called soft tissue sarcomas. They arise in the extraskeletal supportive and connective tissues: the muscles, tendons, synovial tissues, fat, the endothelium of blood and lymphatic channels, and the mesothelium of visceral organs. These tumors of mesenchymal origin can occur in any anatomic site (Table 17–1), but they arise most commonly in the extremities.

While soft tissue sarcomas are heterogeneous, they are grouped together because of similarities in pathologic appearance, clinical presentation, and natural history. The following are some features common to soft tissue sarcomas: (1) enlargement in a centrifugal fashion; (2) presence of a mesenchymal pseudocapsule; (3) microprotrusions of tumor through the pseudocapsule; (4) hematogenous metastatic spread with lung as the most common site; (5) uncommon lymph node metastases (except for rhabdomyosarcoma and epithelioid sarcoma); and (6) direct extension from one major anatomic compartment to another.

INCIDENCE

Approximately 5900 new cases of soft tissue sarcoma and 3300 deaths from this disease will occur in the United States in 1992. Soft tissue sarcomas comprise about 0.7% of all malignancies but about 6.5% of all malignancies in children younger than 15. The median age of patients with sarcoma is 45 years, significantly younger than that of patients with carcinoma.

Table 17–2 lists the most common histologic types of soft tissue sarcomas. Recently, the incidence of Kaposi's sarcoma has risen dramatically in association with the acquired immune deficiency syndrome (AIDS) (Chap. 29). Clinical features of the soft tissue sarcomas can be quite characteristic (Table 17–3).

ETIOLOGY

Viruses and chemical carcinogens cause soft tissue sarcomas in laboratory animals. The etiologic data concerning human soft tissue sarcomas are less clear. The human immunodeficiency virus (HIV) contributes to the development of Kaposi's sarcoma in AIDS patients, but it is not directly causative. Herbicides (e.g., Agent Orange) and wood preservatives may increase the incidence of human sarcomas, but the data are conflicting. Thorium dioxide (Thorotrast) and vinyl chloride significantly increase the incidence of hepatic angiosarcomas, and asbestos increases the incidence of mesotheliomas. Bone sarcomas and to a lesser extent soft tissue sarcomas can represent late complications of radiation therapy.

Genetic factors are important in some soft tissue sarcomas. Patients with neurofibromatosis, tuberous sclerosis, Gardener's syndrome, and the Li-Fraumeni syndrome are at increased risk of soft tissue sarcomas. Numerous distinctive chromosomal abnormalities exist for different sarcomas (Table 17–4). Among them is the retinoblastoma gene on chromosome 13q14, which functions as a tumor suppressor gene. Deletions or mutations of both copies of this gene result in retinoblastomas as well as later osteosarcomas and soft tissue sarcomas.

PATHOLOGY

The cell of origin determines the classification of the soft tissue sarcomas. Specialized techniques such as immunohistochemical staining, electron microscopy, cytogenetic analysis, and flow cytometry help to categorize the sarcomas. However, the size of the primary

Table 17–1. **SITES OF SOFT TISSUE SARCOMAS**

Site	%
Head and neck	9%
Trunk/retroperitoneum	32%
Upper extremity	14%
Lower extremity	45%

From Chang AE, Rosenberg SA, Glatstein EJ, Antman KH: Sarcomas of soft tissues. *In* DeVita VT, Hellman S, Rosenberg SA (eds): Cancer: Principles and Practice of Oncology. 3rd ed. Philadelphia, JB Lippincott, 1989, p 1347.

Table 17–2. **RELATIVE INCIDENCE OF SOFT TISSUE SARCOMAS**

Type	%
Liposarcoma	34%
Malignant fibrous histiocytoma	15%
Tendosynovial sarcoma	13%
Fibrosarcoma	12%
Malignant peripheral nerve sarcoma	8%
Pleomorphic rhabdomyosarcoma	7%
Leiomyosarcoma	4%
Others	7%

Modified from Collin C, Hadju SI, Godbold J, et al: Localized, operable soft tissue sarcoma of the lower extremity. Arch Surg 121:1425–1433, 1986. Copyright 1986, American Medical Association.

Table 17–3. **CLINICAL FEATURES OF SOFT TISSUE SARCOMAS**

HISTOLOGIC TYPE	TISSUE OF ORIGIN	AGE	USUAL SITE	COMMENTS
Fibrosarcoma	Connective tissue, nerve sheath	All	Lower limb, trunk	One of the two most common types in adults
Liposarcoma	Adipose tissue	All	Lower limb, retroperitoneum	One of the two most common types in adults
Rhabdomyosarcoma	Striated muscle	All	Popliteal, gluteal, intrascapular, orbit	Most common in children
Synoviosarcoma	Synovium	Young adults	Knee, ankle	Often painful
Angiosarcoma	Blood vessels	Adults	Subcutaneous tissue, muscles	Previous chronic lymphedema
Malignant fibrous histiocytoma	Unknown	Adults	Trunk, extremities	Increasingly recognized subtype

Table 17–4. **CHROMOSOMAL CHANGES IN SARCOMA**

TUMOR	CHROMOSOME CHANGE
Synovial cell	t(X;18)(p11.2;q11.2)
Ewing's sarcoma	t(11;22)(q24;q12)
Peripheral neuroepithelioma	t(11;22)(q24;q12)
Neuroblastoma	del(1)(p32p36)
Liposarcoma (myxoid)	t(12;16)(q13;p11)
Retinoblastoma	del(13)(q14)
Rhabdomyosarcoma (alveolar)	t(2;13)(q37;q14)
Extraskeletal myxoid chondrosarcoma	t(9;15;22)(q31;q25;q12.2)
Esthesioneuroblastoma	t(11;22)(q24;q12)

From McClay EF: Epidemiology of bone and soft tissue sarcomas. Semin Oncol 16:264–272, 1989.

tumor and its histologic grade are better predictors of the metastatic propensity than the presumed cell of origin.

DIAGNOSIS AND STAGING

These tumors can be morphologically heterogeneous; therefore, adequate sampling is necessary. The appropriate diagnostic surgical technique for any suspected soft tissue sarcoma greater than 3 cm in diameter is incisional biopsy. Since the goal of treatment is to achieve local control while preserving function, evaluation prior to the biopsy by an experienced surgeon and a radiotherapist is optimal. The biopsy incision should be parallel to the long axis of the extremity, so the subsequent wide resection of the sarcoma can encompass the biopsy site while preserving lymphatic drainage of the distal portion of the extremity. Excisional biopsy and "shelling out" of a soft tissue sarcoma are inappropriate.

Optimal management of soft tissue sarcomas depends on accurate delineation of tumor extent. The complete diagnostic work-up includes history and physical examination, soft tissue x-ray of the affected part, computed tomography (CT) scan or preferably magnetic resonance imaging (MRI) of the anatomic region, and chest x-ray and chest CT scan. An arteriogram is often helpful in delineating the vascular supply for (1) feasibility of limb-sparing surgery; (2) assessment of vascular invasion; (3) determination of the venous drainage, which must be controlled intraoperatively to reduce the likelihood of tumor embolization; and (4) possible intra-arterial chemotherapy. A bone scan may be helpful in sarcomas that invade the periosteum or the bone.

The prognosis of patients with soft tissue sarcoma varies with histologic grade and size as well as primary site (proximal versus distal), lymph node involvement, and metastases (Table 17–5). The age and sex of the patient and the specific histologic subtype have less prognostic significance. More than 60% of patients present with either stage III or IV disease.

TREATMENT

Surgery

Complete surgical resection of soft tissue sarcomas, with microscopic tumor-free margins, is essential for optimal control. Local excision results in a local recurrence rate of 60 to 80%. With radical surgery (removal of an entire muscle group or involved anatomic compartment) or amputation, local recurrence rates drop to the 20% range. However, wide local resections or amputations result in significant functional and cosmetic disabilities. Current surgical techniques emphasize highly specialized but more conservative surgery that frequently avoids amputation but maintains adequate local control with the addition of radiation therapy. Involvement of the neurovascular structures or joint space by the tumor generally precludes limb-sparing surgery.

Radiotherapy

The purpose of surgery is to remove all evident tumor at the initial site of disease; radiation then eliminates any microscopic extensions into or beyond the pseudocapsule.

Table 17–5. **SOFT TISSUE SARCOMA: CLINICOPATHOLOGIC STAGING AND PROGNOSIS**

STAGE	COMMENTS	5-YEAR SURVIVAL (%)
1	Low grade (<1 mitoses/10 HPF*)	76
2	Intermediate grade (1–4 mitoses/10 HPF)	56
3	High grade (>5 mitoses/10 HPF)	26
4A†	Gross invasion of bone, major vessel, or nerve	
4B	Metastases	4

From Antman KH, Eilber FR, Shiu MH: Soft tissue sarcomas: Current trends in diagnosis and management. Curr Prob Cancer 13:340–367, 1989.

*HPF: High power field

†Lesion size: A <5 cm, grades 1–3; B >5 cm, grades 1–3.

With this approach, recurrence rates for lesions of the distal extremity range from 5 to 13%, and the functional and cosmetic results are excellent. Seventy-five percent of patients retain a useful limb, free of pain and edema. More proximal lesions show poorer rates of local control.

Radiation therapy may be given preoperatively or postoperatively. The usual dose of postoperative radiation is 60 Gy in 6 weeks for low-grade lesions and 65 Gy in 6½ weeks for high-grade lesions. Some institutions prefer preoperative radiation therapy at doses of 50 to 60 Gy over 5 to 6 weeks followed in 2 to 3 weeks by conservative resection of tumor. The advantages of preoperative radiotherapy are (1) reduction in the risk of intraoperative contamination of vascular spaces by viable tumor cells, (2) possibly a decreased volume of tissue to be irradiated, and (3) the lesser tumor bulk may allow an easier, more conservative surgery. Radiation without surgery is used in patients with inoperable disease or for those who refuse surgery. Local recurrence rates are higher than with the combined approach, but a small proportion of patients may be cured.

Adjuvant Chemotherapy

With appropriate combinations of surgery and radiation therapy, local control rates for extremity sarcomas are >90%; for truncal sarcomas, 50 to 75%; and for retroperitoneal sarcomas, 30 to 50%. Despite local control, the 5-year survival rate for adults with high-grade soft tissue sarcomas is only 40 to 60%. Virtually all deaths are due to metastatic disease. Numerous trials of adjuvant chemotherapy have attempted to improve survival in patients presenting with localized soft tissue sarcomas. Adjuvant studies have used single-agent Adriamycin (doxorubicin), with a response rate of 26% in advanced disease, or Adriamycin-based combination regimens. Comparisons with historical controls have shown improved disease-free and overall survival rates, particularly in patients with extremity lesions and significantly less so for truncal and head and neck lesions. However, randomized trials, for the most part, have failed to confirm these results.

Ten prospectively randomized trials of adjuvant chemotherapy with observation-only control arms used either single-agent Adriamycin or Adriamycin combinations (Table 17–6). Of the 10 trials, only 1 reported prolongation in both disease-free and overall survival, and the follow-up has been short (28 months). The National Cancer Institute trial comparing cyclophosphamide plus Adriamycin/methotrexate initially reported prolongation of disease-free and overall survival. With additional follow-up, the survival is no longer significantly different. This study resulted in a 56% incidence of abnormal cardiac function and a 14% incidence of overt clinical congestive heart failure. The 10 randomized studies of adjuvant chemotherapy did demonstrate a prolonged disease-free survival in the treated patients. A Mayo Clinic study showed that chemotherapy may also reduce the number of pulmonary metastases.

Table 17–6. **ADJUVANT CHEMOTHERAPY TRIALS FOR SOFT TISSUE SARCOMAS OF THE EXTREMITY**

		DISEASE-FREE SURVIVAL (%)		OVERALL SURVIVAL (%)	
INSTITUTION	**DRUGS**	**Obs**	**Chemo**	**Obs**	**Chemo**
Rizzoli Institute	Adriamycin	45	73*	70	91*
DCFI/MGH	Adriamycin	81	89	81	88
ECOG	Adriamycin	71	72	71	64
ISSG	Adriamycin	53	79	76	79
UCLA	Adriamycin	58	58	75	78
SCAND	Adriamycin	55	52	44	40
NCI	ACM	28	54	60	54
MD Anderson	ACVAd	35	55	57	65
MAYO	AVDAd	67	88	83	63
EORTC	ACVD	66	77	74	81

Modified from Elias AD, Antman KH: Adjuvant chemotherapy for soft tissue sarcoma: An approach in search of an effective regimen. Semin Oncol 16:305–311, 1989.

Abbreviations: Obs, observation only; Chemo, chemotherapy; A, Adriamycin; C, cyclophosphamide; M, methotrexate; V, vincristine; Ad, dactinomycin; D, DTIC.

*p <.05.

Because of its failure to achieve statistically significant improvement in overall survival, adjuvant chemotherapy of soft tissue sarcomas remains investigational. Randomized clinical trials that include a "no treatment" control arm continue, and patients with soft tissue sarcomas should be offered the opportunity to participate.

These conclusions regarding adjuvant chemotherapy pertain to adult soft tissue sarcomas and not to childhood disease. Childhood sarcomas are more responsive to chemotherapy, and adjuvant chemotherapy is standard treatment for most childhood sarcomas. The discussion of the management of pediatric malignancies is beyond the scope of this book.

Chemotherapy for Advanced Disease

Approximately 10% of patients with soft tissue sarcomas present with disseminated disease, and another 40 to 50% develop distant metastases within 5 years of initial diagnosis. Systemic chemotherapy for soft tissue sarcomas first demonstrated benefit in children with rhabdomyosarcoma. Vincristine, actinomycin D, and cyclophosphamide (VAC) produced response rates of 80% in children. Adult sarcomas do not respond as often or as completely to chemotherapy as childhood sarcomas. The VAC regimen produces only a 20% response rate in adult sarcomas and no improvement in survival. Adriamycin is the most active single agent, with a dose-response relationship requiring doses of 20 to 25 mg/m²/week for response rates of >20%. Continuous intravenous infusion of Adriamycin has comparable activity to bolus administration but reduced cardiac toxicity.

All the multidrug combinations currently in use employ Adriamycin (Table 17–7). Other active agents include DTIC (dacarbazine), ifosfamide (along with the uroepithelial protective agent mesna), cyclophosphamide, methotrexate, actinomycin D, and the nitrosoureas. Prospectively randomized trials comparing combination chemotherapy (Adriamycin plus DTIC, or cyclophosphamide, vincristine, Adriamycin plus DTIC) to single-agent Adriamycin have not demonstrated any advantage in overall survival for the combination regimens. The combinations produce higher response rates, but only at the cost of greater toxicity.

A combination of mesna, Adriamycin, ifosfamide, and dacarbazine (MAID) achieves a response rate of 47%, including 10% complete responses. The median duration of response is 10 months. Neutropenic fevers requiring hospitalization occur in 25% of the courses. MAID is currently under investigation as an adjuvant regimen in adult soft tissue sarcomas.

Surgery for Metastatic Disease

Continued, aggressive, surgical excision of local recurrences and accessible metastatic disease may improve survival. In a Mayo Clinic report of adjuvant chemotherapy, patients with soft tissue sarcomas entered on study after surgery for locally recurrent disease had almost the same survival as those entered after surgery for primary disease. An alternative approach is to administer two cycles of Adriamycin-based chemotherapy to establish drug sensitivity preoperatively. Postoperative chemotherapy is administered if the metastases were sensitive preoperatively.

Table 17–7. **CHEMOTHERAPY REGIMENS FOR SOFT TISSUE SARCOMAS**

AGENTS	DOSE	INTERVAL
Adriamycin	60–75 mg/m² IV	3 weeks
ADIC		
Adriamycin	60 mg/m² IV, day 1	3 weeks
Dacarbazine	250 mg/m² IV, days 1–5	
MAID		
Mesna	2500 mg/m² day CIV,* days 1–4	3 weeks
Adriamycin	20 mg/m²/day CIV, days 1–3	
Ifosfamide	2500 mg/m²/day CIV, days 1–3	
Dacarbazine	300 mg/m²/day CIV, days 1–3	

*CIV: continuous intravenous infusion.

REFERENCES

Eilber FR, Huth JF, Mirra J, Rosen G: Progress in the recognition and treatment of soft tissue sarcomas. Cancer 65:660–666, 1990.
Elias AD, Ryan L, Sulks A, et al: Response to mesna, Adriamycin, ifosfamide, and dacarbazine in 108 patients with metastatic or unresectable sarcoma and no prior chemotherapy. J Clin Oncol 7:1208–1216, 1989.
Mazanet R, Antman KH: Sarcomas of soft tissue and bone. Cancer 68:463–473, 1991.
Kane MJ: Chemotherapy for advanced soft tissue and osteosarcoma. Semin Oncol 16:297–304, 1989.
Tepper J: Role of radiation therapy in the management of patients with bone and soft tissue sarcomas. Semin Oncol 16:281–288, 1989.
Yang JC, Rosenberg SA: Surgery for adult patients with soft tissue sarcomas. Semin Oncol 16:289–296, 1989.

OSTEOGENIC SARCOMA

INCIDENCE AND ETIOLOGY

Osteogenic sarcoma is the most common primary bone malignancy, with about 900 new cases reported in the United States each year. The disease affects males 1.6 times as often as females, and the peak incidence occurs in the 10- to 25-year age group. It represents 5% of all childhood cancers. Virtually any bone may be involved, but most tumors arise in the femur, tibia, and humerus. Primary osteosarcomas of the axial skeleton account for less than 10% of cases.

Paget's disease of bone and high-dose radiation therapy are the only known predisposing conditions. About 5% of patients with Paget's disease develop osteosarcoma, and the prognosis for these tumors is worse than that of osteosarcoma arising in normal bone. Patients with retinoblastoma are at increased risk for osteogenic sarcomas. Both malignancies share deletions of the retinoblastoma (tumor suppressor) gene on chromosome 13.

CLINICAL MANIFESTATIONS

Osteogenic sarcomas extend locally beyond the intramedullary cavity to produce cortical destruction, involvement of adjacent soft tissues, and consequent pain and swelling. X-ray findings include periosteal reaction and elevation in the characteristic sunburst or onion-skin appearance. The lesion itself usually combines lytic and blastic features. Diagnosis requires an open biopsy with meticulous technique to permit subsequent limb-sparing, curative resection.

Laboratory evaluation reveals elevation of the serum alkaline phosphatase in about half of all patients. CT scan or MRI of the affected bone is necessary to detect skip lesions that occur at a distance from the primary tumor. Magnetic resonance imaging provides more detailed information about involvement of neurovascular bundles, joints, and soft tissues. Chest x-ray and chest CT scan are essential for detection of pulmonary metastases. Arteriography may help in the selection of the appropriate primary surgical procedure. A bone survey and radionuclide bone scan may disclose the rare instances of multifocal primary osteogenic sarcoma. Table 17–8 shows the TNM staging system for bone sarcomas.

Periosteal and paraosteal osteogenic sarcomas have a more favorable prognosis than the more common central tumors. Osteosarcomas arising in the extremities have a better outlook than axial tumors, and patients with tibial lesions have a better survival than those with distal femur lesions. Poor histologic differentiation correlates with poor prognosis.

TREATMENT

Surgery

Selected patients now undergo limb-sparing surgery rather than amputation with equivalent survival. Limb-sparing procedures preserve the function of the affected limb and maintain or improve the rate of local control by using specialized, conservative surgery and chemotherapy. Only those tumors that can be resected with clear surgical margins are candidates for limb-sparing surgery. Reconstruction follows tumor resection and

Table 17–8. **STAGING FOR OSTEOSARCOMA**

HISTOPATHOLOGIC GRADE (G)				
G1	Well differentiated			
G2	Moderately differentiated			
G3	Poorly differentiated			
G4	Undifferentiated			
PRIMARY TUMOR (T)				
T0	No evidence of primary tumor			
T1	Tumor confined within the cortex			
T2	Tumor invades beyond the cortex			
REGIONAL LYMPH NODES (N)				
N0	No regional lymph node metastasis			
N1	Regional lymph node metastasis			
DISTANT METASTASIS (M)				
MX	Presence of distant metastasis cannot be assessed			
M0	No distant metastasis			
M1	Distant metastasis			
STAGE GROUPING				
Stage IA	G 1,2	T1	N0	M0
Stage IB	G 1,2	T2	N0	M0
Stage IIA	G 3,4	T1	N0	M0
Stage IIB	G 3,4	T2	N0	M0
Stage III		Not defined		
Stage IVA	Any G	Any T	N1	M0
Stage IVB	Any G	Any T	Any N	M1

From American Joint Committee on Cancer: Beahrs OH, Henson DE, Hutter RVP, Myers MH (eds): Manual for Staging of Cancer. 3rd edition. Philadelphia, JB Lippincott, 1988.

provides limb function superior to or (at least) equal to a postamputation prosthesis. Preoperative chemotherapy may allow limb-sparing procedures in some patients who were initially not suitable candidates. The optimal limb-sparing treatment strategy varies, and patients must be carefully selected and treated at facilities with the required expertise.

Complete resection of pulmonary metastases achieves long-term control in approximately 30 to 40% of patients with resectable lung metastases. Some patients undergo multiple thoracotomies with reported long-term survival. Because of the possibility of surgical "salvage" therapy, postprimary treatment follow-up includes 2 years of monthly chest x-rays with chest CT scans and bone scans every 6 months.

Chemotherapy for Advanced Disease

Systemic chemotherapy is standard for unresectable, metastatic, or recurrent osteogenic sarcoma. Response rates for active agents include Adriamycin, 20 to 25%; high-dose methotrexate with leucovorin rescue, 30 to 40%; and cisplatin 20 to 25%. Combinations of bleomycin, cyclophosphamide, and actinomycin D (BCD) and ifosfamide plus etoposide are also quite active. However, there is no single best regimen, and patients should be offered participation in clinical trials.

Eighty percent of osteosarcoma relapses occur in the lung, and 90% of relapses occur within 2 years of diagnosis. Pulmonary metastases are aggressively resected whenever possible. It is not clear whether chemotherapy provides additional benefit in these patients. Pulmonary recurrences in patients treated with initial adjuvant chemotherapy develop later and in smaller numbers than in patients treated initially with surgery alone.

Adjuvant Chemotherapy

With active chemotherapy available for advanced disease and an 80% relapse rate following surgery alone, a great deal of clinical investigation has focused on adjuvant chemotherapy for osteosarcoma. Initial studies demonstrated improvement in disease-free and overall survival using Adriamycin or high-dose methotrexate. However, the validity of these studies was debated because only historical controls were used, and some felt the improvement in survival was due to more aggressive surgical management of metastatic disease rather than to the effects of adjuvant chemotherapy.

Three randomized, controlled studies of adjuvant chemotherapy for osteosarcoma have produced conflicting results. The earliest trial conducted at the Mayo Clinic did not find benefit for adjuvant, high-dose methotrexate compared with surgery alone. Two later trials compared BCD plus high-dose methotrexate and Adriamycin plus or minus cisplatin with surgical controls, and both demonstrated statistically significant improvement in disease-free survival and one in overall survival. Therefore, most centers routinely treat osteosarcoma patients with adjuvant chemotherapy. Recently, a comparison of BCD plus high-dose methotrexate versus the same drugs plus Adriamycin and cisplatin concluded that six drugs were superior to four. Both groups received preoperative chemotherapy.

Neoadjuvant Chemotherapy

Preoperative (neoadjuvant) systemic or intra-arterial chemotherapy has potential advantages over the more common postoperative regimens. Neoadjuvant treatment avoids delay in initiation of chemotherapy while awaiting surgery. Response to neoadjuvant treatment may allow less aggressive, limb-sparing surgery for patients initially not candidates for this operation. Neoadjuvant treatment also permits an assessment of treatment efficacy against each individual tumor, allowing alteration in the chemotherapy regimen postoperatively in cases of tumor resistance (the concept of *tailored* chemotherapy). These promising results need confirmation in cooperative group settings. Therefore, neoadjuvant chemotherapy remains investigational.

REFERENCES

Consensus Conference: Limb-sparing treatment of adult soft-tissue sarcomas and osteosarcomas. JAMA 254:1791–1794, 1985.
Eilber FR, Rosen G: Adjuvant chemotherapy for osteosarcoma. Semin Oncol 16:312–323, 1989.
Link M, Goorin A, Miser A, et al: The role of adjuvant chemotherapy in the treatment of osteosarcoma of the extremity. N Engl J Med 314:1600–1606, 1986.
Taylor WF, Ivins JC, Unni KK, et al: Prognostic variables in osteosarcoma: A multiinstitutional study. J Natl Cancer Inst 81:21–30, 1989.
Winkler K, Bielack S, Bieling P: Osteosarcoma. Curr Opin Oncol 2:486–490, 1990.

EWING'S SARCOMA

Ewing's sarcoma is a highly malignant small round cell tumor of bone occurring in children and adolescents. The disease is uncommon below age 5 and above age 30; peak incidence is in the late teens. Ewing's sarcoma occurs more often in males than in females and is much more common in whites than in blacks. The etiology is unknown.

PATHOLOGY

Pathologic examination reveals sheets of uniform small round blue cells. Differential diagnosis includes lymphoma, neuroblastoma, rhabdomyosarcoma, primitive neuroectodermal tumors (PNET), and peripheral neuroepithelioma. Special tests such as immunohistochemical staining, electron microscopy for evaluation of ultrastructure, and cytogenetic analysis to detect the 11:22 translocation are helpful in diagnosis.

CLINICAL MANIFESTATIONS

Ewing's sarcoma may arise in any bone but occurs most often in the pelvic bones, femur, humerus, and ribs. Pain and swelling represent the usual initial complaints; fever, weight loss, and fatigue are often present as well. About 25% of patients have metastatic disease (to bone or lung) at the time of diagnosis. Characteristic radiologic features (not always present) include extensive permeation of the bone and laminated periosteal elevation (onionskin appearance). MRI provides the best delineation of bone cortex penetration and soft tissue involvement. Diagnosis requires biopsy.

TREATMENT

Pretreatment evaluation for patients with Ewing's sarcoma is similar to that for osteogenic sarcoma with the addition of a bone marrow biopsy. No generally accepted staging classification for Ewing's sarcoma exists. Factors indicating a poor prognosis include a proximal or axial skeleton primary tumor, large size of the primary tumor, elevated serum LDH level, and metastatic disease. With local therapy alone (excisional biopsy or biopsy and radiation), 10% of patients with Ewing's sarcoma will survive.

Preoperative and/or postoperative systemic chemotherapy significantly improves survival. Combined modality treatment consists of chemotherapy, including vincristine, Adriamycin, cyclophosphamide, and dactinomycin together with radiotherapy (30 to 55 Gy). With this approach, 5-year survival for patients with nonmetastatic Ewing's sarcoma is 80%. Metastatic Ewing's sarcoma is incurable with conventional approaches, but the 5-year survival is 20 to 30%. High-dose chemotherapy plus total body irradiation followed by autologous bone marrow transplantation may cure some patients with pulmonary metastases, but patient numbers are small and follow-up brief. Intensive chemotherapy regimens with ifosfamide and etoposide are under investigation.

REFERENCES

Grier HE: Ewing's sarcoma of bone. Curr Opin Oncol 2:491–494, 1990.

Hayes FA, Thompson EI, Meyer WH, et al: Therapy for localized Ewing's sarcoma of bone. J Clin Oncol 7:208–213, 1989.

Hayes FA, Thompson EI, Parvey L, et al: Metastatic Ewing's sarcoma: Remission induction and survival. J Clin Oncol 5:1199–1204, 1987.

Horowitz ME: Ewing's sarcoma: Current status of diagnosis and treatment. Oncology 3:101–109, 1989.

Jurgens H, Exner U, Gadner H, et al: Multidisciplinary treatment of primary Ewing's sarcoma of bone. Cancer 61:23–32, 1988.

18
CANCERS OF THE HEAD AND NECK

Kishan J. Pandya

INCIDENCE, ETIOLOGY, AND EPIDEMIOLOGY

Head and neck cancers include tumors arising in the oral cavity, pharynx (oropharynx, nasopharynx, and hypopharynx), larynx, nasal fossa, and paranasal sinuses. Tumors of the salivary glands are also included in this chapter. Approximately 42,800 new cases of head and neck cancer will be diagnosed in the United States in 1992, resulting in approximately 11,600 deaths (Table 18–1). While head and neck cancers account for less than 3% of cancer deaths in the United States, in Southeast Asia these tumors are responsible for 15 to 20% of all cancer deaths.

The incidence of head and neck cancer is about three times higher in males than in females and increases with age. Several risk factors associated with head and neck cancer have been identified: poor oral hygiene, chronic irritation such as from ill-fitting dentures, tobacco smoking, tobacco chewing, and the use of betel nut. Heavy use of alcohol is also an important risk factor. It is estimated that at least 90% of head and neck cancers arise as a result of exposure to known environmental factors. Nasopharyngeal cancer, a relatively common tumor in the countries of Southeast Asia, appears to have an association with the Epstein-Barr virus.

PATHOLOGY

The great majority of head and neck cancers are squamous or epidermoid carcinomas of varying degrees of differentiation. As a general rule, epidermoid carcinomas arising from the lip and buccal mucosa tend to be better differentiated than carcinomas arising farther posteriorly. A correlation exists between the degree of differentiation and the aggressiveness of the tumor.

Nonepidermoid tumors are chiefly derived from glandular tissues. Salivary gland tumors exhibit a variety of histopathologies and arise predominantly from the parotids. Adenocarcinomas may originate from the nasopharynx, maxillary sinus, and nose. Other malignancies encountered in the head and neck region include lymphomas arising from the tonsil, nasal fossa, and nasopharynx and sarcomas arising from the mandible and the maxillary sinus.

CLINICAL FEATURES

A large number of vital structures are present in limited space in the head and neck region, and therefore tumors arising from these structures usually produce early symptoms. However, since the population at risk is largely composed of elderly men who are usually

Table 18–1. **HEAD AND NECK CANCER INCIDENCE AND MORTALITY, 1991**

	ESTIMATED NEW CASES			ESTIMATED DEATHS		
SITE	**Male**	**Female**	**Total**	**Male**	**Female**	**Total**
Lip	3100	500	3600	75	25	100
Tongue	3900	2300	6200	1200	650	1850
Pharynx	6700	2700	9400	2600	1200	3800
Mouth	6900	4700	11,600	1400	1000	2400
Larynx	10,000	2500	12,500	2900	750	3650
TOTAL	30,600	12,700	43,300	8175	3625	11,800

From Boring CC, Squires TS, Tong T: Cancer statistics, 1991. CA 41:19–36, 1991.

addicted to tobacco and alcohol, warning symptoms may not be heeded, and lesions are often far advanced at the time of first presentation. In some cases, presenting symptoms may be insidious. Symptoms due to tumor in the nasal chamber and the paranasal sinuses may be attributed to chronic inflammatory conditions. Pain in the ear or hearing loss may be the presenting symptom of tumors in the nasopharynx and pharynx. Pain and difficulty in swallowing may be produced by tumors of the oral cavity, hypopharynx, or larynx. A common symptom of laryngeal lesions is a change in voice or hoarseness.

Although most head and neck cancers remain localized and produce the vast majority of their clinical manifestations from local and regional disease, distant metastases do occur. Cancers of the larynx and hypopharynx have a greater tendency to metastasize than cancers of the oral cavity. Cancers of the true vocal cords rarely metastasize, however. Locally advanced tumors and those with extensive nodal involvement are much more likely to spread than small, well-circumscribed cancers. Lung, liver, and bone comprise the most common metastatic sites. However, a solitary pulmonary nodule in a patient with head and neck cancer is more likely to represent a second primary cancer of the lung than a metastasis from the head and neck tumor.

DIAGNOSIS

A complete and careful history, with particular attention to symptoms pertaining to the head and neck region, accompanied by a thorough physical examination, forms the basis of the diagnostic evaluation. A complete examination must include palpation of the floor of the mouth, base of the tongue, and entire oral cavity. Palpation of the region also includes salivary glands and regional lymph nodes. A thorough examination of the nasopharynx, hypopharynx, and larynx requires the use of direct or indirect laryngoscopy. Cranial nerves should also be examined, including both sensory and motor functions.

Radiologic procedures such as plain films, computed tomography (CT) scans, magnetic resonance imaging (MRI), and polytomograms should be performed as indicated. Finally, tissue must be obtained by appropriate biopsy techniques.

STAGING

The treatment of head and neck tumors varies considerably according to the site of origin and extent of disease. Appropriate pretreatment evaluation and staging are therefore of paramount importance. A comparison of different treatments is greatly facilitated by a uniform system of classification and staging. The TNM system includes standard classifications for cancers of the oral cavity, pharynx, larynx, paranasal sinuses, and salivary glands. The tumor (T) classifications for each anatomic site are roughly similar, with higher T levels indicating larger tumor size and/or greater depth of invasion into adjacent structures. However, the T classifications vary in specific detail because of differences in anatomic areas; the individual T classifications for each site will be found in standard references. Classification with respect to regional nodes (N) and distant metastasis (M) is common to all sites and is shown in Table 18–2. The stage grouping of head and neck cancers based on the TNM classification is also included.

TREATMENT

A multidisciplinary approach is essential to the planning and execution of treatment for cancers of the head and neck. It should enlist the joint cooperative efforts of the surgeon, pathologist, radiotherapist, and medical oncologist. A rehabilitation team consisting of a maxillofacial prosthodontist, speech therapist, psychologist, and social worker should also be available.

SURGERY AND RADIOTHERAPY

Surgery and radiotherapy are the two primary modalities for local treatment of cancers of the head and neck. In general, small lesions in accessible sites can be treated either

Table 18–2. **TNM CLASSIFICATION OF HEAD AND NECK CANCERS**

PRIMARY TUMOR (T)			
Specific classification for each head neck site			
LYMPH NODE (N)			
NX	Regional lymph nodes cannot be assessed		
NO	No regional lymph node metastasis		
N1	Metastasis in a single ipsilateral lymph node, 3 cm or less in greatest dimension		
N2	Metastasis in a single ipsilateral lymph node, more than 3 cm but not more than 6 cm in greatest dimension or in multiple ipsilateral lymph nodes, none more than 6 cm in greatest dimension; or in bilateral or contralateral lymph nodes, none more than 6 cm in greatest dimension.		
N3	Metastasis in a lymph node more than 6 cm in greatest dimension		
DISTANT METASTASIS (M)			
MX	Presence of distant metastasis cannot be assessed		
M0	No distant metastasis		
M1	Distant metastasis		
STAGE GROUPING			
Stage 0	Tis	N0	M0
Stage I	T1	N0	M0
Stage II	T2	N0	M0
Stage III	T3	N0	M0
	T1–T3	N1	M0
Stage IV	T4	N0, N1	M0
	Any T	N2, N3	M0
	Any T	Any N	M1

From American Joint Committee on Cancer: Beahrs OH, Henson DE, Hutter RVP, Myers MH (eds): Manual for Staging Cancer. 3rd edition. Philadelphia, JB Lippincott, 1988.

with surgery or radiotherapy with equally good results. The choice of therapy in these cases depends on tumor location, patient preference, and available expertise. Five-year disease-free survivals of 80 to 90% are commonly achieved with T1 lesions of the lip or larynx. Larger, more invasive lesions, particularly those associated with positive regional nodes, usually require a combination of surgery and radiotherapy. There is no agreement on the proper extent of each modality and the optimal sequence of treatment. Tumors arising in inaccessible locations (i.e., nasopharynx) receive radiotherapy regardless of extent. Tumors in some sites—hypopharynx and pyriform sinus, for example—present with bulky disease and have a high incidence of involved nodes at diagnosis; in other sites such as larynx, anterior tongue, and lip, tumors are often detected when small. Prognosis is closely related to stage.

Overall, about 60 to 65% of patients with head and neck cancer will be cured with surgery, radiotherapy, or both. The remainder, however, who present with advanced disease or develop locoregional recurrences with or without distant metastases following initial treatment will require additional therapy. The majority of deaths from head and neck cancer occur as a result of uncontrolled locoregional disease.

CHEMOTHERAPY

Traditionally, the role of chemotherapy in head and neck cancer has been a palliative one, administered to bedridden patients in poor nutritional state with recurrent or metastatic carcinoma at the end stage of the disease. Not surprisingly, the benefit of chemotherapy to such patients has been minimal. Response rates to single-agent chemotherapy in such patients have been low and response durations very brief. Higher response rates have been reported with several combination chemotherapy regimens, and in recent years systemic treatment has been increasingly employed before local treatment of large invasive lesions (see below). Despite improved response rates, randomized trials to date have failed to confirm any survival advantage for combination chemotherapy over single-agent treatment in patients with recurrent or metastatic head and neck cancers.

In general, patients with prior surgery and/or radiotherapy do not respond as well to chemotherapy as those without prior treatment. Patients with better nutritional and performance status have better response rates and survivals. It is important, therefore, to improve the nutritional status of these patients and to include nutritional support in the overall management plan.

Single-Agent Chemotherapy

Several single agents have activity, including methotrexate, bleomycin, cisplatin, and 5-fluorouracil (5-FU). Methotrexate is the most extensively studied single agent and produces an overall response rate of about 30% (Table 18–3). The median duration of response is 3 to 5 months. Weekly or biweekly regimens using dosages of 40 to 60 mg/m^2 appear to achieve the best results with minimum toxicity. Myelosuppression and mucositis are the major dose-limiting toxicities and are particularly troublesome in debilitated patients with impaired hepatic and renal function. Intra-arterial therapy may be used for developing high regional concentrations of the drug, but overall response rates attained with this method are no higher than with systemic administration. Toxicities and complications with intra-arterial therapy are much greater; therefore, this approach is unwarranted for routine (nonexperimental) use. Methotrexate has also been used in high doses with leucovorin rescue. However, several trials failed to demonstrate any advantage for the high-dose methotrexate regimen over the conventional-dose standard treatment; therefore, the high-dose program is not recommended.

Bleomycin has been extensively studied in head and neck cancer and produces response rates of 20%. Response durations are usually brief. Because this agent causes negligible myelosuppression, it is frequently used in combination regimens. However, other side effects of bleomycin, including pulmonary toxicity and mucositis, may be severe.

Cisplatin is also active in the treatment of head and neck cancers, with response rates in patients with advanced disease ranging from 16 to 40%. Although many believe that this drug does have a dose-response curve, a recent randomized study revealed no evidence of dose dependency of cisplatin activity in head and neck cancer. Cisplatin is most commonly given as a daily dose of 20 mg/m^2 for 5 days or as a single dose of 100 mg/m^2, both used in combination with a 96-hour infusion of 5-FU.

5-FU produces a response rate ranging from 15 to 20%. There are at least four doses and schedules in clinical use; the most commonly used regimen is a 96-hour infusion combined with cisplatin (see below).

Other cytotoxic agents with activity against head and neck cancer include carboplatin, hydroxyurea, cyclophosphamide, vinca alkaloids, BCNU, Adriamycin (doxorubicin), and mitomycin C.

Combination Chemotherapy

Results of numerous combination chemotherapy regimens in patients with recurrent or metastatic head and neck cancers have been reported. While higher response rates are generally seen with combination chemotherapy, toxicity is greater and no improvement in survival is achieved compared with methotrexate as a single agent. Selected symptomatic patients with good performance status may benefit from the higher response rates produced by combination chemotherapy with the resultant improvement in cancer-related symptoms. The combination of cisplatin and 5-FU infusion for 96 to 120 hours has produced the highest response rates thus far (70 to 84%) and is the most commonly used palliative combination chemotherapy. This and other combinations reported in the literature are shown in Table 18–4.

Table 18–3. **SINGLE-AGENT CHEMOTHERAPY FOR HEAD AND NECK CANCERS**

AGENT	DOSE	FREQUENCY	RESPONSE (%)
Methotrexate	40–60 mg/m^2 IV	Weekly	30
Bleomycin	15 U/m^2, IV or IM	Weekly	20
Cisplatin	80–120 mg/m^2 IV	Every 3 weeks	30
5-Fluorouracil	400–500 mg/m^2, IV, days 1–5	Every 4–5 weeks	
	500–600 mg/m^2, IV	Weekly	15
	800–1500 mg/m^2/24 hr, days 1–5	Every 3–4 weeks	

Table 18–4. **COMBINATION CHEMOTHERAPY FOR HEAD AND NECK CANCERS**

AGENTS	DOSE	FREQUENCY	RESPONSE (%)
Methotrexate	40 mg/m^2, days 1, 15	3 weeks	61
Bleomycin	10 mg, days 1, 8, 15		
Cisplatin	50 mg/m^2, day 4		
Cisplatin	120 mg/m^2, day 6	4 weeks	46
Vincristine	0.5 mg/m^2, days 1, 4		
Bleomycin	30 mg/24 hr, days 1–4		
Cisplatin	100 mg/m^2, day 1	3 weeks	70
5-Fluorouracil	1000 mg/m^2/24 hr, days 1–4		

ADJUVANT CHEMOTHERAPY

Traditional adjuvant chemotherapy, i.e., chemotherapy after locoregional treatment with surgery and/or radiation therapy, has thus far produced no improvement in disease-free or overall survival. Cisplatin-based regimens are currently being evaluated in this setting. In general, postirradiation chemotherapy produces significant toxicity and results in poor patient compliance. To overcome this problem, the Head and Neck Intergroup Study is conducting a randomized trial of conventional postoperative radiation therapy versus cisplatin plus 5-FU infusion for three cycles, followed by radiation therapy.

CONCURRENT CHEMOTHERAPY AND RADIOTHERAPY

Another approach intended to achieve better local as well as systemic control of the disease, especially in patients with locally advanced tumors, is the use of concurrent chemotherapy and radiotherapy. This strategy has resulted in a higher complete response rate as well as prolonged disease-free survival compared with radiation therapy alone but has yet to conclusively demonstrate a prolongation of overall survival. Most commonly employed regimens for this approach include cisplatin either alone or in combination with 5-fluorouracil infusion.

NEOADJUVANT OR INDUCTION CHEMOTHERAPY

Interest and enthusiasm have arisen in recent years in the concept of neoadjuvant or induction chemotherapy—that is, the use of chemotherapy prior to surgery and radiotherapy in patients with locally advanced tumors with a high risk of recurrence. In theory, chemotherapy would debulk the tumor, facilitating surgery and rendering otherwise inoperable lesions operable. By decreasing tumor size, successful chemotherapy might also improve oxygenation, thus improving the effectiveness of radiation. Some chemotherapeutic agents might also serve as radiation sensitizers. In addition, adjuvant chemotherapy would also be expected to perform its traditional role, the destruction of micrometastases.

Numerous trials with a variety of regimens have demonstrated that this approach is feasible and that locally advanced lesions can be improved and in some cases eradicated by preoperative chemotherapy in a majority of patients. Response rates are high (70 to 80% in many series), and complete response rates are also substantial (about 20%). Randomized trials to date have demonstrated no improvement in survival with this approach, but a decrease in relapses and distant metastases is seen. In addition, some responding patients have been treated with definitive radiation therapy and have avoided surgery, thus preserving their organs (particularly the larynx). These findings have provided the impetus for continued clinical trials in this area.

SALIVARY GLAND CANCERS

Parotid tumors account for roughly 80% of all salivary gland tumors, with the submandibular, sublingual, and minor salivary glands comprising the rest. While only 20% of parotid tumors are malignant, more than 50% of the tumors arising from the other salivary glands are cancers. Tumors of the salivary glands exhibit a variety of histopathologies.

Most patients present with a mass near the ear, which, if associated with ulceration, fixation, or facial nerve involvement, is highly suggestive of malignancy. Primary treatment consists of surgery, which may include partial mandibulectomy and radical neck dissection in advanced cases. Radiotherapy is often utilized for residual or recurrent tumor. A retrospective report suggests that a combined modality approach with surgery plus radiotherapy may be superior to surgery alone.

Very limited data exist on the role of chemotherapy in salivary gland tumors. A variety of single agents appears to have activity, and a combination of cisplatin, Adriamycin, and cyclophosphamide seems promising on the basis of small numbers of patients.

REFERENCES

Brady LM (ed): Head and neck cancer. Semin Oncol 15:1–102, 1988.

Clark JR, Dreyfuss A: The role of cisplatin in treatment regimens for squamous cell carcinoma of the head and neck. Semin Oncol 18(suppl 3):34–48, 1991.

Decker J, Goldstein JC: Risk factors in head and neck cancer. N Engl J Med 30:1151–1155, 1982.

Erwin TJ, Clark JR, Werchselbaum RR, et al: An analysis of induction and adjuvant chemotherapy in the multidisciplinary treatment of squamous cell carcinoma of the head and neck. J Clin Oncol 5:10–20, 1987.

Feder M, Gonzalez MF: Nasopharyngeal carcinoma. Am J Med 79:365–369, 1985.

Jacobs C: The internist in the management of head and neck cancer. Ann Intern Med 113:771–778, 1990.

Johns ME, Goldsmith MM: Current management of salivary gland tumors. Oncology 3:85–91, 1989.

Johns ME, Goldsmith MM: Incidence, diagnosis and classification of salivary gland tumors. Oncology 3:47–58, 1989.

19
MALIGNANT MELANOMA

Craig S. McCune

INCIDENCE AND ETIOLOGY

Melanoma accounts for 3% of all cancers. The National Cancer Institute estimates there will be 32,000 new cases and 6700 deaths from melanoma in the United States in 1992. The incidence is rising sharply at a rate of 4.5% annually, which will double the incidence in less than 20 years. Although definitive proof of causation is lacking, the increased incidence corresponds to greater sun exposure with changes in clothing styles and more leisure time. Melanomas rarely occur in children; the peak incidence occurs in the fifth to seventh decades. The incidence is equal in males and females, but women have a better prognosis, possibly for hormonal reasons. Early detection of melanoma is critical and may account for the improvement in survival figures from 50% in the 1950s to 80% currently.

Exposure to sunlight is the major risk factor for the development of malignant melanoma. Epidemiologic studies consistently demonstrate that the incidence of melanoma is latitude dependent. For example, the incidence among whites in Atlanta, Georgia, is almost twice that in Detroit, Michigan. Areas of skin with the greatest sun exposure have the highest incidence of melanoma, as illustrated by lower leg melanomas occurring much more commonly in women than in men. Individuals with light hair and fair skin are at greatest risk; melanomas are uncommon in blacks. Office workers have a higher incidence than construction workers and farmers, suggesting that intermittent intense sun exposure may be particularly harmful. A sunscreen with a high sun protection factor (SPF) is advisable for primary prevention of melanoma. An SPF of 15 or greater is optimal; reapplication is necessary approximately every 2 hours and after swimming.

DYSPLASTIC NEVI

Dysplastic nevi are present on the skin of 2 to 8% of the American population and are precursors to melanoma. Table 19–1 shows that the lifetime risk of melanoma is much higher for affected individuals than for the general population. There are four risk groups for patients with dysplastic nevi (in order of increasing risk): type A patients have no family history of dysplastic nevi or melanoma; type B have a family history of dysplastic nevi; type C have a family history of melanoma; type D patients have a family history of dysplastic nevi and melanoma. Type D patients with a family history positive for multiple malignant melanomas have a lifetime risk of melanoma that approaches 100%.

Table 19–2 compares the features of dysplastic nevi with those of common acquired nevi. Suspected dysplastic nevi require confirmation by biopsy of one to three lesions, and the frequency of follow-up depends on the familial risk category. Patients at high risk and with many lesions need photographic follow-up of involved skin. Changes suggestive of melanoma necessitate biopsy.

CLINICAL FEATURES

Ninety-five percent of melanomas develop in the skin; the remainder arise as primary lesions in the oral cavity, eye, anus, and genitalia. Most melanomas result from malignant transformation of preexisting nevi or moles. Even experienced clinicians cannot accurately

Table 19–1. **LIFETIME RISK OF MELANOMA**

U.S. Caucasians	1 in 100
Persons with dysplastic nevi	1 in 2–14
Persons with prior melanoma	1 in 10
Persons with family history of dysplastic nevi *and* melanoma	1 in 1

Table 19–2. **CLINICAL CHARACTERISTICS OF COMMON AND DYSPLASTIC NEVI**

COMMON NEVI	DYSPLASTIC NEVI
Round or oval with a smooth border	Irregular border
Sharply demarcated from surrounding skin	Margin is not sharp
Often uniformly pigmented but may be mottled	Mottled mixture of tan, brown, dark brown
Typical size: 4–6 mm	Typical size: 6–15 mm

predict whether a particular lesion is a melanoma or not; excision and histologic examination of any suspicious pigmented lesion are essential.

Table 19–3 classifies primary cutaneous melanomas into four groups based on clinical and histologic characteristics. Except for the nodular type, most melanomas exist for relatively long periods prior to diagnosis, which explains the potential benefit of early detection and excision.

Changes in a nevus suspicious for malignant transformation include sudden increase in size, change in color, ulceration with oozing or bleeding, surrounding erythema or swelling, and development of tenderness or itching. Three characteristics central to the detection of superficial spreading melanomas are:

- Variegated color. The presence of red, white, or blue colors in a pigmented lesion suggests malignancy.
- Irregular border. The presence of indentations or notches in the border of a lesion is suspicious and should lead to biopsy.
- Irregular surface. Visible or palpable irregularities in the surface and absence of skin markings are also suggestive of malignancy.

The less common but more lethal nodular melanomas usually occur as blue-gray or blue-black papules with a smooth surface. Amelanotic nodular melanomas may be extremely difficult to recognize. Malignant melanomas occasionally present with lymphadenopathy or with widespread metastatic disease. Sometimes no primary skin lesion is detected, although careful questioning may elicit a history of previous removal of a "benign" mole.

STAGING AND PROGNOSIS

The clinical stages of melanoma and the corresponding 5-year survival rates are as follows:

Stage I	Localized with thickness less than 1.5 mm	90%
Stage II	Localized with thickness greater than 1.5 mm	70%
Stage III	With involved regional nodes	40%
Stage IV	With distant metastases or advanced regional nodes	<10%

Clearly the presence of involved lymph nodes adversely affects prognosis. The measured thickness of the primary lesion also correlates strongly with prognosis (Table 19–4), and this measurement is a standard procedure in the pathologic evaluation of excised melanomas.

TREATMENT

SURGERY

Table 19–5 summarizes guidelines for surgical management. First, incisional or excisional biopsy establishes the diagnosis. Then a wide excision accomplishes local control at the primary site. Patients with clinically palpable regional lymph nodes, whether detected concurrently with the primary tumor or later, should undergo a therapeutic regional node dissection. Twenty to 30% of pathologically proven stage III patients will achieve a tumor-free survival by this additional procedure. Prophylactic regional lymph node dissection for

Table 19–3. **CHARACTERISTICS OF THE FOUR MAJOR TYPES OF MELANOMA**

TYPE OF MELANOMA	DURATION OF LESION PRIOR TO DIAGNOSIS	RELATIVE INCIDENCE (%)	FEATURES
Superficial spreading	1–5 years	70	Variegated color, irregular border, irregular surface
Nodular	0–2 months	20	Uniform bluish to black color
Lentigo maligna	5–15 years	5	Occurs in the head and neck area of the elderly
Acral lentiginous	Highly variable	5	Palms, soles, and nail beds

Table 19–4. **RELATIONSHIP OF TUMOR THICKNESS TO SURVIVAL**

THICKNESS RANGE (mm)	5-YEAR SURVIVAL (%)
0–0.75	89
0.76–1.49	75
1.5–2.49	58
2.5–3.99	46
>4.0	25

From Balch CM, Soong SJ, Milton GW, et al: A comparison of prognostic factors and surgical results in 1786 patients with localized (stage I) melanoma. Ann Surg 196:677–683, 1982.

patients with clinically negative nodes is controversial. Two prospective randomized studies failed to substantiate the value of this procedure. Several retrospective analyses detected a statistically significant advantage for this surgery for patients with primary melanomas of intermediate thickness. While awaiting the results of additional prospective studies, regional lymph node surgery remains a debatable option for patients with intermediate-thickness melanoma. The procedure is inappropriate for both thin lesions, where the incidence of nodal spread is very low, and thick lesions, where the incidence of systemic spread is very high.

RADIATION

Although melanomas are relatively radioresistant, treatment of symptomatic bone or brain metastases can provide valuable palliation. There may be an advantage to using large daily fractions.

CHEMOTHERAPY

Chemotherapy provides very limited benefit to patients with advanced melanoma. Response rates are very low in patients with a poor performance status or involvement of

Table 19–5. **SURGICAL MANAGEMENT OF MELANOMA**

LOCAL RESECTION OF PRIMARY LESION	
<1.0 mm thick: Wide excision with 1-cm margin	
>1.0 mm thick: Wide excision up to 3-cm margin	
THERAPEUTIC REGIONAL LYMPH NODE DISSECTION	
When clinically palpable lymph nodes are detectable	
PROPHYLACTIC REGIONAL LYMPH NODE DISSECTION	
<1.5 mm thick	Not indicated
>1.5 but <4.0 mm thick	Controversial
>4.0 mm thick	Not indicated

liver or brain; the rates improve slightly when metastases involve skin, lymph nodes, or lungs. The average response duration remains very short (Table 19–6). Combination chemotherapy achieves higher response rates than single-agent therapy but is considerably more toxic.

DTIC is the most active single agent, with a response rate of 20%. BCNU and cisplatin have slightly lower single-agent response rates and are usually part of combination therapy regimens. A regimen combining these three agents plus tamoxifen is popular (see Table 19–6) because of its higher response rate, but there is no proven survival benefit as yet. High-dose treatment with autologous bone marrow rescue produces a still higher rate of remission, but the response duration is brief. The number of patients treated with autologous bone marrow transplantation is very small, and this approach remains investigational.

IMMUNOTHERAPY

Intensive research efforts with biologic agents focus on melanoma and renal carcinoma (Chap. 6). Table 19–6 summarizes the response rates in patients with malignant melanoma. Interferon was the first commercially available biologic and interleukin 2 (IL-2) may soon follow. Both agents produce responses in 15 to 20% of melanoma patients, but these responses occur in only the most favorable patients and each drug has unique, significant side effects. Interferon and IL-2 are treatment options only for patients with excellent performance status and small amounts of symptomatic metastatic disease in the skin, lymph nodes, or lungs, who are ineligible or unwilling to participate in properly conducted research studies.

Several other biologic treatments remain experimental. Adoptive immunotherapy with intravenous infusion of specific immune lymphocytes is one example. The first attempt used tumor-infiltrating lymphocytes (TILs) with IL-2 given to support their activity in vivo. Although the resulting response rate of 50% was remarkable, the duration of responses was disappointing. Monoclonal antibodies directed at melanoma antigens produced some regressions, and current research efforts include conjugating the monoclonal antibodies with toxins or radioisotopes for greater antitumor effect. Vaccines containing intact irradiated melanoma cells or disrupted cells produce remissions in 12 to 20% of patients with metastatic disease. Additional studies of vaccines as adjuvant treatment following excision of the primary lesion and of vaccines combined with cytokines are underway.

POSTSURGICAL ADJUVANT THERAPY

Postoperative adjuvant chemotherapy fails to improve survival for patients with poor prognosis melanoma. Preliminary results of a single, large, phase III randomized study indicate that levamisole may be useful for this purpose. This requires confirmation with additional studies. Trials of adjuvant interferon also continue.

Table 19–6. **CHEMOTHERAPY AND IMMUNOTHERAPY RESULTS FOR METASTATIC MELANOMA**

AGENTS	RESPONSE RATES (%)		MEDIAN DURATION OF RESPONSE (months)
	Complete	Partial	
DTIC	5	15	6
DTIC, BCNU, cisplatin, tamoxifen	10	35	7
High-dose chemotherapy and bone marrow transplant	10	40	4
Alpha interferon	5	10	7
Interleukin 2	5	15	8
Interleukin 2 with specific immune cells	5	45	6
Vaccines	4	12	12

SPECIAL PROBLEMS

Skin metastases are sometimes very painful because of either their location or the associated inflammatory response. Surgical removal, when possible, promptly relieves discomfort in most cases. Radiation therapy is a palliative option for those with painful but inoperable localized disease.

Brain metastases are a common and often devastating complication. Melanoma has the highest frequency of symptomatic brain metastases (35%) of any cancer. Surgery for a resectable solitary brain lesion in the absence of advanced extra–central nervous system disease may be beneficial for selected patients. Corticosteroids and radiation therapy may be worthwhile for symptomatic brain metastases, although the median survival is only 2 to 3 months. Corticosteroid therapy or supportive care alone is a reasonable alternative, and a well-informed patient and family may prefer this conservative care.

In-transit recurrences may develop along the lymphatic drainage of a primary lesion in an extremity. Regional perfusion, particularly with melphalan, may result in regressions, but the complication rate is high. Resection of these lesions is often possible and may be preferable.

REFERENCES

Balch CM: The role of elective lymph node dissection in melanoma: Rationale, results, and controversies. J Clin Oncol 6:163–172, 1988.

Koh HK: Cutaneous melanoma. N Engl J Med 325:171–182, 1991.

Mitchell MS, Harel W, Kempf RA, et al: Active-specific immunotherapy for melanoma. J Clin Oncol 8:856–869, 1990.

Quirt IC, Shelley WE, Pater JL, et al: Improved survival in patients with poor-prognosis malignant melanoma treated with adjuvant levamisole: A phase III study by the National Cancer Institute of Canada Clinical Trials Group. J Clin Oncol 9:729–735, 1991.

Rhodes AR, Weinstock MA, Fitzpatrick TB, Mihm MC, Sober AJ: Risk factors for cutaneous melanoma. A practical method of recognizing predisposed individuals. JAMA 258:3146–3154, 1987.

Rosenberg SA, Packard BS, Aerbersold PM, et al: Use of tumor-infiltrating lymphocytes and interleukin-2 in the immunotherapy of patients with metastatic melanoma. N Engl J Med 3:364–376, 1991.

Veronesi U, Cascinelli N, Adamus J, et al: Thin stage I primary cutaneous malignant melanoma: Comparison of excision with margins of 1 or 3 cm. N Engl J Med 318:1159–1162, 1988.

Wolff SN, Herzig RH, Fay JW, et al: High-dose thiotepa with autologous bone marrow transplantation for metastatic malignant melanoma: Results of phase I and II studies of the North American Bone Marrow Transplantation Group. J Clin Oncol 7:245–249, 1989.

20
MALIGNANT BRAIN TUMORS

Brian D. Smith

INCIDENCE AND ETIOLOGY

The National Cancer Institute estimates that 16,900 new cases of primary brain and spinal cord cancers will be diagnosed in 1992, and 11,800 patients will die from these malignancies. Brain tumors are the most common solid tumors occurring in childhood.

The etiology of malignant brain tumors in humans is unknown, although chemical carcinogens and oncogenic viruses can induce primary brain tumors in laboratory animals. Hereditary factors play a role in the rare cases of gliomas associated with hereditary neurocutaneous syndromes (neurofibromatosis, tuberous sclerosis), and there appears to be a genetic predisposition to medulloblastoma and neuroblastoma, which are predominantly childhood malignancies of the central nervous system (CNS). Chromosomal abnormalities are now being recognized that are characteristic for specific tumor types. An increased incidence of primary CNS lymphomas has been reported in immunocompromised patients such as those with renal transplants, systemic lupus erythematosus, other rheumatic diseases, and acquired immune deficiency syndrome (AIDS).

PATHOLOGY

CNS tumors have been classified by a number of overlapping systems based on cell type, degree of differentiation, and location. While each classification scheme has certain advantages, the simultaneous use of numerous systems of nomenclature makes comparison of data from different institutions very difficult.

The gliomas represent approximately two-thirds of primary CNS malignancies. Most glial tumors arise from one of three neuroglial cell types found in the CNS: astrocytes, oligodendrocytes, and ependymal cells. Astrocytes serve as supporting tissue for neurons and comprise the vast majority of parenchymal brain cells. Oligodendrocytes are associated with the process of myelination, and ependymal cells line ventricular cavities and the central canal of the spinal cord. Neuroglial precursors give rise to medulloblastomas.

The most common gliomas are glioblastomas and astrocytomas. Grades I and II astrocytomas are low grade and less aggressive; grades III and IV astrocytomas are high grade and more lethal. Glioblastomas represent malignant transformation of astrocytic cells; the terms *glioblastoma multiforme, astrocytoma grade IV,* and *malignant glioma* are used interchangeably in the literature.

CLINICAL MANIFESTATIONS

Malignant brain tumors produce symptoms by invasion or compression of adjacent structures, elevation of intracranial pressure, and herniation of uninvolved brain tissue. Most patients with brain tumors complain of headaches at some time during their course. Headaches due to increased intracranial pressure are characteristically bifrontal or bioccipital, occur upon awakening in the morning, recur intermittently during the day, and are occasionally accompanied by vomiting. Increased intracranial pressure may also produce changes in mental function, altered levels of consciousness, and cranial nerve palsies, especially diplopia. Papilledema should be looked for on ophthalmoscopic examination, but its absence does not exclude increased intracranial pressure.

Progressive increase in intracranial pressure may result in herniation of brain tissue through the falx cerebri, foramen magnum, or tentorium cerebelli with life-threatening compression of vital structures. Lumbar puncture, not very useful in the diagnosis of brain tumor in any case, is contraindicated when elevated intracranial pressure is suspected.

Focal neurologic abnormalities usually reflect tumor location. Supratentorial lesions often cause seizures or motor deficits. Frontal and temporal lobe tumors may cause behavioral and emotional changes. Emotional lability, memory loss, personality alteration, intellectual impairment, confusion, and dementia due to brain tumor can be mistaken for a variety of other physical and psychologic problems. Suprasellar tumors may produce visual abnormalities, increased intracranial pressure, and altered hypothalamic function. Posterior fossa tumors present with cerebellar and cranial nerve signs.

Seizures occur in 20 to 50% of brain tumor patients and may precede other signs and symptoms by weeks or months. New onset of seizures in an adult should always suggest brain tumor, even in the absence of localizing neurologic findings.

DIAGNOSIS

The diagnosis of brain tumor depends primarily on recognition of suspicious findings on history and thorough neurologic examination. The most useful tests to confirm the diagnosis are magnetic resonance imaging (MRI) or computed tomography (CT), which have virtually replaced skull films, radionuclide brain scans, and pneumoencephalography in this setting. The MRI is rapidly becoming the diagnostic study of choice. Compared with the CT scan, MRI has greater sensitivity in detecting low-grade astrocytomas, intramedullary and extramedullary spinal cord lesions, and tumors in the posterior fossa or skull base. With gadolinium enhancement, the MRI provides additional sensitivity for differentiating parenchymal disease from surrounding edema. The use of cerebral angiography has diminished but continues to provide important information for tumors adjacent to critical cerebral vessels and for highly vascular tumors.

Occasionally, metastatic disease from an occult extracranial primary presents as an isolated brain tumor (Chap. 22). Therefore, prior to brain biopsy, appropriate history, physical examination, and laboratory evaluation should be performed to exclude primary cancers (lung, breast, hypernephroma, melanoma, gastrointestinal tract, testicle) likely to metastasize to the brain (Fig. 20–1).

Accurate diagnosis and appropriate therapy depend on biopsy of the brain mass. Tumor location dictates the type of neurosurgical procedure required to obtain tissue. Open biopsy with maximal removal of tumor is the preferred approach; however, resection may be impossible when the lesion is deep in the brain or in an especially critical area. In these circumstances, needle biopsy must be employed. The CT-guided stereotactic biopsy has become the standard for accurate and safe diagnosis of surgically inaccessible masses. With CT guidance, the biopsy instrument is directed through a burr hole to the target. Representative tissue is obtained in more than 90% of procedures, and complications such as hemorrhage are rare.

TREATMENT

Symptomatic treatment for the secondary effects of central nervous system tumors includes dexamethasone, 10 mg, initially followed by 4 mg every 6 hours to reduce cerebral edema, and phenytoin or phenobarbital in patients who present with seizures.

SURGERY

Neurosurgical exploration with maximal removal of tumor when possible is the treatment of choice for malignant brain tumors. Excision of tumor provides a definite histologic diagnosis, decompresses the brain, and, in severely compromised patients, reduces the tumor burden, allowing time for the subsequent use of radiotherapy. Surgery may be curative for low-grade malignancies, but the median survival for patients with high-grade astrocytomas (malignant gliomas) treated with surgery alone is only about 14 weeks.

RADIATION THERAPY

Postoperative radiotherapy results in increased longevity and relief of symptoms. In recent series, patients with malignant gliomas treated with surgery plus irradiation have a median survival of 6 to 12 months. Treatment usually begins 1 to 2 weeks after surgery and consists of 5000 to 6000 cGy to the tumor plus a 2-cm margin around the mass, given

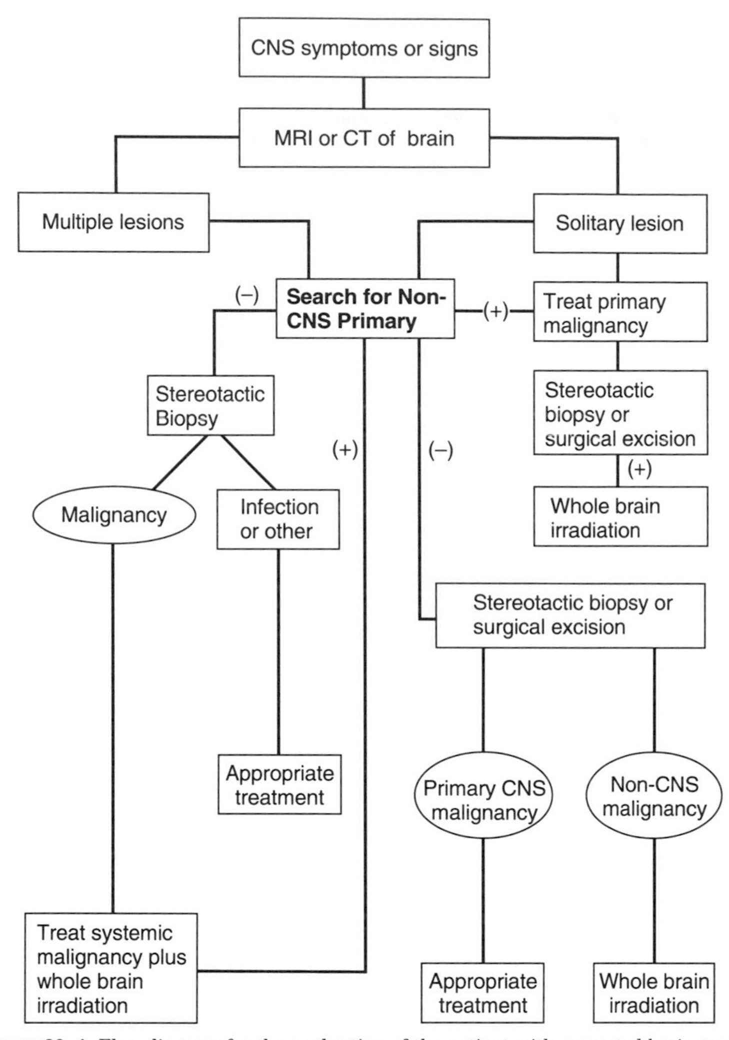

Figure 20–1. Flow diagram for the evaluation of the patient with suspected brain tumor.

over 5 to 7 weeks. Experimental radiation techniques—including hyperfractionation, radiation sensitizers, particle beam irradiation, and hyperbaric oxygen—have not as yet demonstrated any advantage over conventional radiation in the treatment of malignant gliomas.

Adverse effects of cranial irradiation may include cerebral edema during therapy. This problem can be readily controlled with steroids. Late effects occurring months to years following treatment result from brain necrosis and are generally associated with radiation doses in excess of 6000 cGy.

CHEMOTHERAPY

In the past, the blood-brain barrier was thought to prevent the entry of most chemotherapeutic agents into CNS tumors. This concept promoted the development and use of lipid-soluble cytotoxic agents, especially the nitrosoureas, in brain tumor chemotherapy. More recent evidence suggests that breaches in the blood-brain barrier occur within tumor tissue. Many agents, both polar and nonpolar, have been tested, and response rates of 10 to 50% have been reported, as demonstrated by radiologic tumor shrinkage and symptomatic neurologic improvement.

The nitrosoureas have received the most extensive study and are the most active agents. The usual dose of BCNU is 80 mg/m^2 intravenously daily for 3 days, repeated every 6 to 8 weeks. Cumulative doses greater than 1500 mg/m^2 may cause irreversible pulmonary fibrosis. CCNU is given orally in a dose of 100 to 130 mg/m^2 every 6 weeks. Forty to 50% of patients with malignant gliomas respond to nitrosourea therapy, and responses last about 3 to 5 months. Other active agents include procarbazine, dacarbazine, vincristine, and cisplatin. Combination chemotherapy has been employed in several trials, but it appears to offer no advantage over single-agent therapy.

COMBINED MODALITY THERAPY

Many trials have compared radiotherapy alone with radiotherapy plus chemotherapy in malignant glioma patients after surgery. Most of these studies have failed to demonstrate any survival benefit, but the small numbers of patients involved have raised the likelihood of a type II or β error. In a recent meta-analysis of prospective randomized trials of adjuvant chemotherapy in malignant glioma, a statistically significant survival benefit was found; the 12-month survival for patients receiving chemotherapy was 53.5%, versus 41.2% for patients receiving radiation therapy only, and the 24-month survival was 23.4%, versus 15.9% for controls. More substantial survival gains, however, must await the introduction of more effective cytotoxic agents.

NEW TREATMENT APPROACHES

Innovative approaches to the treatment of malignant brain tumors seem long overdue. Currently, several new technologies are being applied and initial results are promising.

Interstitial brachytherapy utilizes temporary implantation of high-activity radiation sources within brain tumors. It has proven effective in treating recurrent malignancies and is now being tried as additional boost therapy in the initial treatment plan at some research institutions. The tumor mass is precisely localized by CT scan; then a stereotactic (3-D) apparatus is attached to the skull using a local anesthetic. Burr holes are made and cannulas are positioned in the tumor and loaded with a radiation source such as high-activity iodine 125. Total dose delivered to the tumor ranges from 5000 to 7500 cGy. The treatment, with or without additional hyperthermia, generally results in excellent local control. The principal side effect is radiation necrosis, which occurs in a small percentage of patients and may require surgical excision.

Stereotactic radiosurgery is a noninvasive technique that is available in only a limited number of referral centers. Narrow beams of ionizing radiation are delivered from many different points on the surface of the skull such that they all converge on the tumor mass. The total tumor dose ranges from 900 to 2500 cGy and is focused and delivered to a precisely circumscribed target; this treatment controls tumor growth in 80 to 90% of cases. Once the stereotactic guidance system is set up, this single-treatment technique requires 30 to 45 minutes to complete and does not necessitate hospital admission.

Biotherapy utilizes the patient's immune system to selectively destroy residual tumor cells without affecting normal cells (Chap. 6). The specific immune cells involved are lymphokine-activated killer cells (LAKs), tumor-infiltrating lymphocytes (TILs), and cytotoxic T lymphocytes (CTLs). Tumor cells are singled out as targets by their unique surface antigens. Tumor tissue removed at initial surgery is analyzed for identifying surface antigens; then monoclonal antibodies to these antigens are developed. Bispecific monoclonal antibodies directed against both target antigens and effector cell antigens serve to cross-link immune cytotoxic cells and their tumor cell targets. Effector cell cytotoxicity and target cell antigen visibility are increased by immune stimulators called lymphokines. Thus residual tumor cells may be lysed by infusing immune effector cells, monoclonal antibodies, and lymphokines. Preliminary studies in patients with gliomas suggest that biotherapy may be a promising new approach to treating primary brain malignancies.

Laser microsurgery may be useful for very small lesions located in critical brain areas not accessible to traditional surgical removal. The use of the laser depends on contrast-enhanced CT scans to outline the tumor in stereotactic space. Then, after standard neurosurgical exposure, the tumor is vaporized by a CT-guided carbon dioxide laser.

Intracarotid infusion of chemotherapy utilizes specially designed catheters to deliver higher peak concentrations of drug within the tumor. Chemotherapeutic agents such as cisplatin, BCNU, and VM-26 have been used with modest improvements in response rates. Adverse effects include seizures, transient motor weakness, and retinal toxicity.

The ultimate role of these new techniques will require further investigation. Physicians are encouraged to enroll patients in controlled clinical studies utilizing these state of the art technologies in order to expedite development of new treatments that may prolong patient survival.

PRIMARY LYMPHOMA OF BRAIN

Primary CNS lymphoma, although uncommon, deserves special attention. Survival without treatment is 3 months; with surgery, survival is 4 to 5 months; and with surgery plus radiotherapy, median survival is 15 months. Unfortunately, the majority of patients die of local recurrence despite high doses of radiation. The addition of chemotherapy, both systemic and intrathecal, has improved median survival in some small studies.

REFERENCES

Black PM: Brain tumors. N Engl J Med 324:1471–1476, 1555–1564, 1991.
Kelly PS, Earnest F, Kall BA, et al: Surgical options for patients with deep-seated brain tumors: Computer assisted stereotactic biopsy. Mayo Clin Proc 60:223–229, 1985.
Nitta T: Preliminary trial of specific targeting therapy against malignant glioma. Lancet 335:368–376, 1990.
O'Neill BP, Illig JJ: Primary central nervous system lymphoma. Mayo Clin Proc 64:1005–1020, 1989.
Shapiro WR (ed): Brain tumors. Semin Oncol 13:1–122, 1986.

BRAIN METASTASES

INCIDENCE AND ETIOLOGY

Brain metastases are a frequent and devastating consequence of systemic cancer. For some primary tumors such as melanoma and lung cancer, the risk of developing symptomatic brain metastases is very high (Table 20–1). The development of brain metastases depends on the ability of blood-borne malignant cells to survive the trauma of the microcirculation and localize in the CNS. The predilection for some cells to home into the CNS and subsequently develop into viable tumor masses is likely the result of tumor cell and brain endothelium receptors, a favorable microenvironment for growth, and a sanctuary from most systemic chemotherapeutics.

CLINICAL MANIFESTATIONS

The classic symptoms of headache, nausea, vomiting, and lethargy may be attributed to the patient's underlying systemic disease, thus delaying definitive diagnosis. Any CNS symptoms in a cancer patient should prompt careful neurological evaluation. Cognitive

Table 20–1. **INCIDENCE OF SYMPTOMATIC BRAIN METASTASES FOR SELECTED PRIMARY TUMOR SITES**

Primary Site	Incidence
Melanoma	33%
Lung	25%
Breast	15%
Kidney, bladder	10%
Colon, pancreas	5%
Liver, prostate	5%
Testicular, lymphoma	5%

deficiencies are frequently demonstrated; localized motor, sensory, or cerebellar deficits are less common. Papilledema, reflecting increased intracranial pressure, may not be seen at initial presentation.

DIAGNOSIS

In patients with known primary malignancies and new CNS symptoms, urgent brain MRI or CT scan is indicated. If multiple masses are identified, then appropriate treatment may be initiated. When a single lesion is found, a stereotactic biopsy should be considered to confirm the diagnosis (see Fig. 20–1). In patients with meningeal symptoms and normal imaging studies, a lumbar puncture is performed for cytology, chemistries, and cultures.

TREATMENT

Decadron (dexamethasone) is given to reduce intracranial pressure from tumor-associated edema. The standard initial dose is 10 mg followed by 4 mg every 6 hours. Decadron is tapered off after 14 to 21 days, but with recurrence of symptoms, longer courses are sometimes required and are attended by the morbidity commonly seen with chronic steroid use.

The use of prophylactic anticonvulsants in patients with newly diagnosed brain metastases is discouraged. One large retrospective study showed no benefit from initiating treatment prior to the first seizure. Anticoagulation in patients with brain metastases who develop a deep venous thrombosis or pulmonary embolus is relatively contraindicated because of the risk of hemorrhage in the tumor. Vena caval interruption is the preferred treatment.

Radiation Therapy

The standard treatment for brain metastases is whole brain irradiation. A total dose of 3000 to 4000 cGy is given over 2 to 4 weeks. A higher additional dose (boost) may be given to the area of disease.

Solitary Metastasis to Brain

Approximately 50% of patients presenting with brain metastases have a single lesion. Surgical resection should be pursued if the tumor is accessible, the systemic disease is controlled, and the patient has a good performance status. These criteria are met in approximately 50% of patients with solitary metastases. Surgical resection is followed by whole brain radiation. If the patient's systemic disease is well controlled but he/she is not a surgical candidate, stereotactic biopsy should be considered to rule out a nonmalignant cause such as abscess or inflammation or to identify a new primary CNS malignancy.

Stereotactic radiosurgery and interstitial brachytherapy, discussed above, are effective treatments for some patients who develop a local recurrence after previous surgical excision or whole brain radiation therapy. Some centers are beginning to use these modalities as a boost to initial whole brain radiation therapy in surgically inaccessible lesions.

SURVIVAL

In the majority of patients, brain metastases occur in the setting of advanced systemic disease and poor performance status or as inoperable lesions. Median survival for patients with brain metastases is 1 month without treatment, 2 months with steroids, and 3 to 6 months with whole brain radiation therapy. For a small subset of patients with a good performance status, a solitary metastasis that is surgically accessible, and controlled systemic disease, treatment with surgery followed by radiation therapy gives a median survival of 9 to 18 months with an occasional long-term survivor.

REFERENCES

Cohen N, Strauss G, Lew R, et al: Should prophylactic anticonvulsants be administered to patients with newly diagnosed cerebral metastases? A retrospective analysis. J Clin Oncol 6:1621–1624, 1988.

Loeffler JS, Kooy HM, Wen PY, et al: The treatment of recurrent brain metastases with stereotactic radiosurgery. J Clin Oncol 8:576–582, 1990.
Patchell RA, Tibbs PA, Walsh JW, et al: A randomized trial of surgery in the treatment of single metastases to the brain. N Engl J Med 322:494–500, 1990.
Prados M: Interstitial brachytherapy for metastatic brain tumors. Cancer 63:657–660, 1989.
Weissman DE: Glucocorticoid treatment for brain metastases and epidural spinal cord compression: A review. J Clin Oncol 6:543–551, 1988.

21
ENDOCRINE MALIGNANCIES

Brian D. Smith

The National Cancer Institute estimates that there will be 13,900 new cases of endocrine malignancies in the United States in 1992, representing just over 1% of all anticipated diagnoses of cancer for that year. The number of estimated deaths from malignant endocrine tumors for 1992 is 1675.

Malignant tumors of the endocrine glands may present special problems for the medical oncologist. These tumors produce symptoms not only by local extension and distant metastasis, but also in many cases by excess production of biologically active hormones and other agents. Successful treatment of such tumors must therefore include measures to control or ameliorate the endocrine syndromes caused by hormone overproduction as well as the more conventional modalities directed against the tumor itself.

THYROID CARCINOMA

Thyroid carcinoma acounts for 89% of endocrine malignancies. In most cases, the cause of thyroid carcinoma is unknown, but radiation to the head and neck region has been recognized as an important risk factor. The disease occurs more than twice as often in women as in men; most cases are detected in patients between ages 25 and 65.

Histologically, thyroid carcinomas are classified as differentiated (papillary and follicular), medullary, and anaplastic. The prognosis for the vast majority of patients with differentiated thyroid carcinomas is extremely favorable, and 10-year survival rates exceeding 80 to 90% have been reported in many series. Medullary carcinoma, comprising 5 to 8% of all thyroid cancers, has a variable prognosis, but in many patients the diagnosis is compatible with survival of 5 to 10 years or more. Anaplastic carcinoma, on the other hand, is a highly virulent malignancy; regardless of treatment, death follows diagnosis within just a few months. Fortunately, the incidence of this type of thyroid cancer is low (10 to 15% of thyroid cancers).

CLINICAL FEATURES

Most patients with differentiated thyroid carcinoma present with a painless mass in the neck, often detected on routine physical examination. In a patient with a multinodular goiter, rapid growth of the goiter, hard consistency of a nodule, fixation to adjacent structures, and the presence of cervical lymphadenopathy or hoarse voice (indicating involvement of the recurrent laryngeal nerve with consequent vocal cord paralysis) are highly suspicious for cancer. Radionuclide imaging demonstrates a hypofunctioning or nonfunctioning nodule in most cases of thyroid carcinoma.

Anaplastic thyroid carcinomas present as rapidly growing bulky masses distorting the normal contour of the neck and often causing obstruction of the airway or esophagus. Medullary thyroid carcinomas may secrete various hormones (calcitonin, prostaglandins, vasoactive intestinal polypeptide [VIP], adrenocorticotropic hormone [ACTH]) and may occur on a familial basis associated with bilateral pheochromocytomas and parathyroid hyperplasia or adenomas (multiple endocrine neoplasia [MEN] type II); this phenomenon may lead to the recognition of medullary carcinomas in asymptomatic family members through screening for elevated serum calcitonin levels.

DIAGNOSIS

Thyroid carcinomas almost invariably appear hypofunctional ("cold") on radionuclide scanning with ^{131}I. A hyperfunctional ("hot") nodule essentially excludes the diagnosis of cancer, but hypofunctional nodules may represent cysts, adenomas, and other benign processes as well as cancer. Ultrasonography reliably distinguishes cystic from solid lesions. Thyroid cysts are almost always benign.

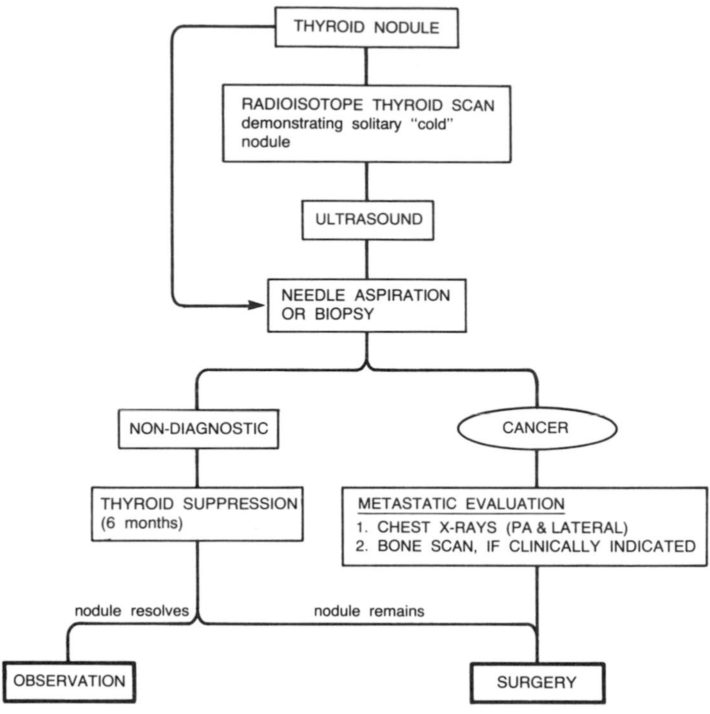

Figure 21–1. Flow diagram for evaluation of the patient with suspected thyroid carcinoma. (*From* Borg SA, Rosenthal S: Handbook of Cancer Diagnosis and Staging. A Clinical Atlas. New York, John Wiley & Sons, 1984. Copyright © 1984. Reprinted by permission.)

Fine needle aspiration of thyroid nodules has become a safe, reliable, and popular technique for cytologic examination and diagnosis. In many centers, fine needle aspiration is employed as the initial diagnostic study, bypassing the thyroid scan and ultrasound. Used properly, fine needle aspiration allows better selection of patients with thyroid nodules for surgery (Fig. 21–1).

Total body radioiodine scanning provides the best method for early detection of local recurrence or distant spread of differentiated thyroid carcinoma. The technique requires that all functioning thyroid tissue be ablated, and that thyroid hormone replacement be discontinued prior to study to allow thyroid-stimulating hormone (TSH) levels to rise. Measurement of serum levels of thyroglobulin is another useful test for recurrence of differentiated thyroid carcinoma, but use of this marker is also limited to patients who have had total removal of all thyroid tissue.

TREATMENT

General Considerations

Surgery and radiation therapy (with radioiodine) provide the mainstay of treatment for differentiated thyroid carcinoma. The extent of surgery—lobectomy, subtotal thyroidectomy, or total thyroidectomy—and the exact indications for radioiodine treatment are controversial. Recurrence rates following total thyroidectomy or lesser surgery followed by radioiodine treatment are almost certainly lower than with less aggressive therapy, but survival may not be affected. Total thyroidectomy carries a greater risk of serious complications, including damage to the recurrent laryngeal nerve and permanent hypoparathyroidism. The low incidence of the disease and its indolent course have prevented prospective studies comparing various forms of therapy, so that overall agreement regarding optimal management may never be achieved. All authorities agree, however, that suppressive therapy with thyroid hormone should be given after treatment of the primary tumor with any method.

Locally recurrent or metastatic disease also responds to treatment with ^{131}I in many cases. Neck dissection and external radiation can be used for troublesome local recurrences; these modalities are also employed in cases of anaplastic carcinoma.

Chemotherapy

Because survival in most cases of differentiated thyroid carcinoma is so high and ^{131}I is available to treat those cases of metastatic disease that do occur, experience with conventional cytotoxic chemotherapy is limited. Methotrexate, cisplatin, bleomycin, and melphalan have shown activity in anecdotal reports. Adriamycin (doxorubicin), however, appears to be the most useful agent; in a series of 30 patients with metastatic thyroid cancer, adriamycin, in a dose of 45 to 75 mg/m^2 every 3 weeks, produced a 37% response rate, and responses occurred in each histologic type. Recently, small studies employing cisplatin plus adriamycin have produced encouraging preliminary results.

REFERENCES

Brennan MD, Bergstralh EJ, van Heerden JA, et al: Follicular thyroid cancer treated at the Mayo Clinic, 1946 through 1970: Initial manifestations, pathologic findings, therapy, and outcome. Mayo Clin Proc 66:11–22, 1991.

Aiello DP, Manni A: Thyroglobulin measurement vs iodine 131 total-body scan for follow-up of well-differentiated thyroid cancer. Arch Intern Med 150:437–439, 1990.

Nel CJ, Heerden JA, Goellner JR, et al: Anaplastic carcinoma of the thyroid: A clinicopathologic study of 82 cases. Mayo Clin Proc 60:51–58, 1985.

McConahey WM, Hay ID, Woolner LB, et al: Papillary thyroid cancer treated at the Mayo Clinic, 1946 through 1970: Initial manifestations, pathologic findings, therapy and outcome. Mayo Clin Proc 61:978–996, 1986.

Ross DS: Long-term managment of differentiated thyroid cancer. Endocrinol Metab Clin North Am 19:719–739, 1990.

Schlumberger M, Parmentier C, Delisle MJ, et al: Combination therapy for anaplastic giant cell thyroid carcinoma. Cancer 67:564–566, 1991.

ADRENOCORTICAL CARCINOMA

Adrenocortical carcinoma is a rare tumor with an incidence of about 0.5 to 2.0 per million population, representing 0.2% of deaths due to cancer in the United States. It may occur at any age and with equal frequency in men and women. The outlook for patients with this tumor is poor; the median survival is about 14 months and less than 25% survive for 5 years.

CLINICAL FEATURES

The clinical manifestations of adrenocortical carcinoma may derive from excessive steroid hormone production by the tumor or from effects due to local invasion or distant metastasis of the cancer itself. In most cases, the tumor is locally invasive or metastatic at the time of diagnosis. A palpable abdominal mass is present in more than 50% of patients. Retroperitoneal invasion may cause abdominal and back pain, and the presence of a large left upper quadrant mass may interfere with digestive function.

Although nonfunctioning adrenocortical carcinomas occur, the majority of patients present with endocrine manifestations (Table 21–1). The typical syndromes may overlap with one another, and Cushing's syndrome accompanied by virilization and striking elevations in urinary 17-ketosteroids is highly characteristic of adrenal carcinoma.

The diagnosis of adrenal carcinoma depends on recognition of the endocrine manifestations and demonstration of an adrenal mass, usually by computed tomography (CT) or magnetic resonance imaging (MRI) (Fig. 21–2). Exploratory laparotomy is generally necessary to establish a tissue diagnosis and determine resectability. The most common metastatic sites include lung, lymph nodes, liver, and bone.

Table 21–1. **ENDOCRINE SYNDROMES ASSOCIATED WITH ADRENOCORTICAL CARCINOMA**

MAJOR SYNDROMES	UNCOMMON SYNDROMES
Cushing's syndrome	Hypoglycemia
Virilization of women	Polycythemia
Feminization of men	Inappropriate ADH secretion
Precocious puberty in children	Hypermineralocorticism

TREATMENT

Surgery

If at all possible, an en bloc resection of the tumor should be performed. Palliative resections may be worthwhile, even in the presence of locally advanced or metastatic disease, in order to reduce excessive hormone levels and ameliorate local symptoms. Patients may require intraoperative and postoperative corticosteroid replacement therapy to avoid adrenal insufficiency. Palliative radiation therapy is frequently successful in relieving pain and reducing tumor bulk in cases of unresectable disease. Following surgical resection, monthly steroid levels should be followed to detect recurrence early.

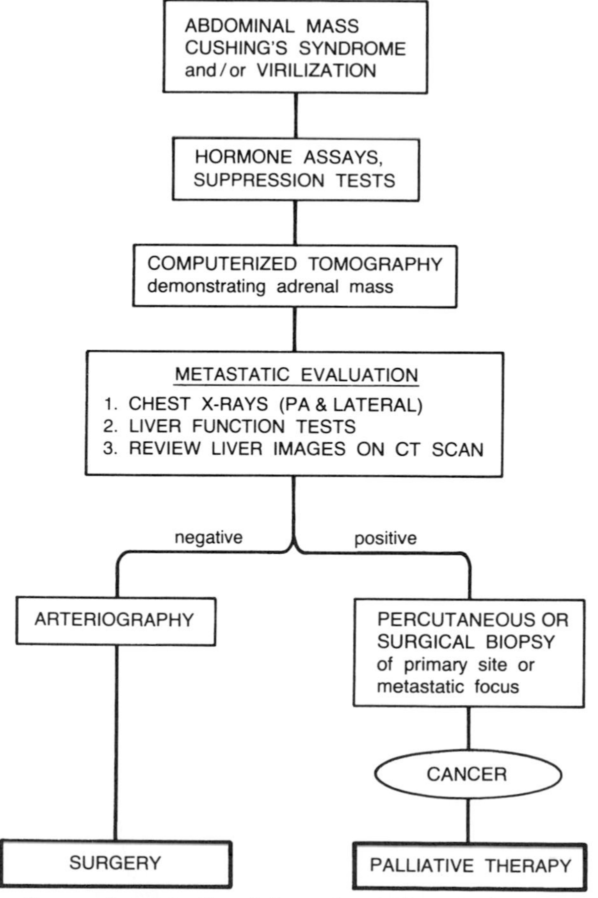

Figure 21–2. Flow diagram for evaluation of the patient with suspected adrenocortical carcinoma. (*From* Borg SA, Rosenthal S: Handbook of Cancer Diagnosis and Staging. A Clinical Atlas. New York, John Wiley & Sons, 1984. Copyright © 1984. Reprinted by permission.)

Chemotherapy

There is no organized experience with conventional chemotherapy in adrenal cancer. Mitotane (ortho,para-DDD), (o,p'DDD), an adrenolytic agent derived from an insecticide, may cause tumor regression and decrease hormone synthesis in patients with unresectable or metastatic tumor. The toxicity, especially gastrointestinal and neuromuscular, is severe. Approximately 25 to 30% of patients demonstrate objective tumor regressions, and twice as many have reductions in hormone levels and improvement in endocrine symptoms. Some patients, despite reductions in hormone levels, have tumor progression while taking mitotane. The use of mitotane as a surgical adjuvant has been advocated in the hope of preventing or delaying recurrent disease. The role of mitotane in this setting and its use in advanced disease are highly controversial; some investigators have found no benefit from its use, while others report long remissions and even cures.

The most common regimen begins with 2 to 6 g of mitotane daily in divided doses, increased gradually to 8 to 10 g per day. Treatment is continued at this level until toxicity develops, at which point the dose is cut by one-third to one-half and continued until progression or regression. Generally, an 8-week course is recommended. It is usually not possible to stop drug treatment after regression occurs, although in some cases the dose may be reduced.

Metyrapone and aminoglutethimide, inhibitors of corticosteroid synthesis, and RU-486, a new glucocorticoid receptor antagonist, have also been used but without much success in attempts to control the manifestations of hypercortisolism in these patients.

REFERENCES

Luton JP, Cerdas S, Lillaud L, et al: Clinical features of adrenocortical carcinoma, prognostic factors, and the effect of mitotane therapy. N Engl J Med 322:1195–1201, 1990.

Thompson NW, Cheung PS: Diagnosis and treatment of functioning and non-functioning adrenocortical neoplasms and incidentalomas. Surg Clin North Am 67:423–436, 1987.

Venkatesh S, Hickey RC, Sellin RV, et al: Adrenal cortical carcinoma. Cancer 64:765–769, 1989.

PHEOCHROMOCYTOMA

Pheochromocytomas are usually tumors of the adrenal medulla, although 10 to 15% occur ectopically in extra-adrenal chromaffin tissues, primarily abdominal sympathetic ganglia. Only about 10% are malignant, and 15 to 20% are multiple. Pheochromocytomas often occur as part of familial syndromes, including neurofibromatosis, multiple endocrine neoplasia type II (MEN II), and von Hippel-Lindau disease.

The clinical manifestations of pheochromocytoma result from excessive secretion of catecholamines (epinephrine and/or norepinephrine). Hypertension, either sustained or paroxysmal, is the most common feature. Severe paroxysms of hypertension accompanied by palpitations, diaphoresis, headache, and occasionally seizures and cardiac arrhythmias occur in some patients. Physical examination is usually normal but may reveal an abdominal mass or hepatomegaly if liver metastases are present. The diagnosis requires evidence of elevated urinary or plasma catecholamines (epinephrine, norepinephrine, or dopamine) or their metabolites (vanillylmandelic acid and total metanephrines). Pharmacologic provocative tests are dangerous and rarely necessary. Computed tomographic scanning demonstrates the tumor in almost all cases, making selective angiography necessary in only a few.

The treatment of pheochromocytoma is surgical. Preoperative management must include pharmacologic control of the symptoms of catecholamine excess with alpha and beta blockers such as labetalol. If metastatic disease is present, aggressive surgical attempts to remove as much tumor as possible are justified. Tumor recurrences should also be treated surgically.

Palliative radiation is indicated for painful bone metastases. No other role for radiation therapy in this disease has been described. Little experience with antitumor agents in the management of malignant pheochromocytoma has been reported, but a recent trial using cyclophosphamide, vincristine, and dacarbazine in patients with this tumor yielded a response rate of 57% and a median duration of response of 21 months. Management of inoperable or unresectable symptomatic disease should include pharmacologic control of excessive catecholamine effects either with alpha and/or beta blockers or with alpha-methylparatyrosine, an inhibitor of catecholamine synthesis.

REFERENCES

Averbuch SD, Steakley CS, Young RC, et al: Malignant pheochromocytoma: Effective treatment with a combination of cyclophosphamide, vincristine, and dacarbazine. Ann Intern Med 109:267–273, 1988.

Duncan MW, Compton P, Lazarus L, Smythe GA: Measurement of norepinephrine and 3,4 dihydroxyphenylglycol in urine and plasma for the diagnosis of pheochromocytoma. N Engl J Med 319:136–142, 1988.

Samaan NA, Hickey RC, Shutts PE: Diagnosis, localization, and managment of pheochromocytoma. Cancer 62:2451–2460, 1988.

Sheps SG, Jiang NS, Klee GG, Heerden JA: Recent developments in the diagnosis and treatment of pheochromocytoma. Mayo Clin Proc 65:88–95, 1990.

CARCINOID TUMORS

CLINICAL FEATURES

Carcinoid tumors, members of the APUD or neuroendocrine system, arise in the gastrointestinal tract, bronchi, ovaries, pancreas, thymus, and many other sites. They are rare, with an annual incidence rate of 0.3 per 100,000 population. Most are benign and are discovered as incidental findings at surgery or postmortem examination. Gastrointestinal carcinoids are found in 0.2 to 1.1% of patients at autopsy. Occasionally, gastrointestinal carcinoids will produce abdominal pain, nausea, vomiting, or small bowel obstruction requiring surgery. A carcinoid tumor is found incidentally in every 200 to 300 appendectomies.

Tumor size correlates closely with malignancy; carcinoids less than 1 cm in diameter are rarely if ever malignant, whereas those measuring 2 cm or greater have a substantial tendency to metastasize. These cases may present with symptoms related to metastatic disease: hepatomegaly, painful bone lesions, or dyspnea due to pulmonary involvement. In more than half the cases with liver involvement, the well-known carcinoid syndrome occurs (Table 21–2). This syndrome, caused by excessive production of serotonin and other bioactive substances, usually consists of flushing, diarrhea, wheezing, and endocardial lesions. Urinary levels of 5-hydroxyindoleacetic acid (5-HIAA), a metabolic product of serotonin, are almost invariably elevated in cases of carcinoid syndrome and correlate to some extent with the severity of its manifestations.

Malignant carcinoid tumors often behave in a very indolent fashion. Median survival from the onset of the carcinoid syndrome is more than 3 years, with 25% of patients alive at 6 years. Although most patients eventually die of widespread tumor, some patients with metastatic carcinoid may live many years without treatment and succumb to an unrelated disease. Cardiac failure may be the cause of death in those with severe tricuspid and pulmonic valve damage from the endocardial lesions of carcinoid syndrome.

TREATMENT

Surgery

Surgery with removal of the primary tumor and, if possible, with resection of bulky metastatic disease, including isolated metastatic lesions in the liver, represents the best initial therapy for patients with or without the carcinoid syndrome. Because of the indolent nature of the disease and the morbidity caused by the production of the various biologically

Table 21–2. **FEATURES OF THE CARCINOID SYNDROME**

Flushing	Endocardial lesions
Telangiectasias	Retroperitoneal fibrosis
Asthma	Pellagra
Diarrhea	

Table 21–3. **DRUGS USED TO TREAT CARCINOID SYNDROME**

Somatostatin	Theophylline sodium glycinate (Cinaphyl)
Histamine-receptor blockers	Chlorpromazine
Methysergide	Corticosteroids
Cyproheptadine	Isoniazid
Alphamethyldopa	Parachlorophenylalanine

active amines, debulking surgery may produce significant palliation in selected patients, including those with extensive metastases. Surgery should be undertaken with great caution in patients with carcinoid syndrome; a number of anesthetic agents can trigger severe episodes of bronchoconstriction and hypotension. Pharmacologic pretreatment prior to surgery can help to avoid or minimize a "carcinoid crisis" due to the sudden lysis of tumor cells and consequent release of their contents.

Pharmacologic Therapy

Several approaches are available to control symptoms of the carcinoid syndrome (Table 21–3). Parachlorophenylalanine, an inhibitor of serotonin synthesis, is effective in reducing diarrhea, but serious side effects, including dizziness, headache, hypothermia, and allergic reactions, severely limit its usefulness. Serotonin antagonists—methysergide (Sansert) and cyproheptadine (Periactin)—and alpha- and beta-adrenergic blockers, alphamethyldopa, chlorpromazine, and adrenocortical steroids produce variable and unpredictable effects in only a small number of patients and are usually accompanied by disturbing side effects of their own. A combination of diphenhydramine and cimetidine (H_1 and H_2 histamine-receptor antagonists, respectively) has been reported to block the carcinoid flush.

The development of a relatively long-acting somatostatin analogue (octreotide, Sandostatin), however, has revolutionized the pharmacologic management of carcinoid syndrome as well as some of the endocrine manifestations of pancreatic islet cell tumors. Natural somatostatin, a peptide synthesized in many tissues, inhibits hormone secretion from the pituitary gland, pancreatic islets, and gastrointestinal tract. Subcutaneous administration of octreotide in a dose of 150 μg (occasionally more) every 8 hours produces marked improvement in flushing and diarrhea in almost all treated patients. Side effects are uncommon, although glucose intolerance, malabsorption, and gallstone development are potential complications of long-term use.

Chemotherapy

Antitumor chemotherapy of malignant carcinoid tumor has received relatively little attention in the literature. Several single agents appear to have activity, and some experience with combination regimens has been reported (Table 21–4). Responses to chemotherapy and to interferon tend to be brief and side effects substantial, and there is little evidence that treatment improves survival. At present, no chemotherapy program can be considered standard treatment for metastatic carcinoid tumor. An aggressive experimental approach employed at the Mayo Clinic for patients with carcinoid syndrome includes hepatic artery ligation for tumor debulking, followed by chemotherapy with

Table 21–4. **CHEMOTHERAPY OF CARCINOID TUMOR**

DRUG(S)	OBJECTIVE RESPONSE RATE (%)
Adriamycin	21
5-Fluorouracil (5-FU)	26
Dacarbazine	13
5-FU + streptozocin	22
5-FU + cyclophosphamide	26
Interferon	20

dacarbazine plus Adriamycin alternating with 5-FU (5-fluorouracil) plus streptozocin (STZ). Preliminary results are favorable.

REFERENCES

Creutzfeld W, Stockmann F: Carcinoids and the carcinoid syndrome. Am J Med 82(supp 5B):4–16, 1987.

Gorden P, Comi RJ, Maton PN, Go VL: Somatostatin and somatostatin analogue (SMS 201–995) in treatment of hormone-secreting tumors of the pituitary and gastrointestinal tract and non-neoplastic diseases of the gut. Ann Intern Med 110:35–50, 1989.

Kvols LK, Buck M: Chemotherapy of endocrine malignancies: a review. Semin Oncol 14:343–353, 1987.

Moertel CG: An odyssey in the land of small tumors. J Clin Oncol 5:1503–1522, 1987.

Valimaki M, Jarvinem H, Salmela P, et al: Is the treament of metastatic carcinoid tumor with interferon not as successful as suggested? Cancer 67:547–549, 1991.

PANCREATIC ISLET CELL TUMORS

Islet cell carcinomas are estimated to occur in fewer than one person per 100,000 population. Despite their rarity, these tumors have been extensively studied and reviewed in the medical literature, owing in large part to the interesting and often devastating endocrine syndromes that they produce. Islet cell carcinomas may occur at any age but the peak incidence is between age 40 and 70. They may involve any portion of the pancreas, and multiple tumors occur in 10 to 20% of cases. Almost all islet cell adenomas and about 80% of the carcinomas produce endocrine syndromes. The hormones responsible include those produced by normal islet cells (e.g., insulin, glucagon) as well as others (ACTH, melanocyte-stimuating hormone [MSH], serotonin) produced ectopically. The functioning islet cell tumors are listed in Table 21–5.

INSULINOMA

Clinical Features

Most patients with insulinoma present with symptoms related to the hypersecretion of insulin. Hypoglycemic manifestations include confusion, headache, blurred vision, stupor, coma, and bizarre behavior that may simulate psychiatric disorders or the effects of alcohol or drugs. Compensatory sympathetic stimulation causes tremor, tachycardia, sweating, and anxiety. Occasionally, patients with malignant insulinoma first present with symptoms related to the tumor and its metastases, i.e., jaundice, hepatomegaly, and abdominal pain.

The diagnosis of insulinoma depends on the demonstration of inappropriately high serum insulin levels during hypoglycemia. Simultaneous glucose and insulin levels are determined during a 72-hour fast. Provocative tests are rarely necessary. An elevated ratio of proinsulin to insulin is often found, particularly in the 10% of cases of malignant insulinomas. Computed tomography or selective angiography usually demonstrates a pancreatic tumor with or without liver metastases. Pathologic examination of tissue obtained at laparotomy or by biopsy of liver metastases, if present, reveals the distinctive features of islet cell tumor, but determination of malignancy depends on the demonstration of local invasion or metastatic spread.

Treatment

Surgery. Surgery with excision of a solitary adenoma is curative in the majority of cases. Malignant insulinomas should also be resected if possible, even in the presence of

Table 21–5. **ISLET CELL TUMORS**

TUMOR	% MALIGNANT	MAJOR MANIFESTATION
Insulinoma	10	Hypoglycemia
Gastrinoma	60	Peptic ulcer, diarrhea
Glucagonoma	60	Diabetes, skin rash
Pancreatic cholera (VIPoma)	60	Watery diarrhea
Somatostatinoma	80	Cholelithiasis, diabetes

hepatic metastases, since such surgical debulking may allow easier control of hypoglycemia.

Antihormone Therapy. In many patients, tumor growth is indolent and the major morbidity of the condition derives from excessive insulin secretion. Therefore, successful management of recurrent hypoglycemia in patients with unresectable or metastatic insulinoma results in worthwhile palliation. Diazoxide, the antihypertensive benzothiadiazine, directly inhibits insulin release. Glucocorticoids and glucagon have been used for their hyperglycemic action but are rarely satisfactory. Recently, long-acting somatostatin analogues have been developed, and these drugs represent a promising avenue of therapy for suppression of insulin secretion. Antihormonal treatment, however, has no effect on tumor growth.

Chemotherapy. Because of the relative rarity of islet cell carcinomas, very few of the conventional chemotherapeutic agents have had adequate trials against these tumors. Streptozocin, an antitumor antibiotic of the nitrosourea class, was found to be diabetogenic in both animals and humans. For this reason, the activity of streptozocin against insulinomas and malignant islet cell tumors in general has been extensively explored. In most series, about 50% of patients with insulinomas respond with an objective reduction in tumor mass, and about 60% will have improvement in insulin levels and hypoglycemia. Both tumor and hormone responses last about 1 year. Interestingly, the activity of streptozocin is not limited to beta cell tumors (insulinomas); the drug is active against non–beta islet cell malignancies (e.g., gastrinomas, glucagonomas) and nonfunctioning islet cell carcinomas as well (see below).

In a randomized prospective study in patients with metastatic islet cell carcinomas, streptozocin alone (500 mg/m^2 IV, daily for 5 days) has been compared with streptozocin at the same dose plus 5-fluorouracil (400 mg/m^2 IV, daily for 5 days). The combination regimen produced a greater response rate (63% versus 34%, $p = .01$) and a greater complete response rate (33% versus 12%, $p < .05$) in all types of islet cell carcinomas, including nonfunctioning tumors. The median survival of patients treated with streptozocin alone was 16 months, whereas patients who received the combination had a median survival of 26 months. The toxicity of the combined regimen was not severe.

In a more recent prospective randomized study in patients with islet cell carcinomas of all types, 5-fluorouracil plus streptozocin was compared with Adriamycin plus streptozocin and with chlorozotocin (an investigational streptozocin analogue with less toxicity) as a single agent. The overall response rate was 47% for all 145 patients, and the median survival was 1.6 years. Patients receiving Adriamycin plus streptozocin had a significantly higher response rate (69%) and a longer median survival (2.2 years) than patients receiving either of the other two regimens. The major toxicity consisted of moderately severe nausea and myelosuppression.

REFERENCES

Boden G: Insulinoma and glucagonoma. Semin Oncol 14:253–262, 1987.

Fraker DL, Norton JA: Localization and resection of insulinomas and gastrinomas. JAMA 259:3601–3605, 1988.

Kvols LK, Buck M: Chemotherapy of endocrine malignancies: a review. Semin Oncol 14:343–353, 1987.

Moertel CG, Lefkopoulo M, Lipsitz S, et al: Streptozocin-doxorubicin, streptozocin-fluorouracil, or chlorozotocin in the treatment of advanced islet-cell carcinoma. N Engl J Med 326:519–523, 1992.

Vinik AI, Delbridge L, Moattari R, et al: Transhepatic portal vein catheterization and localization of insulinomas: A ten year experience. Surgery 109:1–11, 1991.

GASTRINOMA (ZOLLINGER-ELLISON SYNDROME)

Clinical Features

The original description of the Zollinger-Ellison syndrome in 1955 consisted of ulcer disease, massive gastric hypersecretion, and pancreatic islet cell tumor. With increased experience (over 10,000 cases have been reported), the clinical picture of the syndrome has expanded, and at present none of these features is required for the diagnosis.

Most patients with gastrinoma present with ulcer symptoms that are indistinguishable from those seen in patients with ordinary peptic ulcer disease. Many patients with gastrinoma complain of diarrhea, and the association of peptic disease with diarrhea should suggest the possibility of gastrinoma. Multiple ulcers, recurrent ulceration following surgery, ulceration of the distal duodenum or jejunum, and the presence of multiple endocrine neoplasia (MEN) type I in either the patient or family members should raise suspicion of Zollinger-Ellison syndrome. However, 20 to 25% of patients with the Zollinger-Ellison syndrome have no detectable ulcer at the time of initial presentation.

The diagnosis of gastrinoma depends on the finding of an elevated fasting serum gastrin level in the absence of other conditions associated with hypergastrinemia (i.e., achlorhydria, retained gastric antrum, chronic gastric outlet obstruction). Patients with the Zollinger-Ellison syndrome usually have gastrin levels above 200 pg/mL, and levels above 1000 pg/mL are virtually diagnostic of the syndrome, but gastrin levels in the normal range occasionally may be seen. In equivocal cases, provocative tests with secretin, calcium, or glucagon are necessary. The intravenous secretin test is the easiest and most reliable of these. Since the advent of readily available, highly reliable radioimmunoassays for gastrin, measurements of gastric acid output are no longer commonly needed to make the diagnosis of Zollinger-Ellison syndrome.

Treatment

Surgery. Surgical excision of a gastrinoma (located usually in the pancreas but occasionally in the duodenal wall) should be considered in patients with the Zollinger-Ellison syndrome. Most patients, however, are not surgical candidates because the disease is either metastatic at the time of diagnosis (15 to 20%), multiple, or not evident at the time of exploration. The initial imaging procedure should be the CT scan followed by selective angiography if further definition of the tumor is required. MRI and selective venous sampling for gastrin do not provide useful additional information in most cases. Surgical morbidity and mortality from extensive surgical procedures such as pancreatectomy or pancreaticoduodenectomy are substantial.

Therefore, in most patients treatment is directed toward control of gastric acid secretion. Until the past decade, this was usually accomplished by total gastrectomy. With the advent of powerful new agents to suppress gastric acid secretion, gastrectomy for Zollinger-Ellison syndrome is now rarely necessary.

Antihormone Treatment. Histamine H_2-receptor antagonists such as cimetidine, ranitidine, and famotidine suppress gastric acid secretion in over 80% of patients, resulting in diminished symptoms and ulcer healing. However, large doses are required at frequent intervals, and dose escalation is necessary in many patients. In resistant cases, the addition of an anticholinergic drug or parietal cell vagotomy may be necessary. The recent availability of omeprazole, a drug that inhibits hydrogen ion secretion in the gastric parietal cell, has made gastric acid inhibition even more effective. Omeprazole is given orally once daily and is safe and more effective than the H_2-receptor antagonists; omeprazole has therefore become the drug of choice for patients with the Zollinger-Ellison syndrome. Somatostatin analogues are also effective, but their exact role in the managment of gastrinoma remains to be defined.

Chemotherapy. Streptozocin is effective in 30 to 40% of metastatic gastrinomas, but the combination of streptozocin plus Adriamycin is superior. Interferon may also have some activity.

REFERENCES

Andersen DK: Current diagnosis and management of Zollinger-Ellison syndrome. Ann Surg 210:685–703, 1989.

Maton PN, Vinayek R, Frucht H, et al: Long term efficacy and safety of omeprazole in patients with Zollinger-Ellison syndrome: A prospective study. Gastroenterology 97:827–836, 1989.

Wank SA, Doppman JL, Miller DL, et al: Prospective study of the ability of computerized axial tomography to localize gastrinomas in patients with Zollinger-Ellison syndrome. Gastroenterology 92:905–912, 1987.

Wolfe MM, Jensen RT: Zollinger-Ellison syndrome. N Engl J Med 317:1200–1209, 1987.

GLUCAGONOMA

Clinical Features

Glucagon-secreting tumors of the pancreatic alpha cell occur at a female to male ratio of 2:1 and at a mean age of 55 years. A characteristic skin rash, necrolytic migratory erythema, often first brings the patient to medical attention. The pathogenesis of the skin rash remains obscure. Neither the presence nor the severity of the skin disease is correlated with the plasma glucagon level. Amino acid deficiency, zinc deficiency, and fatty acid deficiency have all been put forth as the possible cause of the rash. Glucose intolerance is almost invariably present, but overt diabetes occurs in only about 50% of patients. Anemia, weight loss, glossitis, angular stomatitis, depression, and deep venous thrombosis are common features.

The diagnosis of glucagonoma rests on the characteristic clinical picture, the demonstration of a pancreatic tumor, and the finding of an elevated plasma or tissue glucagon level. Glucagonoma may occur as part of the multiple endocrine neoplasia (MEN) type I syndrome.

Treatment

Curative surgery is possible in fewer than half the cases but, if accomplished, results in clearing of the skin lesions, return to normal glucose tolerance, and correction of all other manifestations. Long-acting somatostatin analogues that inhibit glucagon secretion have been used prior to surgery to prepare cachectic patients for operation.

Streptozocin alone or in combination with 5-fluorouracil or Adriamycin results in tumor shrinkage, clearing of skin lesions, and a drop in glucagon levels. Excellent partial remissions with dacarbazine chemotherapy have also been achieved. The skin disease, which is often extremely severe, has been treated with tetracycline, topical steroids, zinc, and parenteral nutrition. Because of the variable natural history of the eruption, it is difficult to evaluate the effectiveness of these interventions. Liver metastases may be controlled by hepatic artery embolization. Somatostatin analogues are effective in clearing the skin rash as well as in improving other features of the disease.

REFERENCES

Bloom SR, Polak JM: Glucagonoma syndrome. Am J Med 82:25–36, 1987.

Boden G, Ryan IG, Eisenschmid BL, et al: Treatment of inoperable glucagonoma with the long-acting somatostatin analogue SMS 201–995. N Engl J Med 314:1686–1688, 1986.

Freimann J, Pazdure R: Hepatic artery embolization for treatment of glucagonomas: Antineoplastic and palliative benefits. Am J Clin Oncol 13:271–275, 1990.

PANCREATIC CHOLERA: VIPOMA

Clinical Features

Profuse watery diarrhea with consequent dehydration and electrolyte abnormalities is the hallmark of the pancreatic cholera syndrome, produced in many but not all cases by hypersecretion of vasoactive intestinal polypeptide (VIP) from a pancreatic islet cell tumor. Fluid losses may excede 5 L daily in severe cases. Gastric hypochlorhydria, hypercalcemia, and hyperglycemia also occur in many patients. The diagnosis requires the clinical triad of profuse watery diarrhea, an islet cell tumor, and the absence of gastric hypersecretion (ruling out gastrinoma). Elevated blood or tissue levels of VIP are helpful but not necessary for diagnosis. Rarely, the pancreatic cholera syndrome occurs in association with extra-pancreatic tumors of neural crest origin (pheochromocytoma, ganglioneuroblastoma, and bronchogenic carcinoma).

Treatment

Partial pancreatectomy is useful in patients with localized disease, but at least 50% of patients have metastases at the time of diagnosis. Streptozocin alone or in combination with 5-FU or Adriamycin has produced excellent subjective and objective remissions. Corticosteroids and prostaglandin inhibitors (indomethacin, nutmeg) have been used to control the diarrhea in some patients. Metoclopramide, clonidine, trifluoperazine, and lithium have also been tried with some success, but a somatostatin analogue (octreotide) is now the treatment of choice for diarrhea in patients with VIPomas.

REFERENCES

Krejs GJ: VIPoma syndrome. Am J Med 82 (suppl 5B):37–48, 1987.
O'Dorisio TM, Mekhjian HS, Gaginella TS: Medical therapy of VIPomas. Endocrinol Metab Clin North Am 18:545–556, 1989.

SOMATOSTATINOMA

Somatostatin is a 14–amino acid polypeptide that inhibits the secretion of numerous pituitary, pancreatic, and gastrointestinal hormones. Islet cell tumors secreting excessive amounts of somatostatin produce cholelithiasis (cholecystokinin suppression), mild diabetes mellitus (insulin suppression), steatorrhea (cholecystokinin and pancreozymin suppression), hypochlorhydria, and occasionally anemia. The clinical manifestations are so nonspecific that several cases have been discovered serendipitously at exploration for gallstones.

The diagnosis of somatostatinoma should be considered in patients with diabetes and an islet cell tumor. The finding of an elevated serum somatostatin level is diagnostic. Because only a handful of cases have been reported, conclusions regarding treatment are premature. Nevertheless, good responses have been seen following surgery (Whipple procedure) and chemotherapy with streptozocin.

REFERENCES

Harris GJ, Tio F, Cruz AB: Somatostatinoma: A case report and review of the literature. J Surg Oncol 36:8–16, 1987.
Vinik AI, Strodel WE, Eckhouse FE, et al: Somatostatinomas, PPomas, neurotensinomas. Semin Oncol 14:263–281, 1987.

22
CANCER OF UNKNOWN PRIMARY ORIGIN

Julia L. Smith

Metastatic cancer presenting without an apparent primary lesion represents a common problem in oncologic practice, accounting for up to 10% of cases. The clinician may be faced with malignant hepatomegaly, multiple pulmonary nodules, malignant pleural effusion, or metastases to lymph nodes, bone, brain, skin, or other sites in a patient without previous history of malignant disease and without evidence of primary site of origin on routine evaluation. The first step in the investigation of this problem should be biopsy of the most accessible metastatic lesion.

PATHOLOGY

Biopsy and tissue diagnosis should precede attempts to locate a primary site, since pathologic examination may obviate the need for a search (in melanoma, for example) or may provide clues to direct the search more effectively. If the pathologist identifies squamous cell carcinoma, an origin in the upper aerodigestive tract, lung, or uterine cervix is most likely. A diagnosis of lymphoma demands a staging evaluation, but a search for a primary is unnecessary. Often the pathologist simply diagnoses poorly differentiated tumor or undifferentiated malignancy because of an inability to distinguish carcinoma from melanoma, sarcoma, or lymphoma. Adenocarcinoma is the most common histologic diagnosis in this setting and indicates a possible origin in numerous sites, including gastrointestinal tract, lung, breast, prostate, kidney, gynecologic organs, and others. Careful review of the material with the pathologist is critical, since clinical details may stimulate additional pathologic suggestions. Under ordinary light microscopy, the pathologist may be able to select certain primary sites that would be more likely than others. With the use of special stains for keratin, mucin, glycogen, melanin, and other cellular components, the pathologist can offer further information. In especially difficult cases, rebiopsy may be advisable to obtain adequate tissue for sophisticated studies, including electron microscopy, immunohistochemistry, cell membrane markers, and hormone receptors. These studies can provide definite pathologic diagnoses in cases that remained obscure under routine examination.

Immunohistochemistry often proves especially helpful. The technique employs immunoperoxidase-labeled monoclonal antibodies directed against particular cellular constituents. The most commonly used antibodies identify cytokeratin antigens found in carcinomas, common leukocyte antigen in lymphoid and hematologic malignancies, S-100 commonly found in melanoma, and prostate-specific antigen in prostate cancers. Numerous other monoclonal antibodies are available for immunohistochemical studies as well. On occasion, electron microscopy provides definite pathologic diagnoses in obscure cases. With electron microscopy, the pathologist may be able to identify premelanosomes, indicating melanoma; neurosecretory granules, suggesting small cell carcinoma; microvilli and junctional complexes, indicating adenocarcinoma; or tonofilaments, indicating squamous cell carcinoma.

CLINICAL PRESENTATION

Patients with metastatic disease of unknown primary origin may present with metastases involving almost any site. Patients with unknown primaries whose primary site is ultimately identified manifest an atypical pattern of metastatic spread (Table 22–1). This may account in part for the difficulty in determining the primary site. For example, known primary lung and breast cancers frequently metastasize to bone, whereas occult primary lung and breast cancers involve bone much less often. Another difference is the incidence of unknown versus known primary malignancies. Cancer of the pancreas is among the most frequent primary sites identified in patients who present with unknown primary

Table 22–1. **PERCENT OF METASTATIC INVOLVEMENT: UNKNOWN PRIMARY (A) VERSUS KNOWN PRIMARY (B)**

PRIMARY TUMOR	METASTATIC SITE							
	Bone		Lung		Liver		Brain	
	A	*B*	*A*	*B*	*A*	*B*	*A*	*B*
Lung	4	30–50	90	34	36	30–50	21	15–30
Breast	33	50–85	66	60	60	45–60	33	15–25
Thyroid	0	39	100	65	50	60	0	1
Pancreas	28	5–10	31	25–40	72	50–70	3	1–4
Liver	31	8	19	20	100	—	6	0
Colorectal	13	5–10	40	25–40	87	71	0	1
Gastric	9	5–10	18	20–30	36	35–50	9	1–4
Renal	66	30–50	77	50–75	33	35–40	0	7–8
Ovary	0	2–6	25	10	25	10–15	0	1
Prostate	25	50–75	75	13–53	50	13	25	2

From Neumann KH, Nystrom JS: Metastatic cancer of unknown origin: Nonsquamous cell type. Semin Oncol 9:427–434, 1982.

cancer, but it is relatively less frequent in cancer registries. Cancers of the lung, liver, and kidney are also overrepresented among patients with unknown primaries, whereas cancers of the breast and prostate are markedly underrepresented in comparison with the general population of cancer patients.

Some clues as to site of origin may be derived from tumor site at diagnosis; patients presenting with disease above the diaphragm most often are found to have lung primaries, whereas those with tumor below the diaphragm are more likely to harbor occult pancreatic carcinomas. Cervical lymph node presentations most often represent metastases from head and neck primaries. A supraclavicular node containing adenocarcinoma (Virchow's node) often indicates an intra-abdominal primary tumor, especially gastric carcinoma. Malignant axillary node involvement in a woman strongly suggests occult breast cancer, and if estrogen receptor is present in the tumor, a diagnosis of metastatic breast cancer should be made, even if a breast mass cannot be demonstrated. Metastatic cancer in inguinal lymph nodes suggests a primary site in the pelvis or lower extremities. Metastatic tumor in the skin is most likely to derive from melanoma or cancers of the lung, breast, or kidney.

CLINICAL EVALUATION

The approach to a patient with metastatic carcinoma of unknown origin should concentrate on evaluation for treatable sources. These include breast, ovarian, prostate, and thyroid adenocarcinomas, malignant germ cell tumors, and lymphomas. A prudent workup should include a meticulous history and physical examination and limited diagnostic evaluations. Specific inquiries should be made regarding specific symptoms, smoking history, asbestos and toxin exposure, past removal of pigmented skin lesions, biopsy or excision of "benign" tumor in the past, and vaginal bleeding in postmenopausal women. The physical examination should include a thorough survey of the skin, including subungual areas, pelvic and rectal examinations including fecal occult blood testing, and careful evaluation of the optic fundi, oral cavity, lymph nodes, breasts, testes, prostate, and thyroid gland. In cases of cervical adenopathy or supradiaphragmatic squamous cell carcinoma, a full evaluation of the head and neck by an experienced otolaryngologist is required.

Screening laboratory studies should be confined to complete blood count, urinalysis, chemistry panel, and chest x-ray. Further studies should be guided by clues derived from the clinical evaluation and pathologic findings. The appropriate extent of additional investigative studies is difficult to prescribe, but several observations are revelant to this issue:

- In most patients, the primary site will not be discovered during life, no matter how extensive the evaluation.

Table 22–2. **TREATABLE METASTATIC CANCERS**

TYPE	KEY DIAGNOSTIC FEATURES
Curable Cancers	
Lymphomas	Immunohistochemistry
Germ cell tumors	Alpha-fetoprotein and β-HCG
Cancers with >50% Response Rate	
Breast cancer	Physical examination, mammography
Prostate cancer	Digital examination, PSA
Ovarian cancer	CA-125
Small cell lung cancer	Electron microscopy, immunohistochemistry
Thyroid cancer	Physical examination
Endometrial cancer	History of bleeding, endometrial biopsy
Head and neck cancer	Indirect laryngoscopy

- In a substantial number the primary will not be found, even at autopsy.
- The median survival of these patients is about 3 to 7 months, with less than 25% alive at 1 year and less than 10% at 5 years.
- With the exception of lymphomas and germ cell tumors, these cancers are not curable, and useful palliative therapy can be offered only to a minority (Table 22–2). In most patients, discovery of the primary tumor will have no therapeutic implications.

In the past, extensive searches for occult primary tumors were carried out in order to discover treatable diseases and to identify untreatable lesions and thus avoid futile and toxic therapy. Many recognized that the hazard and expense of such searches were staggering and that the information derived was often misleading and of little use in improving the length or the quality of the patient's survival. This led to a more focused approach: given the short survival of these patients, extensive diagnostic studies are unjustified, frequently inaccurate (Table 22–3), and inhumane.

The best course is a compromise—a limited, thoughtful search to discover treatable tumors, to evaluate patient signs and symptoms, and to offer palliative therapy. This approach requires judicious restraint in the use of diagnostic procedures; studies are performed only when their results will change the management of the patient. For example, in a woman with metastatic adenocarcinoma, a mammogram is indicated, since the diagnosis of breast cancer would permit the use of specific chemotherapy or hormonal therapy that is likely to have an impact on the course of the disease. In a man with metastatic adenocarcinoma, in addition to a digital prostate examination, serum acid phosphatase and prostate-specific antigen (PSA) may support a diagnosis of prostate cancer and lead to hormonal manipulation. On the other hand, upper gastrointestinal (GI) series, barium enema, GI endoscopy, and endoscopic retrograde cholangiopancreatography (ERCP) are inappropriate in a patient who presents with metastatic adenocarcinoma and who has no signs or symptoms suggesting a bowel or pancreatic tumor. In this case, the finding of an occult primary tumor in the GI tract would have no implications for management,

Table 22–3. **RESULTS OF CONTRAST ROENTGENOGRAPHY**

	UGIS	BARIUM ENEMA	IVP	TOTAL
Number of cases	218	198	187	603
Number positive for carcinoma	14	17	16	47
Number true positive	8	9	5	22
Number false positive	6	8	11	25
Number false negative	4	6	4	14

From Nystrom JS, Weiner JM, Wolf RM, et al: Identifying the primary site in metastatic cancer of unknown origin. JAMA 241:381–383, 1979. Copyright 1979, American Medical Association.

Abbreviations: UGIS, upper gastrointestinal tract contrast radiograph; IVP, intravenous pyelogram.

Roentgenographically positive study results include all examinations thought to be positive by the radiologist for a primary cancer site. True positive studies were confirmed by a second procedure or necropsy. False-positive and false-negative results were verified by necropsy.

since no useful systemic therapy exists for these cancers. Likewise intravenous urography should be performed only if hematuria and symptoms referable to the kidneys are present. Furthermore, the number of false-positive examinations is high, and a substantial number of occult primary tumors will actually be missed (see Table 22–3).

Several authors have suggested that abdominal computed tomography (CT) scans should be performed in patients with metastatic cancer of unknown primary origin, particularly in patients with abdominal symptoms. Since pancreatic cancer accounts for a large fraction of unknown primary cancers, this recommendation very likely will lead to the identification of the primary in an increased percentage of cases. However, in the absence of effective systemic therapy for metastatic pancreatic cancer or for other primaries detectable by abdominal CT (e.g., renal, liver, adrenal, gallbladder), the utility of this approach can be questioned.

If the initial biopsy reveals a squamous cell cancer, the evaluation differs. If the presentation is supradiaphragmatic, head and neck, lung, and esophageal cancers should be sought. If the metastases are below the diaphragm, the likely sources are anal and, in women, cervical or labial cancers.

SPECIAL SITUATIONS

Several groups of patients with cancers of unknown primary origin deserve special consideration. Patients with "poorly differentiated adenocarcinoma" or "undifferentiated carcinoma" with pulmonary, mediastinal, or paraaortic nodal disease may actually have occult extragonadal germ cell cancers. This is particularly true if the patient is young and male. Serum marker levels for alpha-fetoprotein and beta human chorionic gonadotropin (β-HCG) should be obtained, and if possible immunohistochemical studies should be performed on the tumor tissue in an attempt to detect these markers in the tumor cells. Such patients frequently respond to cisplatin-based combination chemotherapy regimens, even in the absence of a firm histologic diagnosis of germ cell tumor (Chap. 15). The prognosis of this group is somewhat worse than that of patients with testicular cancers, probably due to the large tumor volume at diagnosis.

Another important subset of patients comprises women who present with intra-abdominal adenocarcinoma without evidence of primary site. The cancers in these patients often behave like ovarian carcinomas and may respond to cisplatin-based chemotherapy. Poorly differentiated tumors with neuroendocrine features by light or electron microscopy also have high response rates to chemotherapy and in some instances to local treatment with surgery or radiation therapy.

TREATMENT

If a treatable tumor (see Table 22–2) can be identified, then the choice of therapy is straightforward. If the focused work-up reveals one of the responsive tumors, appropriate therapy should be started immediately.

If no primary is found and no presumptive diagnosis of a treatable malignancy can be made, then therapy should be directed toward relief of symptoms. Tube thoracostomy for malignant pleural effusion, LeVeen shunt for malignant ascites, radiotherapy for painful bone metastates, nutritional counseling, narcotic analgesics, and a variety of other measures may be remarkably rewarding. Asymptomatic patients require no palliation. If the pattern of disease falls into one of the special cases outlined above, antineoplastic therapy is warranted if the patient can tolerate it. Otherwise, in some cases, a brief trial of palliative chemotherapy directed against the most likely treatable tumor types is reasonable, but responses are rare and brief. Patients with widespread disease with poor performance status should receive supportive care only.

SUMMARY

Patients with metastatic disease without apparent primary tumor should undergo biopsy of a metastatic lesion prior to further radiologic or endoscopic search for an occult primary cancer. The pathologist, not the radiologist, should be the clinician's major ally in these cases. Careful review of the specimen and performance of special studies may produce a definite diagnosis or helpful clues in previously puzzling material.

Meticulous history and physical examination, with attention to areas frequently overlooked (lymph nodes, pelvic examination, prostate, testes, head and neck area), may yield unexpected and useful information. Routine screening tests (e.g., urinalysis, chest x-ray) may provide clues that guide further studies. Clinical indications deserve further evaluation, and screening tests for likely treatable tumors (see Table 22–2) should follow. The indiscriminate diagnostic "fishing expedition" can only be condemned, however.

REFERENCES

Altman E, Cadman E: An analysis of 1539 patients with cancer of unknown primary site. Cancer 57:120–124, 1986.

Greco FA, Vaughn SK, Hainsworth JD: Advanced poorly differentiated carcinoma of unknown primary site: Recognition of a treatable syndrome. Ann Intern Med 104:547–553, 1986.

Hainsworth JD, Johnson DH, Greco FA: Poorly differentiated neuroendocrine carcinoma of unknown primary site. A newly recognized clinicopathologic entity. Ann Intern Med 109:364–371, 1988.

Haskell CM, Cochran AJ, Barsky SH, Steckel RJ: Metastasis of unknown origin. Curr Prob Cancer 12:4–58, 1988.

Johnston WW: The malignant pleural effusion. Cancer 56:905–909, 1985.

Karsell PR, Sheedy PF, O'Connell MJ: Computed tomography in search of cancer of unknown origin. JAMA 248:340–343, 1982.

Kirsten F, Chi CH, Leary JA, et al: Metastatic adeno or undifferentiated carcinoma from an unknown primary site—Natural history and guidelines for identification of treatable subsets. Q J Med 62:143–161, 1987.

Silverman C, Marks JE: Metastatic cancer of unknown origin: Epidermoid and undifferentiated carcinomas. Semin Oncol 9:435–441, 1982.

Steckel RJ, Kagan AR: Diagnostic persistence in working up metastatic cancer with an unknown primary site. Radiology 134:367–369, 1980.

Strnad CM, Grosh WW, Baxter J, et al: Peritoneal carcinomatosis of unknown primary site in women. Ann Intern Med 111:213–217, 1989.

23
ONCOLOGIC EMERGENCIES

Timothy J. Woodlock

Interference with the normal function of vital organ systems can occur in cancer patients as a result of tumor growth or metabolic products produced by tumors, or from side effects of therapy. When normal physiology is severely compromised, emergency situations develop. Prompt recognition and appropriate treatment of these oncologic emergencies may significantly reduce morbidity and mortality.

HEMATOLOGIC EMERGENCIES

THERAPY-INDUCED CYTOPENIAS

Suppression of hematopoiesis is a common side effect of cytotoxic therapy with drugs and/or radiation, and the consequent decrease in peripheral blood counts may alter normal blood function. A decrease in all forms of blood cells may occur, although of particular concern are granulocytopenia (neutropenia) and thrombocytopenia, which limit the patient's ability to control acute infection and bleeding. The risks of morbidity and mortality increase with the extent of cytopenia, and patients with granulocyte counts less than 500/mm^3 and platelet counts less than 20,000/mm^3 are at highest risk. Marrow infiltration by cancer, immune destruction of blood cells, hypersplenism, and consumption coagulopathies can also cause cytopenias of clinical significance. A detailed discussion of the approach to fever and neutropenia is found in Chapter 28. Effective management generally requires prompt diagnostic studies and initiation of broad-spectrum antibiotic treatment, including coverage for *Pseudomonas* species.

Management of thrombocytopenia involves the consideration of many factors, including platelet count, absence or presence of comorbid illness, concurrent therapy with any drugs that affect platelet function, and the absence or presence of clinical bleeding. Patients must be managed on an individual basis, and clinical judgment is the best guide to the use and timing of platelet transfusions or other interventions. Many physicians recommend prophylactic transfusion of random donor platelets if the platelet count is less than 20,000/mm^3. The quantity transfused is commonly 3 U/m^2 body surface area or 0.1 U/kg body weight, with each unit containing 40 to 60 mL of plasma in addition to platelets. The posttransfusion increment in platelet count varies with individual circumstances, and some patients become refractory to random donor platelets and require serologically compatible single-donor platelets. Recipients of platelet transfusions should have three platelet counts: one immediately prior to platelet transfusion, the second 1 hour after administration of the platelet concentrate, and the third the next morning (8 to 24 hours later). This serial recording of the platelet counts allows the determination of peak recovery and survival of transfused platelets.

Patients with fever and sepsis, coexisting coagulation abnormalities, or gastrointestinal (GI) ulceration are more likely to have internal bleeding and may benefit from maintaining the platelet count at a threshold higher than 20,000/mm^3. Many drugs affect platelet function, although aspirin has the most marked clinical effect; aspirin and aspirin-containing medications should be avoided in thrombocytopenic patients. Patients with clinical bleeding that persists despite platelet transfusion may benefit from epsilon-aminocaproic acid (Amicar), 3 to 5 g every 6 hours given by the intravenous or oral route.

Platelet transfusion reactions are most often due to sensitization to histocompatibility (HLA) antigens or ABO antigens. They commonly occur either during or shortly after the infusion and are characterized by chills and fevers with or without urticaria. Premedication with antihistamines, corticosteroids, and acetaminophen may ameliorate these reactions, but premedication need not be routinely administered to the majority of patients. New blood product filters are available that can remove granulocytes and may be used to avoid some platelet transfusion reactions.

REFERENCES

Consensus Conference: Platelet transfusion therapy. JAMA 257:1777–1780, 1987.
George JN, Shattil SJ: The clinical importance of acquired abnormalities of platelet function. N Engl J Med 324:27–39, 1991.
Heyman MR, Schiffer CA: Platelet transfusion therapy for the cancer patient. Semin Oncol 16:198–209, 1990.
Kickler TS, Bell W, Ness PM, Drew H, Pall D: Depletion of white cells from platelet concentrates with a new absorption filter. Transfusion 29:411–414, 1989.
McCullough J, Steeper TA, Connelly DP, et al: Platelet transfusion in a university hospital. JAMA 259:2414–2418, 1988.

DISSEMINATED INTRAVASCULAR COAGULATION (CONSUMPTION COAGULOPATHY)

Disturbances in coagulation leading to clinical emergencies are frequent in patients with acute progranulocytic leukemia and are occasionally seen in prostatic carcinoma and other solid tumors. Clotting factors are activated when tumor cells produce procoagulant material, stimulate platelet-aggregating activity, or promote increased generation of tissue factor activity by monocytes. The resultant widespread clotting in the microcirculation consumes available coagulation factors and platelets, resulting in a bleeding diathesis. The widespread fibrin deposition may cause microangiopathic hemolytic anemia. Migratory thrombophlebitis and marantic endocarditis with arterial embolization may also occur. The process may be exacerbated by cytotoxic therapy, presumably because treatment-induced cell destruction increases release of procoagulant materials from neoplastic cells. Surgical manipulation of tumors and overwhelming infection are other common causes of coagulopathies in cancer patients.

Signs of a bleeding diathesis include oozing from venipuncture sites and gingiva, ecchymoses, petechiae, epistaxis, GI bleeding, and hematuria. Signs of thrombosis in the microvasculature include azotemia, oliguria, focal ischemia and superficial gangrene in the skin, delirium, coma, acute ulceration in the GI tract, and acute respiratory distress syndrome.

Diagnosis

Fulminant disseminated intravascular coagulation (DIC) produces a severe hemorrhagic diathesis with or without clinical evidence of thrombotic disease. Laboratory data reveal a prolonged prothrombin time, prolonged activated partial thromboplastin time, thrombocytopenia, hypofibrinogenemia, and elevated fibrin-fibrinogen degradation products. The peripheral blood smear often shows microangiopathic changes with red blood cell fragments. Subclinical DIC often occurs in cancer patients and may cause mild bleeding with abnormalities in some of the above-mentioned parameters.

Treatment

Long-term control of DIC depends on adequate therapy for the underlying disease. In the solid tumor patient with a severe bleeding diathesis, fresh frozen plasma and platelets should be transfused generously to replace both clotting factors and platelets, which are being consumed at a rapid rate. In patients who demonstrate clinical evidence of thrombosis as well as bleeding, heparin is given initially to interrupt the clotting cascade, then immediately followed by fresh frozen plasma and platelets. Patients with acute progranulocytic leukemia may present with mild degrees of intravascular coagulation, and therapy may stimulate further factor consumption. Such patients should be considered for possible prophylactic continuous heparin therapy before and during the first 10 to 14 days of treatment.

Patients with prostate carcinoma and possibly other tumors may develop a bleeding syndrome that is clinically similar to DIC, but with no evidence of thrombosis, clotting factor consumption, or thrombocytopenia. This condition is due to primary fibrinolysis, where fibrin and fibrinogen are rapidly degraded because of tumor-induced release of plasminogen activators. Patients with primary fibrinolysis and clinically severe bleeding should be considered for possible treatment with antifibrinolytic drugs such as epilson-aminocaproic acid (Amicar).

REFERENCES

Baker WF: Clinical aspects of disseminated intravascular coagulation: A clinician's point of view. Semin Thromb Hemost 15:1–57, 1989.

Bick RL: Disseminated intravascular coagulation and related syndromes: A clinical review. Semin Thromb Hemost 14:299–338, 1988.

Colman RW, Rubin RN: Disseminated intravascular coagulation due to malignancy. Semin Oncol 17:172–186, 1990.

LEUKOSTASIS

In patients with acute leukemias and circulating blast cell counts in excess of 50,000/mm^3, blood flow in the microcirculation is compromised. Patients with chronic myelogenous leukemia with white cell counts greater than 150,000/mm^3 also have an increased incidence of leukostasis. Elevated white blood cell counts result in a measurable leukocrit that is proportional to the number of white cells and the mean white cell volume. Chronic lymphocytic leukemia lymphocytes have an MCV of 200 μm^3 compared with 300 μm^3 for lymphoblasts of acute lymphoblastic leukemia and 400 μm^3 for myeloblasts of acute myeloblastic leukemia. The difference in cell volume plus cell membrane characteristics help explain why patients with chronic lymphocytic leukemia with very high white cell counts do not develop leukostasis.

Signs and symptoms of leukostasis include visual blurring, dizziness, dyspnea, stupor, delirium, hypoxia, and intracranial hemorrhage. The primary problem appears to be the formation of leukostatic plugs in the microcirculation with subsequent hemorrhagic infarctions in the circulation of the lung, brain, and other organs.

In acute leukemias, a blast cell count greater than 50,000/mm^3 requires prompt treatment to decrease the cell count. Two methods are commonly employed: leukapheresis and/or hydroxyurea. Leukapheresis rapidly reduces the white cell count with the advantage of removing the leukocytes intact; thus the renal system is spared toxic cell breakdown products. Hydroxyurea provides rapid cytolytic therapy for chronic myelogenous leukemia. It is often used in acute nonlymphocytic leukemia with blast counts greater than 100,000/mm^3 prior to initiating standard induction therapy. In order to avoid the complication of hyperviscosity, patients with very high white counts and anemia should not receive red cell transfusions until the leukocyte count has been reduced.

REFERENCES

Dutcher JP, Schiffer CA, Wiernik PH: Hyperleukocytosis in acute nonlymphocytic leukemia: Impact on remission rate and duration and survival. J Clin Oncol 5:1364–1372, 1987.

Gerson SL, Lazarus HM: Hematopoietic emergencies. Semin Oncol 16:532–535, 1989.

OBSTRUCTIVE EMERGENCIES

SPINAL CORD COMPRESSION

Spinal cord compression develops in 1 to 5% of patients with systemic cancer. Ninety-five percent of spinal cord tumors are extradural. Most result from metastatic spread to one or more vertebral bodies, with subsequent extension into the epidural space. Some may result from paraspinal soft tissue tumors that extend directly into the spinal canal. Intramedullary metastases account for only 3 to 4% of spinal cord compressions. The primary tumors most commonly responsible for spinal cord compressions are lymphoma, myeloma, and cancers of the lung, breast, prostate, and kidney. The thoracic spinal cord is involved in approximately 75% of cases, the cervical cord in 15%, and the lumbosacral cord and roots in the remainder of cases. Because the devastating effects of spinal cord compression may include irreversible paraplegia and loss of bowel and bladder control, prompt diagnosis, evaluation, and treatment are essential.

Clinical Presentation

Back pain usually precedes weakness, autonomic dysfunction, and sensory loss. The overwhelming majority of patients have local or radicular pain, which may precede other symptoms by several weeks. The presence of unexplained persistent back pain or back pain with an abnormal plain film of the spine is sufficient evidence to pursue further diagnostic studies. In a recent series, 52% of cancer patients with back pain alone had epidural masses, some of which produced greater than a 75% block on myelogram.

Weakness is present at the time of diagnosis in about 87% of patients, and bowel and bladder dysfunction in about 50 to 60%. If appropriate diagnostic and therapeutic maneuvers are delayed until neurologic findings are severe, the majority of patients will be unable to walk at the end of therapy. Patients who are ambulatory when treatment begins are likely to remain ambulatory, whereas those who are unable to walk initially have a very poor prognosis.

Diagnosis

Initial evaluation of cancer patients with back pain should include a careful neurologic history and physical examination, plain films of the spine, and bone scan. If radiologic evidence (paraspinal mass, loss of a pedicle) of vertebral metastasis is present, further evaluation should follow. A complete myelographic study can document the full cephalad and caudad extent of the block, although with the possible risk of neurologic worsening. With the advent of CT of the spine and more recently magnetic resonance imaging (MRI), myelography can be avoided where these technologies and the appropriate expertise are available.

Treatment

Radiation treatment to the level of the block, plus one or two vertebral body lengths above and below the block, is standard therapy. Total doses for spinal cord compression are in the range of 3000 to 4000 cGy delivered over a 2- to 4-week period. Corticosteroids may help decrease edema and relieve signs and symptoms. The standard dose is 10 mg of dexamethasone followed by 4 mg every 6 hours; however, some neurologists recommend use of up to 10-fold higher doses. For patients with rapid progression of findings, emergency laminectomy should be considered. The following are indications for surgery: (1) requirement of tissue for diagnosis, (2) structurally unstable spine that requires orthopedic intervention, (3) previous radiation to cord tolerance or known radioresistant tumor, (4) progressive deterioration in spite of steroids and radiation, and (5) to rule out epidural abscess or hematoma. Radiation therapy can produce an outcome as good as that with surgery or surgery plus radiation therapy. Prognosis after therapy depends on tumor type, duration of symptoms, extent of signs, and tumor location. Those patients with highly radioresponsive tumors (seminoma, lymphoma, myeloma, Ewing's sarcoma) whose symptoms are of short duration, whose lesions are in the lower as compared with the upper thoracic spine, and who have no evidence of myelopathy have the best response to therapy.

REFERENCES

Sarpel S, Sarpel G, Yu E, et al: Early diagnosis of spinal-epidural metastasis by magnetic resonance imaging. Cancer 59:1112–1116, 1987.

Willson JKV, Masaryk TJ: Neurologic emergencies in the cancer patient. Semin Oncol 16:490–503, 1989.

SUPERIOR VENA CAVA SYNDROME

Occlusion of the superior vena cava causes an increase in upper body venous pressure and forces blood from this region to return to the right atrium via collateral venous channels. The most common cause of this syndrome is mediastinal adenopathy or an expanding mediastinal tumor mass. Lung cancers and lymphomas are most frequently responsible. Symptoms include shortness of breath made worse on recumbency, a feeling of fullness in the head, lethargy, cough, and dysphagia. Although symptoms may develop within a few days, often weeks or months may intervene between onset of symptoms and initiation of therapy. Physical findings include thoracic and neck vein distention, edema of the face with cyanosis, tachycardia, and edema of the upper extremities. Autopsy series indicate that one-half to one-third of patients with superior vena cava syndrome have an associated thrombosis within the superior vena cava itself.

Diagnosis

A chest x-ray or CT scan reveals a mass in the superior mediastinum in the majority of patients. A radionuclide superior vena cavagram can document the site and extent of occlusion. If there is doubt as to the malignant etiology of the obstruction, and if the patient is not in extremis, an attempt should be made to obtain a histologic diagnosis. Relatively safe procedures such as sputum cytology or biopsy of an accessible, abnormal lymph node should be pursued. Because therapy, prognosis, and future management depend on the histologic type and anatomic site of the primary tumor, invasive diagnostic procedures such as bronchoscopy, esophagoscopy, and mediastinoscopy are warranted. A diagnosis should be deferred in favor of immediate therapy if the clinical condition is unstable.

Treatment

Treatment most often consists of radiation therapy (3000 to 4000 cGy). Most patients respond within 3 to 4 days. In patients who have previously received maximum doses of radiation and who have responsive tumors (small cell carcinoma of the lung, lymphoma), superior vena cava obstruction is generally relieved with systemic chemotherapy. Diuretic therapy provides symptomatic relief of edema. Survival after treatment depends on the underlying diagnosis. A recent study reports that 45% of lymphoma patients with superior vena cava syndrome survived 30 months in comparison with only 10% of patients with lung cancer.

REFERENCES

Ahmann FR: A reassessment of the clinical implications of the superior vena caval syndrome. J Clin Oncol 2:961–969, 1984.
Helms SR, Carlson MD: Cardiovascular emergencies. Semin Oncol 16:463–470, 1989.

UPPER AIRWAY OBSTRUCTION

The most common malignancies causing upper airway obstruction include thyroid carcinomas, head and neck carcinomas, esophageal cancer, and superior mediastinal tumors (lymphomas and lung cancers), all of which can compress the trachea. Obstruction of a mainstem bronchus is most commonly caused by bronchogenic carcinoma. Occasionally, metastatic disease to the peribronchial lymph nodes and/or the pulmonary parenchyma surrounding the mainstem bronchi can produce obstruction.

An early symptom of upper airway obstruction is shortness of breath, especially with exercise. Because the obstruction usually progresses slowly, orthopnea, cough, wheezing, and stridor develop gradually. Patients rarely decompensate suddenly because of acute narrowing of the hypopharynx, pharynx, or upper airway. Diagnosis can be made with plain x-rays of the neck and chest; bilateral oblique views of the chest give full-length tracheal contours. Chest x-ray often demonstrates a mediastinal mass and may show narrowing or displacement of the tracheal air column. CT scan of the neck and upper chest provides useful views of the obstructing lesion and gives the radiation therapist information needed for proper treatment planning. If there is no tissue diagnosis, bronchoscopy and biopsy should be done but with caution.

For a rapidly progressive proximal obstructing lesion, a tracheostomy may be lifesaving. Under most circumstances, however, emergency radiation therapy provides effective treatment. Bronchoscopic laser treatment for malignant airway obstruction has recently shown promising short-term results. Complications include severe hemorrhage and damage to normal tissues. Following partial resection by laser, focal obstructive lesions may be palliated by endobronchial brachyradiotherapy. In chemotherapy-responsive malignancies, systemic cytotoxic treatment should be initiated as soon as possible.

REFERENCES

Gelb AF, Epstein JD: Neodymium-yttrium-aluminum-garnet laser in lung cancer. Ann Thorac Surg 43:164–167, 1987.
Spain RC, Whittlesey D: Respiratory emergencies. Semin Oncol 16:471–489, 1989.
Unger M: Neodymium:YAG laser therapy for malignant and benign endobronchial obstructions. Clin Chest Med 6:277–290, 1985.

BILATERAL URETERAL OBSTRUCTION

Pelvic tumors such as bladder, rectosigmoid, prostate, cervical, and ovarian carcinomas and retroperitoneal tumors, especially malignant lymphomas, may cause bilateral ureteral obstruction. A history of oliguria or anuria is obtained, and occasionally patients describe nonspecific pain in the abdomen, flank, or back. Symptoms vary with the degree of uremia, ranging from nausea and lethargy to frank coma. Uremia may develop insidiously and occasionally may be the presenting symptom of these diseases. Obstruction-induced hydronephrosis predisposes to pyelonephritis; thus flank pain, fever, chills, and dysuria may be the initial complaints.

Blood chemistries reveal the typical abnormalities of uremia. Either renal ultrasonography or CT scan of the abdomen may be useful in making the diagnosis. Bilateral retrograde ureterography may be necessary to establish the existence of obstruction and to demonstrate the site.

If uremia is severe and if prospects for therapy of the underlying malignancy are reasonably good, placement of ureteral catheters or bilateral percutaneous nephrostomies will relieve obstruction while antitumor therapy is undertaken. In selected cases, ureteral diversion to an ileal or colonic bladder or cutaneous ureterostomy may be advisable. Emergency hemodialysis can be performed in cases of life-threatening uremia when prospects for treatment of the underlying malignancy are favorable, as in the case of malignant lymphoma and ovarian cancer.

REFERENCES

Bodner D, Kursh ED, Resnick MI: Palliative nephrostomy for relief of ureteral obstruction secondary to malignancy. Urology 24:8–10, 1984.
Greenfield A, Resnick MI: Genitourinary emergencies. Semin Oncol 16:516–520, 1989.

INCREASED PRESSURE/FLUID ACCUMULATION

INCREASED INTRACRANIAL PRESSURE

Increased intracranial pressure in the cancer patient occurs most often as a result of intracerebral metastases. The most common primary sites of tumors that metastasize to brain include lung, breast, and melanoma. Primary brain tumors (Chap. 20) also cause increased intracranial pressure. Rapid diagnosis and quick intervention are essential to prevent irreversible neurologic deficits or death.

Clinical Presentation

The clinical presentation depends on the location(s) of the lesion(s) and the presence of associated edema. Symptoms include headache, behavioral and mental changes, cerebellar dysfunction, lethargy, and seizures. The most common signs are hemiparesis, impaired cognitive function, unilateral sensory loss, cranial nerve palsies, papilledema, ataxia, and aphasia. Nausea and vomiting may precede a change in the level of consciousness or focal neurologic symptoms. The differential diagnosis includes intracerebral hemorrhage, subdural hematoma, brain abscess, hydrocephalus (especially with posterior fossa lesions), and radiation necrosis.

Diagnosis

CT scan of the brain with contrast demonstrates metastatic lesions and differentiates tumor from infarction, abscess, or radiation necrosis in most cases. An MRI scan can be obtained when uncertainty exists, and many believe MRI is the initial study of choice. The presence of a mass in the brain produces a shift in the intracranial contents, and depending on the location of the tumor, frank herniation may follow. A sudden change in the level of consciousness with associated findings (ipsilateral dilated pupil) plus respiratory and motor deficits is a neurologic emergency.

If symptoms and signs suggesting central nervous system tumor are present but the CT scan is negative, the spinal fluid should be examined. Lumbar puncture should not be performed prior to CT scan when the possibility of increased intracranial pressure exists. A diagnosis of carcinomatous meningitis is made when cytologic analysis of the cerebrospinal fluid reveals malignant cells.

Treatment

Patients with evidence of increased intracranial pressure should receive 10 mg of dexamethasone initially, followed by 4 mg every 6 hours. Prophylactic phenytoin (Dilantin), 300 mg daily, should not be used unless a seizure has occurred. Whole brain radiation therapy is the principal treatment. Ambulatory patients without evidence of metastatic disease outside the brain with solitary metastatic lesions in accessible and "silent areas" benefit from neurosurgical resection followed by radiotherapy. Patients who present with a solitary brain lesion without other evidence of malignancy should undergo resection for both diagnostic and therapeutic purposes. Patients with multiple metastatic lesions have a poor prognosis, but most improve functionally and neurologically following therapy. Median survival for patients with metastatic cancer to the brain ranges from 3 to 8 months.

REFERENCES

Patchell RA, Tibbs PA, Walsh JW, et al: A randomized trial of surgery in the treatment of single metastases to the brain. N Engl J Med 322:494–500, 1990.

Weissman DE: Glucocorticoid treatment for brain metastases and epidural spinal cord compression: A review. J Clin Oncol 6:543–551, 1988.

Willson JKV, Masaryk TJ: Neurologic emergencies in the cancer patient. Semin Oncol 16:490–503, 1989.

PERICARDIAL TAMPONADE

In published series, 0.1 to 21% of autopsied cancer patients have pericardial involvement by tumor. Clinical syndromes include acute effusive pericarditis, constrictive pericarditis, and neoplastic cardiac tamponade. Cardiac tamponade most often results from pericardial invasion by breast and lung cancers, leukemia, lymphoma, malignant melanoma, and GI tumors. Malignant pericardial effusions tend to develop rapidly, causing orthopnea, chest pain, and decreased exercise tolerance. Clinical signs include peripheral edema, hypotension, significant pulsus paradoxus, increased jugular venous pressure, softened heart sounds, and pericardial friction rub (less than 5%). Chest x-ray usually shows an enlarged cardiac silhouette. Electrocardiographic changes include low QRS amplitude and nonspecific ST-T wave changes. Echocardiogram is the most reliable test for detection of pericardial effusion.

Management of neoplastic acute pericardial tamponade depends on the histologic diagnosis, cardiovascular status, and prior therapy. If the patient is hemodynamically unstable or has had prior chest irradiation, pericardiocentesis is the therapy of choice. Cytologic study of pericardial fluid is diagnostic for malignancy in over 80% of cases. For recurrent pericardial effusions, obliteration of the pericardial space with instillation of a pericardial irritant such as tetracycline, nitrogen mustard, or thiotepa is often effective. Another option is a pericardiotomy (pericardial window) to allow external or internal drainage of the accumulated fluid. If the patient has had no prior cardiac irradiation and is hemodynamically stable, local irradiation (2000 to 3000 cGy) controls the effusion in 60% of cases, with the highest responses in patients with lymphomas. When these therapeutic modalities are successful, survival depends on the natural history of the underlying disease.

REFERENCES

Alcan KE, Zabetakis PM, Marino ND et al: Management of acute cardiac tamponade by subxiphoid pericardiotomy. JAMA 247:1143–1148, 1982.
Davis S, Rambott P, Grignani F: Intrapericardial tetracycline sclerosis in the treatment of malignant pericardial effusion: An analysis of 33 cases. J Clin Oncol 2:631–636, 1984.
Helms SR, Carlson MD: Cardiovascular emergencies. Semin Oncol 16:463–470, 1989.
Posner MR, Cohen GI, Skarin AT: Pericardial disease in patients with cancer. Am J Med 71:407–413, 1981.

MALIGNANT PLEURAL EFFUSION

Accumulation of fluid in the pleural space is a common occurrence in the cancer patient and is most often caused by breast, lung, and ovarian carcinomas as well as lymphomas. Intrathoracic malignancy can cause pleural effusion in several ways—inflammatory response to malignant cells in the pleura produces increased capillary permeability; obstruction of lymphatic channels impairs pleural reabsorption of fluid and protein; and increased pulmonary venous pressure increases capillary pressure in the visceral pleura, causing transudation of fluid. Restriction of lung expansion by pleural fluid accumulation predisposes to atelectasis, hypoxia, and infection.

Common symptoms include progressive dyspnea and pain on the affected side. Physical examination reveals dullness to percussion, decreased breath sounds, and absent vocal fremitus. The trachea may be pushed to the unaffected side. Chest x-ray reveals opacification of the pleural space, and lateral decubitus films confirm the existence of free-flowing fluid. Malignant pleural fluid characteristically has a protein concentration greater than 3 g/dL, a glucose concentration lower than blood glucose level, and a cytology positive for tumor cells.

Thoracentesis should be the initial therapy in a patient with an effusion. Some patients are relieved after the first thoracentesis and require no further local therapy. In patients who have rapid reaccumulation of pleural fluid, chest tube drainage with subsequent instillation of a sclerosing agent such as tetracycline or bleomycin is employed. Systemic chemotherapy for the underlying malignancy, particularly malignant lymphomas, ovarian cancer, and breast cancer, may cause resolution of the effusion. In the patient with effusion caused by blockage of lymph channels, radiation therapy to the mediastinum is often effective.

REFERENCES

Hausheer FH, Yarbro JW: Diagnosis and treatment of malignant pleural effusions. Semin Oncol 12:54–75, 1985.
Moores DWO: Malignant pleural effusions. Semin Oncol 18(suppl 2):59–61, 1991.
Ruckdeschel JC: Management of malignant pleural effusions. Semin Oncol 15(suppl 3):24–28, 1988.

METABOLIC EMERGENCIES

HYPERCALCEMIA

Hypercalcemia occurs in a variety of malignancies, either from the local effect of extensive bone involvement by tumor or from the systemic effect of various humoral factors produced by tumors. Hypercalcemia is most often seen in breast carcinoma, lung carcinoma (particularly squamous cell), multiple myeloma, and T-cell lymphomas. Patients with renal cell carcinoma, ovarian carcinoma, and other lymphomas occasionally develop hypercalcemia, and the risk is lower but not absent in other malignancies. Substantial evidence supports the role of parathyroidlike hormones, prostaglandins, and osteoclast-activating factor (in multiple myeloma) in the pathogenesis of some cases of hypercalcemia.

Clinical Presentation

Hypercalcemia must be considered in the differential diagnosis of progressive fatigue and weakness where no other cause is obvious. Other common symptoms include nausea and vomiting, anorexia, constipation, and urinary frequency. As hypercalcemia advances, increasing confusion, lethargy, and eventually coma and death result. The syndrome should be considered in any confused or comatose cancer patient. Signs of hypercalcemia include dehydration, azotemia, ileus, and ECG changes (QT interval shortening and widening of the T wave). A routine serum calcium above 10.5 mg/dL is generally a sign of abnormal calcium homeostasis, and a serum calcium above 11.0 mg/dL with accompanying signs and symptoms is an indication to begin therapy.

Treatment

If a patient is minimally symptomatic with a calcium level of less than 13 mg/dL, oral hydration plus increasing mobilization may be sufficient to reduce the calcium level. Thiazide diuretics adversely affect hypercalcemia by decreasing urinary calcium excretion and should be avoided if possible. If the patient is a candidate for antitumor therapy, this should be initiated at once, since successful therapy will help control serum calcium.

If the calcium level is above 13 mg/dL, and the patient is moderately symptomatic, vigorous intravenous hydration with normal saline, 6 to 10 L/24 hours, should be instituted. Many physicians add 40 to 80 mg of furosemide every 6 hours for its calciuric effect, but dehydration should be corrected and a saline diuresis established before any furosemide is given. Potassium should be supplemented as needed.

If the calcium level does not decrease after 24 to 36 hours, pharmacologic treatment should be initiated. Currently, several options are available. Plicamycin (Mithracin, formerly mithramycin), a chemotherapeutic agent formerly used to treat testicular tumors, is commonly employed as initial therapy. The dose is 15 to 25 μg/kg intravenously, repeated every 4 to 7 days if necessary. Onset of action is usually within 24 to 48 hours. Plicamycin is often well tolerated when given short term, although the drug has multiple potential toxicities, including nausea and vomiting, thrombocytopenia, coagulation abnormalities, and renal and hepatic toxicity.

Treatment with calcitonin, 4 to 8 MRC U/kg by continuous 24-hour infusion, or the same dose SQ or IM every 6 to 12 hours, is an option with a rapid onset of action. Patients often escape from the effect of calcitonin within 72 hours and may benefit from the addition of corticosteroids.

Another treatment approach employs biphosphonate analogues of endogenous pyrophosphate, which are potent inhibitors of osteoclastic activity. Etidronate disodium (Didronel) is administered at 7.5 mg/kg/day as a 2-hour infusion repeated daily for 3 to 7 days. Pamidronate disodium (Aredia) is given as a 60- to 90-mg infusion over 24 hours. In a recent randomized study, a single infusion of pamidronate proved equally safe and more effective than 3 days of etidronate infusions. Clinical toxicity with both agents is minimal, although fever and transient elevations in serum phosphate and creatinine concentrations can occur.

Gallium nitrate for acute management of hypercalcemia is another effective new therapy. Gallium also inhibits bone resorption. Experience with gallium is limited, although hypocalcemia and elevated serum creatinine are potential toxicities. The recommended dose is 200 mg/m^2 as a continuous infusion daily for 5 days.

Serum calcium, creatinine, electrolytes, magnesium, fluid intake, and urine output should be strictly monitored during therapy for hypercalcemia. If the underlying disease is treatable but renal dysfunction prohibits vigorous hydration, hemodialysis may be used as a temporizing measure to reduce serum calcium. Long-term outpatient management of hypercalcemia is difficult unless the underlying tumor is definitively treated. In patients with breast cancer, myeloma, or lymphoma, corticosteroids may be effective. Other treatments include oral phosphates, 2 g per day in divided doses diluted with water to minimize diarrhea, and indomethacin (a prostaglandin inhibitor), 25 mg every 6 to 8 hours.

REFERENCES

Broadus AE, Mangin M, Ikeda K, et al: Humoral hypercalcemia of cancer: Identification of a novel parathyroid hormone-like peptide. N Engl J Med 319:556–563, 1988.
Gucalp R, Ritch P, Wiernick PH, et al: Comparative study of pamidronate disodium and etidronate disodium in the treatment of cancer-related hypercalcemia. J Clin Oncol 10:134–142, 1992.
Ralston SH, Gallacher SJ, Patel U, et al: Cancer-associated hypercalcemia: Morbidity and mortality. Ann Intern Med 112:499–504, 1990.
Warrell RP, Murphy WK, Schulman P, et al: A randomized double-blind study of gallium nitrate compared with etidronate for acute control of cancer-related hypercalcemia. J Clin Oncol 9:1467–1475, 1991.

HYPERURICEMIA

Elevated serum uric acid levels occur commonly with malignant diseases characterized by rapid cell turnover. The most marked elevations are seen following initial therapy of leukemias, malignant lymphomas, and other very sensitive tumors. Attacks of acute gouty arthritis may be precipitated, but the most severe consequence of markedly elevated serum uric acid levels is acute uric acid nephropathy. Urine in the collecting ducts and ureters is characterized by high acidity, low volume, and high concentration of uric acid, all of which promote precipitation of uric acid crystals and tubular obstruction. Symptoms of hyperuricemia are often those of advancing renal insufficiency. In most patients, oliguria or anuria develop. Renal colic may occur with the formation of uric acid calculi. Laboratory findings include high serum levels of uric acid, hyperuricosuria, and elevated BUN and creatinine.

Treatment

Uric acid is the product of purine nucleotide catabolism. Purine degradation depends on the enzyme xanthine oxidase, which is competitively inhibited by allopurinol. Prior to treating acute leukemias or high-grade lymphomas with combination chemotherapy, patients should receive 600 mg of allopurinol for 1 to 2 days and then 300 mg/day for 1 to 2 weeks until the danger of severe hyperuricemia has passed. Allopurinol is also helpful in patients with chronic myelogenous leukemia with very high white blood counts. If uric acid nephropathy occurs, allopurinol should be supplemented with increased hydration plus urine alkalinization with sodium bicarbonate or carbonic anhydrase inhibitors (acetazolamide, Diamox) in an attempt to solubilize the uric acid crystals. Dialysis has been effective in advanced cases.

TUMOR LYSIS SYNDROME

The syndrome of acute tumor lysis associated with the initiation of chemotherapy has been described in a number of neoplastic disorders, especially lymphomas (particularly Burkitt's lymphoma) and acute leukemias. The syndrome is characterized by hyperuricemia, hypocalcemia, hyperphosphatemia, and hyperkalemia as a consequence of rapid tumor cell lysis following chemotherapy. Renal failure and sudden death can occur as a result of these metabolic disturbances. Clearance of enormous loads of uric acid, potassium, and phosphates depends on renal excretory capabilities, and the syndrome is more severe in patients with preexisting renal insufficiency.

Preventive therapy for patients in whom massive cytolysis is anticipated includes 600 mg daily of allopurinol for 1 to 2 days prior to chemotherapy, with a reduction in dose to 300 mg per day after the third or fourth day of chemotherapy; hydration with 4 to 6 L of fluid per 24 hours during the first few days of therapy; and alkalinization of the urine with sodium bicarbonate or Diamox. Close monitoring of electrolytes, BUN, creatinine, uric acid, calcium, phosphorus, and lactic dehydrogenase (LDH) is imperative. In patients refractory to these measures, hemodialysis may be required. Duration of the metabolic aberration in patients with the tumor lysis syndrome is usually limited to 5 to 7 days.

REFERENCES

Boles JM, Dutel JL, et al: Acute renal failure caused by extreme hyperphosphatemia after chemotherapy of an acute lymphoblastic leukemia. Cancer 53:2425–2429, 1984.
Cohen LF, Balow AE, et al: Acute tumor lysis syndrome: A review of thirty-seven patients with Burkitt's lymphoma. Am J Med 68:486–491, 1980.
Silverman P, Distelhorst CW: Metabolic emergencies in clinical oncology. Semin Oncol 16:504–515, 1989.

HYPOGLYCEMIA

Tumor-associated hypoglycemia may be seen in patients with large mesenchymal tumors (mesothelioma, fibrosarcoma, neurofibrosarcoma, hemangiopericytoma), hepatoma, adrenal carcinoma, islet cell carcinoma of the pancreas (insulinoma), and occasionally other gastrointestinal cancers and lymphomas. The tumors are usually quite large (1 to 10 kg) and often invade the liver. While the exact cause of the hypoglycemia is not clear, a defect in glycogenolysis has been associated with certain hepatomas, and elaboration of an insulinlike hormone (NSILA, nonsuppressible insulinlike activity) has been associated with various other tumors. Insulinomas secrete insulin (and therefore C-peptide) independently of blood glucose concentration.

Signs and symptoms of hypoglycemia are largely independent of the underlying cause. Hypoglycemic stimulation of the autonomic nervous system results in hunger, nervousness, tachycardia, diaphoresis, pallor, and tremulousness. Central nervous system manifestations include headache, lightheadedness, visual disturbances, irritability, lethargy, agitation, confusion, inappropriate behavior, stupor, convulsions, paralysis, and even coma. When these signs and symptoms are accompanied by a blood glucose level of less than 60 mg/dL, further diagnostic work-up is indicated. Testing might include a carefully monitored in-hospital fast with measurements of 24-, 48-, and 72-hour plasma glucose levels along with insulin and C-peptide levels. A persistent increase in both the insulin and the C-peptide levels is diagnostic of insulinoma; a decrease in the insulin level with a concomitant decrease in the C-peptide level is suggestive of tumor-associated hypoglycemia in the cancer patient.

Immediate treatment of symptomatic hypoglycemia consists of the intravenous administration of 50 mL of 50% glucose solution. Tumor-associated hypoglycemia responds to the successful treatment of the responsible malignancy. In the case of an insulin-secreting islet cell carcinoma, surgical excision is the treatment of choice. For metastatic islet cell carcinoma, treatment with systemic chemotherapy may induce a response in the tumor mass as well as the associated hypoglycemic syndrome (Chap. 21). Hyperglycemic agents such as glucagon, high-dose corticosteroids, and diazoxide may also ameliorate symptoms.

REFERENCES

Axelrod L, Ron D: Insulin-like growth factor II and the riddle of tumor-induced hypoglycemia. N Engl J Med 319:1477–1478, 1988.
Daughaday WH, Emanuele MA, Brooks MH, et al: Synthesis and secretion of insulin-like growth factor II by a leiomyosarcoma with associated hypoglycemia. N Engl J Med 319:1434–1440, 1988.
Silverman P, Distelhorst CW: Metabolic emergencies. Semin Oncol 16:504–515, 1989.

24
PSYCHOSOCIAL CARE OF THE CANCER PATIENT

Deborah J. Dudgeon

The diagnosis of cancer is always a traumatic event. It challenges the coping skills of even the best-adjusted person. Despite tremendous efforts at public education, many people believe, incorrectly, that cancer invariably means uncontrolled pain and suffering prior to an inevitable death. Even if the prognosis is good, patients respond with uncertainty and fear as they are suddenly immersed in a world of unfamiliar medical treatments. As the disease progresses, it presents recurring challenges as each successive treatment fails and new physical disabilities diminish the expectation of cure. The diagnosis of cancer leaves even the survivor with a heightened awareness of his or her vulnerability and mortality. Despite the inevitable emotional distress, most patients can muster their inner strengths and external supports to confront the disease and its treatment with little psychological dysfunction. The challenge for the busy professional is to anticipate psychological trouble and recognize early signs of difficulties for which further intervention from the health care system is necessary.

SPOTTING DIFFICULTIES

Higher levels of emotional distress and greater problems with coping should be anticipated in patients who have delayed seeking medical treatment and in those with a previous psychiatric history, little evidence of support from others, or concurrent life crises. Difficulties in coping are more likely shortly after diagnosis, at the completion of active treatment, and when unexpected changes occur in treatment or disease course. Health care professionals should be more vigilant at these times and with these groups of people, since they may need more than the usual supportive care and additional psychotherapeutic, psychopharmacologic, or behavioral interventions.

An unexplained change in attitude, uncontrolled pain, or intolerance of previously well-tolerated symptoms or side effects may reflect psychosocial problems. The physician, nurse, social worker, and other members of the patient care team should explore the possibility that these symptoms may signal psychological or social difficulties. In helping patients cope with their illness, it is often useful to identify and mobilize persons and strategies that they have called upon in the past to deal with previous problems. Identification and evaluation of these resources will also help predict the patient's ability to adapt and the problems that may arise.

Most individuals cope with problems by employing one or more defense mechanisms. Certain defense mechanisms, such as denial, can be maladaptive; nevertheless, they always serve a function and may represent the best response the patient is able to offer at the time. The patient care team should support those defense mechanisms that are adaptive and respect those that are dysfunctional. Challenging maladaptive defenses directly can heighten anxiety and work counterproductively; their loss can create a psychologically perilous situation. If a more supportive environment can be created or the situation redefined, anxiety can be reduced and the patient's sense of control enhanced, thus allowing behavior to change.

COMMUNICATION

Central to the psychosocial care of the cancer patient is a secure, consistent, and trusting relationship with the multidisciplinary health care team. The initial discussions with the patient and family are crucial to subsequent interactions. Early involvement of the family avoids the possibility that the diagnosis or prognosis is withheld, forcing the patient to deal with his or her illness in isolation.

Telling the diagnosis of cancer is always difficult. This task often falls to a physician who does not know the patient well, which can complicate the process and lead to misunderstandings. The primary physician can be a useful resource in learning how best to communicate with a particular patient. The patient should be told in a private setting where he or she can feel free to express emotions. Receiving this diagnosis over the phone or in the recovery room or in a crowded hallway, the patient may (accurately) perceive that the doctor is insensitive and unfeeling. At the time the diagnosis is told, the discussion should include a plan for treatment as well. This gives the patient and family evidence that something can be done and a concrete basis to begin the process of adjustment.

Although the oncologist does not usually tell the diagnosis, he or she is often greeted by an angry, frightened, and confused patient. Patients and families frequently relate to the oncologist their experience with missed or delayed diagnosis, poor telling of the diagnosis, fears of treatment and prognosis, and tales of family or friends with cancer. Communication can be difficult, since the subject is emotionally charged, the information complex, the treatments usually toxic, and the benefits often uncertain. Bringing a friend or family member along to the consultation or tape recording the discussion improves recall and comprehension. Explanations by the physician should be brief and focused, with ample opportunity for questions and discussion. In many cases, a second or third visit will be necessary to clarify the situation and allay fears.

Knowledge is an essential tool in developing a coping strategy. It decreases uncertainty and increases the sense of control. Discussions of treatment should include rationale, potential risks and benefits, and available alternatives. A common ground of understanding facilitates more effective negotiation of treatment goals and methods. Preparatory education decreases emotional distress and treatment-related problems, leading to less disruption in patients' lives. Oncology nurse specialists can be invaluable to the patient and family by reinforcing diagnostic, prognostic, and treatment-related information.

INVESTIGATIONAL THERAPIES

Open discussion is particulary important when the patient is offered participation in an experimental protocol. Experimental treatments may contain unproven drugs or combinations that may have substantial toxicity. Specific regulations protect the rights of individuals who receive experimental treatments. In all hospitals experimental treatments must be approved by an institutional review board composed of physicians, nurses, administrators, and lay individuals. The treating physician must discuss with the patient and present in written form the options available for treatment of the disease, the possible side effects and complications of each, and the expected outcomes. To participate, the patient must sign a consent form that indicates that he or she understands the issues presented and agrees to treatment on protocol. The decision-making picture becomes more complex when two or more treatment options are involved in the protocol; here the patient must decide whether to participate prior to knowing which of several treatment alternatives will be received. Adequate explanation of research protocols requires considerable time and effort, since they are complicated and often confusing to the medically unsophisticated patient. Giving the patient written materials (i.e., brochures, pamphlets, and a copy of the consent form when experimental treatment is proposed) allows the patient and family an opportunity to consider their options in a less stressful environment.

ACTIVE TREATMENT

The period of active treatment carries a considerable impact for the patient's psychosocial adjustment. The nature of the disruption depends partly on tumor type, stage, and treatment. Chemotherapy and hormonal therapy, by producing weight gain and/or hair loss, may lead to marked changes in body image. Surgery can cause disfigurement, alter the route or the means of elimination, or change sexual function. Radiation therapy can cause skin burns, dysphagia, alopecia, or diarrhea. In one study, 75 to 90% of all patients receiving chemotherapy experienced some emotional distress or disruption in their work or social life. Disruption often increases as treatment progresses.

For some patients, the chronic effects of fatigue and weakness produce greater emotional distress than the more acute effects. Younger and better-educated patients seem to have heightened anxiety and are most likely to develop anticipatory side effects (see Chap. 26). Surprisingly, greater emotional distress may result from a more rapid response to treatment. The disappearance of palpable disease can leave the patient with the fear that the cancer is hidden or spreading silently. A lack of evident disease can cause problems with compliance, since the patient may believe that he or she has already been cured. As the completion of active treatment nears, many patients experience heightened anxiety. Frequent visits with the doctor and contacts with the health care team produce a sense of security and provide emotional support. During the observation phase after treatment is completed, the patient's sense that something is being done is removed, leaving a frightening void. The end of active treatment may be as terrifying for the patient as its beginning.

RECURRENT DISEASE

The first recurrence of cancer is probably the most stressful event in the natural history of the disease. It revives all the previous questions and fears that surrounded the initial diagnosis with less promise of successful treatment and less expectation of cure. Under most, but not all, circumstances, the diagnosis of recurrent or metastatic disease shifts the emphasis from cure of disease to palliation of symptoms. This is a difficult transition for patient, family, and health care team. Continued frank but compassionate communication is essential as treatment options are explored. The goals of therapy must be clearly defined so that the patient can make well-informed decisions. It is often helpful to give a time limit to a trial of treatment after which the merits of continuing, changing, or stopping will be assessed. Probably the most important assurance to communicate to the patient and family during this time is that they will not be abandoned.

NEUROBEHAVIORAL DISORDERS

Early detection and accurate diagnosis of behavioral and cognitive disorders in the patient with cancer is a challenging problem. The potential etiologies include disease-related, treatment-related, and psychiatric conditions. Subtle changes in behavior, memory, or attention may represent the first signs of metastatic brain tumor, meningeal disease, or a paraneoplastic syndrome. Confusion or apathy may signal metabolic derangement or major organ failure. Clouding of consciousness or disorientation may be the initial manifestations of infection, hypoxia, or adrenal insufficiency. Clearly, accurate diagnosis is essential to appropriate management of these problems.

Treatment-related neuropsychiatric complications may follow both chemotherapy and radiotherapy. Cranial radiation can cause acute (general malaise and low-grade fever), subacute (transient functional loss 6 to 16 weeks following treatment), and chronic changes (memory loss and mild to severe neuropsychiatric impairment). Behavioral disorders, including personality change and attentional disturbance, can be acute and reversible effects of high-dose methotrexate or cytosine arabinoside chemotherapy. Methotrexate, cytosine arabinoside, BCNU, and thiotepa can cause a delayed leukoencephalopathy manifested by progressive personality change, intellectual decline, and dementia. Both interleukin 2 and interferon have been associated with changes in mental status, hypersomnia, and apathy. Diagnosis of these syndromes should prompt decreases in dose or discontinuation of therapy.

Psychiatric problems are also common in the cancer population. The prevalence of psychiatric disorders in a group of 215 patients receiving cancer treatments in three collaborating cancer centers was 47%. Sixty-eight percent of the diagnoses consisted of adjustment disorders (depression, anxiety, and mixed reactions), which are often responsive to psychological interventions. This high prevalence emphasizes the need for vigilance on the part of the health care team to ensure early diagnosis and appropriate treatment.

Anxiety in the cancer patient can be an acute response to the diagnosis or treatment of the disease or exacerbation of a chronic disorder. It can be aggravated by tests, treatments, drugs, withdrawal from narcotics, or physical problems. Anxiety can sometimes be reduced by giving patients the opportunity to talk, identifying their fears, and developing other strategies for coping. Short-term therapy with anxiolytics is beneficial to many patients and can help them to function more effectively by gaining control of their emotions. Behavioral techniques such as meditation, guided imagery, and progressive relaxation can help those who are highly motivated and able to concentrate. If symptoms are chronic and disabling or interfere with daily functioning, then referral to a psychiatrist is indicated.

Many antianxiety drugs are available, some of which are listed in Table 24–1. Selection among them should be based on concurrent medical problems, side effects, routes of administration, and drug half-life.

Benzodiazepines are most frequently used for the treatment of anxiety. Elderly and debilitated patients are best treated with short-acting drugs such as alprazolam (Xanax), oxazepam (Serax), or lorazepam (Ativan). Patients with liver dysfunction should receive oxazepam or lorazepam, which are short acting, metabolized by conjugation, and excreted by the kidney. Lorazepam produces an antegrade amnesia and is therefore useful in controlling anticipatory nausea and vomiting associated with chemotherapy. Longer-acting drugs are best reserved for patients with chronic anxiety and little comorbidity.

Major tranquilizers are very useful in treating anxiety and do not cause the confusion and agitation that are sometimes seen in elderly patients receiving benzodiazepines. Haloperidol (Haldol) lacks respiratory depressant effects, has a low incidence of cardiovascular and anticholinergic side effects, and is a good antiemetic. It can produce significant extrapyramidal effects, which are controlled with antiparkinson agents (e.g., Cogentin). Thioridazine (Mellaril) is a sedating antipsychotic agent that seldom causes extrapyramidal reactions. It has some antidepressant effect and prominent anticholinergic activity.

Insomnia in the cancer patient can indicate physical or emotional distress. Treatment involves identifying the underlying cause. At times, simple measures such as discussing fears or changing the timing of certain medications (e.g., corticosteroids) are sufficient to achieve a restful night. Medications can be employed, but they rarely provide a long-term solution to the problem.

Hypnotic agents are among the most frequently prescribed psychotropic drugs for hospitalized cancer patients. Flurazepam (Dalmane), triazolam (Halcion), and temazepam (Restoril) are becoming the most popular medications for sleep. Triazolam has the advantages of a very short half-life and no active metabolites, resulting in little morning hangover and relative safety in patients with hepatic dysfunction. Disadvantages of triazolam include early morning awakening, rebound insomnia, daytime anxiety, dependence, and withdrawal seizures. Temazepam shares some of the properties of triazolam, and it is absorbed slowly and therefore needs to be taken at least 1 hour before bedtime. Flurazepam and diazepam have longer half-lives and therefore seldom cause early morning awakening or rebound insomnia but are more likely to accumulate and cause drowsiness. Chloral hydrate, hydroxyzine, and diphenhydramine can be useful when respiratory depression must be avoided.

Depression in the cancer patient can be difficult to diagnose. The usual vegetative signs of anorexia, sleep disturbance, loss of libido, weight loss, poor concentration, and fatigue that characterize depression can also represent signs of the underlying cancer. Reactive depression is much more common than psychotic depression in cancer patients. Reactive depression is usually responsive to supportive measures, including attentive listening and consistent emotional support from family, friends, and the health care team. Antidepressant medication and/or psychiatric intervention should be considered if the patient does not respond to these measures or has suicidal ideation or pervasive feelings of hopelessness and worthlessness that interfere with the ability to function. Professional counseling or psychotherapy may also become necessary if the patient's social support network is borderline or if he or she is unable to express feelings.

Table 24–1. **PHARMACOLOGIC AGENTS FOR ANXIETY IN CANCER PATIENTS**

AGENT	ORAL DOSAGE (mg)	HALF-LIFE (hours)
Benzodiazepines		
Lorazepam (Ativan)	0.25–2.0 tid	12–18
Oxazepam (Serax)	7.5–15.0 tid	5–15
Alprazolam (Xanax)	0.25–0.50 tid	12–15
Diazepam (Valium)	2–10 tid	20–50
Major tranquilizers		
Haloperidol (Haldol)	0.5–5.0 qid	
Thioridazine (Mellaril)	10–25 tid	
Chlorpromazine (Thorazine)	10–25 tid	

Antidepressants (Table 24–2) should be chosen to address the target symptoms associated with the depression, avoid adverse effects due to coexisting medical problems, and minimize side effects. If insomnia and loss of appetite are the major problems, then amitriptyline or doxepin given at bedtime is preferable. Desipramine or fluoxetine is indicated in patients with significant psychomotor slowing. The second-generation antidepressants have the advantage of less anticholinergic effects. Fluoxetine, a new antidepressant, does not produce cardiac arrhythmias, orthostasis, or anticholinergic effects. Experience with this drug in patients with multiple medical problems is limited, so it should be instituted cautiously. Desipramine and doxepin are preferred in patients with seizure disorders. A 10- to 14-day course of treatment with any of the antidepressants is required before a therapeutic effect is seen.

The treatment of depression with monoamine oxidase (MAO) inhibitors requires dietary restrictions that are generally not desirable in the cancer population. Dextroamphetamine and methylphenidate are effective in improving mood, activity, and appetite in patients with advanced cancer. They should be not be used in patients with organic brain dysfunction. If anxiety symptoms predominate, then alprazolam (Xanax) should be considered.

ETHICAL ISSUES

The fundamental principle of medical ethics is autonomy—that is, the right of the patient or his or her surrogate to make decisions about health care, including the right to forego potentially life-saving treatments. It is the physician's responsibility to provide adequate information about risks and benefits, alternative treatments, and the probable outcome of receiving no treatment. Coercion (conscious or unconscious) must be avoided. Strongly recommending a treatment, however, is proper if the alternatives are openly and objectively explained. The patient may choose whether or not to follow the physician's recommendations, but a patient cannot force a physician to prescribe treatments that the physician opposes. A physician may withdraw from a case if the patient is given sufficient notice and provided with adequate care from another physician.

A valid consent to treatment requires that the patient has the capacity to understand the implications of the therapeutic options. If the patient lacks "capacity," then consent should be obtained from the person who is legally authorized. When the patient or surrogate makes a decision that is unquestionably irrational, then it is appropriate to obtain consultation from the hospital's ethics committee or to seek legal counsel. In the vast majority of cases, however, careful and repeated explanations offered in a concerned and compassionate manner suffice to resolve differences and disagreements between patients and their physicians.

Table 24–2. **MEDICATIONS FOR TREATMENT OF DEPRESSION IN CANCER PATIENTS**

MEDICATIONS	STARTING DOSE (mg)	THERAPEUTIC DOSE (mg)	SEDATION	ANTI-CHOLINERGIC EFFECTS
Tricyclic antidepressants				
Amitriptyline (Elavil)	25 qhs	75–150	+ + + + +	+ + + + +
Doxepin (Sinequan)	25 qhs	75–150	+ + + + +	+ + + +
Desipramine (Norpramin)	25 qhs	75–150	+ + +	+
Second-generation antidepressants				
Trazodone (Desyrel)	50 qhs	50–300	+ +	+
Fluoxetine (Prozac)	20 qod	20–60	0	0
Benzodiazepines				
Alprazolam (Xanax)	0.25 tid	0.25–2.0	+ +	0
Sympathomimetic stimulants				
Methylphenidate (Ritalin)	2.5 qam	10–15	0	0
Dextroamphetamine (Dexedrine)	2.5–5 qam	15–20	0	0

LIMITING TREATMENT

Advanced cancer forces inevitable choices on the patient, family, and health care team. Modern technology is very capable of prolonging the dying process when little hope for a meaningful recovery exists. Not everything that can be done to or for a patient necessarily should be done. Most serious cancer care decisions can be anticipated and decided in advance. Introducing the topic of cardiopulmonary resuscitation and limiting treatments early in the course of the disease can allow the patient to specify his or her wishes, thereby relieving the family of this burden. Some states recognize living wills or advanced directives that allow patients to outline their wishes should they become mentally incapacitated. When the family must make choices because the patient lacks capacity, then it is important to explain the therapeutic options in the context of the entire illness. An accurate description of the level of discomfort and the risk associated with any anticipated treatment should be given. The surrogate's mandate is to make the choice the patient would have made if he or she were competent to decide. If the surrogate wants to persist with treatment that seems inappropriate, sympathetic discussion that explores underlying feelings will often help to resolve the dilemma. Hospital ethicists and ethics committees can be called upon to mediate serious differences.

SUPPORT GROUPS

Support groups have a definite role in helping some people cope with their illness. A group of people going through similiar experiences can offer tremendous support and creative solutions for many difficult situations. A group provides a sense of connectedness and may impart the courage to look at issues that would be too painful to address by oneself. A support group can relieve some of the pressure on the family that might already be overburdened. A group setting allows the individual to explore his or her particular life situation, receive feedback, and maintain contact with reality. The group can be an instrument of change, exerting pressure on an individual to alter behavior. It can reinforce good coping strategies by indicating to the patient how well he or she managed a particular situation. Groups furnish a forum for expression of feelings and fears that may be taboo in other social situations, serving to counter the alienation and social isolation encountered by many people with cancer.

Two different types of groups exist: self-help and therapeutic. Self-help groups tend to emphasize self-reliance and offer a fellowship network of people with similar problems. Therapeutic groups are led by professionals who direct the dynamics. The self-help groups learn from the empirical experience of the group members themselves. Support groups seem to have a beneficial effect on levels of depression, self-esteem, life satisfaction, and sense of well-being. Studies have shown that participants display decreased anxiety and fewer maladaptive methods of managing stress.

UNPROVEN METHODS OF CANCER TREATMENT

Unorthodox and unproven remedies include nutritional, psychological, medicinal, and ritualized practices (e.g., coffee enemas). Underlying all of them is a desperate person's attempt to gain or maintain control of his or her disease. Studies have shown that it is often the successful, highly educated patient with early disease who seeks unconventional treatments. Conventional therapy is rejected when there is a lack of trust in the medical profession, a sense of abandonment, or anger. Dietary changes, meditation, and mental imagery can improve a patient's quality of life, but no data show that survival is prolonged. Most of the unproven methods have no scientific rationale and fall into the realm of myth and belief. They can have a placebo effect, improve the person's sense of control, and provide a source of hope. Dangers arise when conventional therapy is prematurely abandoned, when toxicity is associated with the treatments, and when money is wasted and guilt fostered when treatments fail. The multidisciplinary health care team can be instrumental in helping people avoid quackery. The most important element of care is never to abandon the patient and the family, but always to be supportive and compassionate, even when the disease is progressing despite treatments. The physician should not participate in unconventional treatments. He or she need not object to such treatments, however, unless they are harmful to the patient; under these circumstances, the physician should vigorously challenge and criticize the therapy.

SURVIVORS

More than 50% of all patients diagnosed with cancer will survive more than 5 years. Studies have shown that most people survive with no evidence of major psychopathology. Survivors can suffer more subtle psychosocial distress, however, from sexual dysfunction, fatigue, infertility, disfigurement, or decreased intellectual ability resulting from previous treatment. Fear of recurrence, years after diagnosis, can affect a survivor's sense of control over life. Visits to the cancer center on the anniversary of diagnosis can reactivate intense feelings of vulnerability and anxiety. Some people experience an incapacitating survival guilt.

Work studies have shown that cancer survivors are no less productive than age-matched controls, but misinformation and prejudice against them can lead to dismissal or demotion. Cancer survivors often stay in undesirable jobs or avoid seeking promotion because of fear of further illness and loss of health insurance benefits.

During courtship, unmarried survivors need to find partners who accept their cancer history and must decide how much of their history to disclose. Cancer survivors may be reluctant to participate in long-term planning, since they may have a tenuous sense of longevity. Physical limitations can interfere with the ability to participate fully in previous activities. The expectations of others can retard integration into normal life.

The health care team can decrease survivor morbidity by informing patients of possible delayed treatment effects, educating them that fear of recurrence and marital stress are common, monitoring their psychosocial adjustment, and suggesting support groups or professional consultation if needed.

SUMMARY

The treatment of cancer involves a process that extends over time, and just as the treatment for the disease itself must be tailored to the specifics of the tumor, so must the psychological support fit the needs of the individual. One of the best sources of support is a doctor-patient relationship that embodies a respect for and an interest in the patient as a person and that encourages the patient to express his or her beliefs and expectations of the disease and its treatment. Patients should be encouraged to use coping strategies and the support of individuals that have helped in the past. Support groups can decrease isolation and enhance the ability to cope.

Adjusting to a disease like cancer is among the greatest challenges faced in life. The more the physician and the health care team can help the patient achieve a sense of control and an interest in life beyond the illness, the less the distress and disability experienced. Psychotropic medications, behavioral modification techniques, and psychiatric interventions may be necessary for some individuals to achieve optimal adjustment. While not always able to treat the cancer successfully, oncologic professionals are seldom unable to reduce the suffering associated with it.

REFERENCES

Billings JA: Outpatient Management of Advanced Cancer. Philadelphia, JB Lippincott, 1985.

Derogatis LR, Morrow GR, Fetting J, et al: The prevalence of psychiatric disorders among cancer patients. JAMA 249:751–757, 1983.

Hermann JF: Psychosocial support: Interventions for the physician. Semin Oncol 12:466–471, 1985.

Holland JC, Rowland JH (eds): Handbook of Psychooncology: Psychological Care of the Patient with Cancer. New York, Oxford University Press, 1989.

Lieberman MA: The role of self-help groups in helping patients and families cope with cancer. CA 38:162–168, 1988.

Meyerowitz BE, Heinrich RL, Coscarelli Schag CA: Helping patients cope with cancer. Oncology 3:120–131, 1989.

Meyers CA, Scheibel RS: Early detection and diagnosis of neurobehavioral disorders associated with cancer and its treatment. Oncology 4:115–130, 1990.

Quill TE, Townsend P: Bad news: Delivery, dialogue, and dilemmas. Arch Intern Med 151:463–468, 1991.

Siminoff LA: Cancer patient and physician communication: progress and continuing problems. Ann Behavioral Med 11:108–112, 1989.

Welch-McCaffrey D, Hoffman B, Leigh SA, et al: Surviving adult cancers. Part 2: Psychosocial implications. Ann Intern Med 111:517–524, 1989.

25
MANAGEMENT OF PAIN IN THE CANCER PATIENT

Richard B. Patt
John E. Loughner

The prospect of suffering from unrelieved pain is one of the most feared aspects of cancer. Comprehensive management involves careful assessment, individualized therapy, and close follow-up. Adequate pain control is achievable in the vast majority of cancer patients. Optimal pain control promotes an enhanced quality of life and better compliance with therapy.

Pain is the most common symptom associated with cancer. Ten to 15% of cancer patients experience significant pain with early, localized disease. With the development of metastases, the incidence of pain increases to 25 to 30%, and in far advanced disease, 60 to 90% of patients report significant pain. For patients with incurable cancer, symptom control is the most important goal of therapy.

PHYSIOLOGY OF PAIN

The predominant mechanism of cancer pain is tumor invasion with consequent tissue damage and activation of peripheral nociceptors (pain receptors). In addition, up to one-third of patients may experience therapy-related pain, such as vinca-induced polyneuropathy, postradiation tissue necrosis, and postsurgical nerve injury, especially after mastectomy or thoracotomy.

Pain occurs because injury to peripheral tissue activates deep and cutaneous nociceptors by both mechanical trauma and the release of biochemical mediators such as prostaglandins, serotonin, and bradykinin. Stimuli travel along afferent pathways to the dorsal root ganglia. After signal modification by input from adjacent neurons, the afferent signal then crosses and ascends in the spinothalamic tracts, which radiate to the medulla, pons, and thalamus where further processing occurs. Finally, the signal travels the neospinothalamic tract, terminates in the postcentral gyrus, and results in the awareness of pain.

Descending signals, which originate in the midbrain and then travel to the dorsal horn via the medial descending pathways, decrease the intensity of incoming painful stimuli. Serotonin, substance P, dopamine, norepinephrine, and other neurotransmitters are all important modulators of the afferent and efferent limbs of pain sensation. Along with the endogenous opioid peptides (enkephalin, beta endorphin, and dynorphin), the neurotransmitters accentuate or diminish the sensation of pain. Additional modulation occurs via the opioid receptors (the principal target for the opioid analgesics), also found within the ascending and descending pathways.

The perception of and reaction to pain vary tremendously from individual to individual. Perceived pain is the product of biochemical physiology and emotional psychology. Thus patients with the same location and extent of disease may experience very different difficulties with pain. These individual differences also have significant impact on patients' tolerance of and need for analgesia. This "total" view of the experience of pain requires careful attention to the patient's description of and reaction to pain in order to devise an optimal, individualized pain management program.

PAIN ASSESSMENT

The evaluation of the patient presenting with cancer-related pain serves multiple purposes. A careful history defines the pain syndrome within the context of the patient's general health, premorbid psychological history, and family concerns. Patients and their families desperately need objective compassion and reassurance; receiving both has definite positive impact on the cancer pain therapy. Input from the primary care physician and limited psychologic testing may also provide a better understanding of the patient's pain.

Since pain is a subjective experience, quantitative measurement necessarily depends on subjective tools. Nevertheless, it is possible to characterize and measure pain in a meaningful and reproducible fashion. This characterization is essential to assessing the efficacy and toxicity of the pain treatment. Multiple instruments exist for these purposes: the most useful are the visual analogue scale, McGill Pain Questionnaire, Brief Pain Inventory, and Memorial Pain Questionnaire. A meticulous physical examination is an essential adjunct to the history for a complete pain assessment. Table 25–1 summarizes the comprehensive evaluation of the patient with cancer pain.

CLASSIFICATIONS OF CANCER PAIN

ACUTE VERSUS CHRONIC

Associated with sympathetic nervous system hyperactivity and extreme distress, acute pain frequently occurs at disease onset, requires transient (but effective) analgesia, and typically resolves with antineoplastic therapy. In contrast, assessment and management of patients with chronic pain is more complex. With time, biologic and behavioral adjustment to symptoms occurs, and associated signs of tachycardia, hypertension, and diaphoresis are often absent. The manifestations of pain (alterations in facial expression, gait, posture, and mood) usually persist throughout the course of the disease. Premorbid chronic nonmalignant pain (e.g., that due to degenerative arthritis or diabetic neuropathy) may further complicate management. Exacerbation of pain in a cancer patient usually signals tumor progression and requires appropriately directed intervention.

PHYSIOLOGIC

Somatic pain results from activation of nociceptors in the skin and deep tissues, may be acute or chronic, and is usually well-localized and aching or gnawing in character.

Visceral pain results from distention or irritation of the bowel or liver. It is characteristically vague in distribution and quality and is often deep, dull, aching or pressure-like. When acute, it may be paroxysmal and colicky and associated with nausea, vomiting, diaphoresis, and alterations in blood pressure and heart rate.

Neuropathic pain results from neural injury and is a spontaneous burning dysesthesia, hyperpathia, and hyperalgesia. This pain is diffuse and excruciating and accompanied by exaggerated skeletal muscle and autonomic responses. Patients may report symptoms ranging from anesthesia to allodynia (pain in response to a stimulus that usually does not provoke pain, e.g., light stroke). An additional characteristic is persistence despite standard analgesic therapy and a tendency for favorable response to tricyclic antidepressants and

Table 25–1. **EVALUATION OF THE CANCER PATIENT WITH PAIN**

I. Review of medical record and radiologic studies
II. Physical examination
III. Review of responses to pain questionnaires
IV. Pain history
   A. Premorbid chronic pain
   B. Premorbid drug or alcohol use
   C. Pain catalogue (number and locations)
   D. For each pain
      1. Onset and evolution
      2. Site and radiation
      3. Pattern (e.g., constant, intermittent, predictable)
      4. Intensity (best, worst, average, current): 0–10 scale
      5. Quality
      6. Exacerbating factors
      7. Relieving factors
      8. How the pain interferes
      9. Neurologic and motor abnormalities
      10. Vasomotor changes
      11. Current analgesics (use, efficacy, and side effects)
      12. Prior analgesics (use, efficacy, and side effects)

anticonvulsant drugs. Examples include phantom limb pain, spinal cord transection, and postherpetic neuralgia.

CANCER PAIN SYNDROMES

Bone pain is the most common cancer pain. Although the majority of skeletal metastases are painless, pain from bony metastases varies tremendously. When present, pain is usually constant but may peak at night and is often worse with movement or weight bearing. Patients may report a dull ache or deep, intense pain, with or without referred pain, muscle spasm, or paroxysms of stabbing pain. Knee pain associated with hip metastases is an important example of referred bony pain.

Spinal cord invasion secondary to vertebral metastases causes spinal and/or radicular pain, often with weakness and paresthesias in a dermatomal pattern. Pain usually precedes neurologic changes, is dull, steady, and aching, and increases gradually over time. Rapid progression of neurologic deficit signals progressive epidural spinal cord compression and warrants urgent intervention.

Plexopathy of the brachial plexus is most common with lung and breast cancer and most frequently damages the lower cord (C8-T1). Distinguishing brachial plexus abnormalities due to radiation fibrosis from those due to tumor invasion is difficult because the clinical findings are similar. Horner's syndrome and severe pain and weakness in the C8-T1 distribution are more common with tumor invasion, whereas weakness of shoulder abduction and arm flexors is more common after radiation injury.

Invasion of the lumbar plexus by cancer causes aching or pressure-like radicular lower extremity pain. Pain is the presenting symptom in most patients, about half of whom later develop significant weakness and numbness. Abnormalities in reflexes and straight leg raising are common early findings. Computed tomography (CT) scans of the pelvis and lumbar spine and diagnostic nerve blocks help to corroborate clinical findings.

Invasion of the sacral plexus causes severe constant lower backache, often with perineal sensory loss and bowel or bladder dysfunction. Plain films, CT scans, and bone scans frequently demonstrate invasion of the sacrum.

CANCER PAIN MANAGEMENT

The most effective treatment for cancer pain is successful treatment of the cancer. This is especially true for painful bone metastases, which often respond promptly and dramatically to a brief course of local radiation therapy. Nevertheless, the majority of patients require primary analgesic therapy, either while awaiting tumor response or because their antitumor therapy is ineffective. When cure is impossible, one of the primary goals of treatment is the successful palliation of pain.

It is vital to tailor the specific analgesic treatment to the needs of the individual patient. Constant and unremitting pain is most amenable to an around-the-clock analgesic dosing schedule. This prevents pain rather than treating it retroactively and works most successfully with long-acting analgesics or infusions of analgesics. Despite a mostly effective around-the-clock analgesic schedule, breakthrough pain is still common. Breakthrough pain refers to intermittent exacerbations of pain occurring spontaneously or in relation to specific activity. Supplemental, rapid-onset, short-duration narcotic analgesics are the most effective treatment for breakthrough pain. If a specific activity (e.g., walking, transferring) incites pain, anticipatory supplemental analgesia may facilitate the function. For patients receiving narcotic infusions (subcutaneous, intravenous, epidural), the addition of patient-controlled analgesia (PCA) supplemental boluses allows the patient to manage breakthrough pain.

ANALGESIC MEDICATIONS

Table 25–2 summarizes the basic guidelines for use of narcotic analgesics for cancer pain. Familiarity with the pharmacology of the individual drugs is essential. Titrating the dose according to the patient's tolerance and requirements is critical to success. Extremely high doses may be necessary for patients on chronic analgesia regimens.

Table 25–2. **GUIDELINES FOR THE USE OF NARCOTIC ANALGESICS IN PAIN MANAGEMENT**

1. Start with a specific drug for a specific type of pain.
2. Know the pharmacology of the drug prescribed.
   a. Duration of the analgesic effect
   b. Pharmacokinetic properties of the drug
   c. Equianalgesic doses for the drug and its route of administration
3. Adjust the route of administration to the patient's needs.
4. Administer the analgesic on a regular basis after initial titration of the dose.
5. Use drug combinations to provide additive analgesia and reduce side effects (e.g., nonsteroidal antiinflammatory drugs, antihistamine [hydroxyzine], amphetamine [Dexedrine]).
6. Avoid drug combinations that increase sedation without enhancing analgesia (e.g., benzodiazepine, phenothiazine).
7. Anticipate and treat side effects.
   a. Sedation
   b. Respiratory distress
   c. Nausea and vomiting
   d. Constipation
8. Watch for the development of tolerance.
   a. Switch to an alternative narcotic analgesic.
   b. Start with one-half the equianalgesic dose and titrate the dose for pain relief.
9. Prevent acute withdrawal.
   a. Taper drugs slowly.
   b. Use diluted doses of naloxone (0.4 mg in 10 mL of saline) to reverse respiratory depression in the physically dependent patient, and administer cautiously.
10. Do not use placebos to assess the nature of the pain.
11. Anticipate and manage complications.
    a. Overdose
    b. Multifocal myoclonus
    c. Seizures

From Foley KM: The treatment of cancer pain. N Engl J Med 313:84–95, 1985.

Anticipating and ameliorating analgesia side effects, especially constipation, may make the difference between analgesic success and failure. Figure 25–1 summarizes a reasonable clinical decision protocol to optimize pain control. With these principles, 70 to 90% of patients achieve acceptable pain control.

Mild Pain

It is possible to control mild pain with regular doses of aspirin, acetaminophen, or nonsteroidal anti-inflammatory drugs (NSAIDs). These agents are unlikely to cause central nervous system toxicity because they work peripherally. Aspirin is relatively contraindicated in some patients because of its antiplatelet and gastrointestinal toxicities. Acetaminophen results in little toxicity, but patients often do not perceive it as a significant analgesic.

The NSAIDs are active by themselves and as adjuncts to narcotics, particularly for bone pain; their drawbacks include high cost and gastrointestinal and renal toxicities. Inhibition of platelet aggregation also occurs but to a lesser degree than with aspirin (Table 25–3). The nonacetylated salicylates (sodium salicylate, choline magnesium trisalicylate) have a particularly favorable toxicity profile (no platelet toxicity, less gastrointestinal bleeding, well tolerated with asthma). In contrast to opioids, there is a ceiling effect, above which dose escalations do not result in more analgesia. Regular use promotes both an anti-inflammatory as well as an analgesic effect.

Moderate Pain

Moderate pain usually requires codeine or oxycodone, which are more effective when combined with aspirin, acetaminophen, or NSAIDs. Commonly used examples of these medications with equivalent efficacy include Tylenol #3, Tylox, Percodan, Percocet, and other brand and generic equivalents. All share the same potential side effects of mild

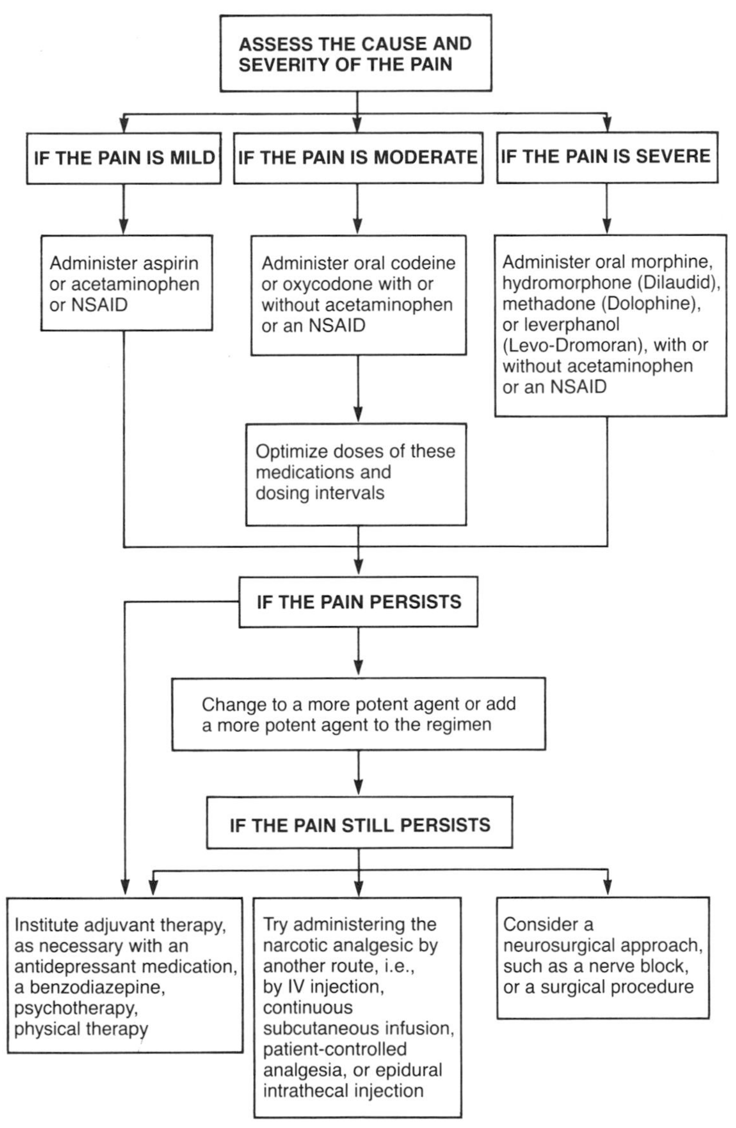

Figure 25–1. Management of chronic cancer pain. (*Modified from* Plezia P, Alberts DS: Integrated approach to cancer pain treatment [editorial]. Hosp Ther 10:20–25, 1985.)

gastrointestinal distress, constipation, and sedation, but prices and patient preferences vary widely (Table 25–4). It is important to administer these medications regularly (not as needed). With time, as patients develop tolerance to initially effective analgesia, dose escalations become necessary to continue the same level of analgesic efficacy.

Analgesics to avoid are pentazocine (Talwin), propoxyphene (Darvon), and oral meperidine (Demerol). Pentazocine (50 mg) is no more effective than aspirin and has significant psychomimetic effects. Propoxyphene (65 mg) is also no more effective than aspirin, and it is metabolized to toxic norpropoxyphene. Oral meperidine is not very effective and has variable gastrointestinal absorption; it also transforms into a neurotoxic metabolite, causing myoclonus and seizures. As a parenteral analgesic, meperidine is effective for only 2 to 3 hours, not the commonly prescribed 4 to 6 hours.

Table 25–3. **ANALGESICS FOR MILD CANCER PAIN**

ANALGESIC AGENT	EQUIANALGESIC DOSE (mg)	DURATION (hr)	APPROXIMATE COST (per week on regular dose)
Aspirin	650–1000	4–6	<$1.00
Acetaminophen	650–1000	4–6	<$1.00
Diflunisal (Dolobid)	500	8–12	$12.90
Ibuprofen (Motrin)	200–600	4–6	$27.00
Naproxen (Naprosyn)	250	6–8	$24.00
Sulindac (Clinoril)	150–200	12	$19.50
Indomethacin (Indocin)	50	6–8	$29.00

The brand names and costs are for comparison only. The cost figures were based on a 33% markup of average wholesale prices in 1991. Generic costs may vary.

Severe Pain

Severe pain requires regular doses of major narcotic analgesics, usually beginning with an oral regimen but sometimes requiring parenteral or rectal administration (Table 25–5). Oral morphine has many advantages. Analgesia is excellent with adequate doses (three to six times parenteral doses). Morphine is available in a variety of forms: liquid (Roxanol), 2 mg/mL and 20 mg/mL; immediate-release tablets, 15 mg and 30 mg; sustained-release forms (MS Contin), 15 mg, 30 mg, 60 mg, and 100 mg; and suppositories (15 mg). Initial treatment should begin with an immediate-release preparation to determine the patient's daily requirement for morphine and subsequently switch to a sustained-release form for dosing convenience (at the same total daily dose). The usual initial dose for oral morphine is 30 to 60 mg every 4 to 6 hours (less in the elderly and debilitated). The "correct" dose of morphine for the management of cancer pain is the dose that effectively relieves the pain without inducing intolerable side effects.

Methadone provides equally good analgesia and is relatively inexpensive. Methadone has a long half-life, however, and causes cumulative toxicity. Careful dose adjustments during the first week on treatment are necessary. Methadone is non–cross-reactive with morphine, so it represents a viable alternative for the morphine-allergic patient.

Hydromorphone (Dilaudid) is in many ways equivalent to morphine. It is also available in oral, parenteral, and rectal suppository forms. Some patients tolerate hydromorphone better than morphine or methadone. However, it is significantly more expensive. Levorphanol (Levodromoran), like methadone, has a long half-life and tends to cause cumulative toxicity. It may also be difficult to obtain, especially in smaller pharmacies.

Fentanyl (Duragesic) is now available as a transdermal patch that reliably releases controlled amounts of fentanyl over a 72-hour period. The advantages of transdermal delivery include consistent blood levels, the convenience of every-3-day dosing, and high patient acceptance. The disadvantages include slow onset of action and persisting drug levels despite removing the patch. Oral or rectal immediate-release analgesia is necessary for breakthrough pain.

Table 25–4. **ANALGESICS FOR MODERATE CANCER PAIN**

ANALGESIC	CONTENT (mg)	DURATION (hr)	APPROXIMATE COST (per week on regular dose)
Acetaminophen and codeine			
Tylenol #3	300/30	4–6	$12.50
Tylenol #4	300/60	4–6	$22.00
Aspirin and codeine			
Empirin #3	325/30	4–6	$15.50
Empirin #4	325/60	4–6	$37.00
Acetaminophen and oxycodone			
Percocet	325/5	4–6	$30.00
Tylox	500/5	4–6	$32.00
Aspirin and oxycodone	325/5	4–6	$32.00

The brand names and costs are for comparison only. The cost figures were based on a 33% markup of average wholesale prices in 1991. Generic costs may vary.

Table 25–5. **ANALGESICS FOR SEVERE CANCER PAIN**

ANALGESIC	EQUIANALGESIC DOSE	DURATION (hr)	APPROXIMATE COST (per week on regular dose)
Morphine			
Oral (immediate release)	30 mg	4–6	$14.00
MS Contin (sustained release)	30 mg	8–12	$28.00
Injectable	10 mg	4–6	$40.00
Hydromorphone (Dilaudid)			
Oral	8 mg	4–6	$54.00
Intramuscular	2 mg	4–5	$56.00
Methadone (Dolophine)			
Oral	10 mg	4–6	$7.30
Intramuscular	5 mg	4–6	$45.00
Fentanyl (Duragesic)	25 μg/hr	72	$25.00

The brand names and costs are for comparison only. The cost figures were based on a 33% markup of average wholesale prices in 1991. Generic costs may vary.

An alternative for patients unable to take oral analgesics is the rectal suppository. Morphine, hydromorphone, and oxymorphone (Numorphan) are all available in rectal suppository form. Table 25–6 compares doses, timing, and approximate costs.

REFRACTORY PAIN

Supplemental Medication

It is possible to control the pain of most cancer patients with a combination of psychologic counseling, reassurance, and the appropriate dose of narcotic analgesic. For those with pain despite this program, supplemental medications may be of value. The most common are the NSAIDs and the antidepressants.

The main indication for antidepressants is neuropathic pain of a sharp, burning, or dysesthetic quality. Specific applications include postherpetic neuralgia, postablative anesthesia dolorosa, posttreatment neuritis, postmastectomy or thoracotomy pain, and invasion of neural structures such as the brachial plexus by tumor. Antidepressants may actually be useful for any cancer patient whose pain is unresponsive to standard pharmacologic management. In addition to their analgesic properties, antidepressants may improve the patient's nighttime sleep and mood. The administration of amitriptyline and other tricyclics begins with low nighttime doses (10 to 25 mg), which are gradually increased with tolerance. The analgesic benefit may not occur until after 2 or 3 weeks of treatment. The common adverse effects of tricyclics—dry mouth and morning drowsiness—are usually mild and tend to resolve over the course of 1 to 2 weeks of regular administration. The elderly and the infirm require dose reductions.

Additionally, therapeutic trials of supplementary benzodiazepines and anticonvulsants may be successful in some patients. Steroids sometimes improve pain control while contributing to a general improvement in "well-being." Behavioral training in "relaxation"

Table 25–6. **ANALGESIC SUPPOSITORIES**

ANALGESIC	EQUIANALGESIC DOSE (mg)	DURATION (hr)	APPROXIMATE COST (per week on regular dose)
Morphine	20	4–6	$67.00
Hydromorphone (Dilaudid)	3	4–6	$100.00
Oxymorphone (Numorphan)	5	4–6	$192.00

The brand names and costs are for comparison only. The cost figures were based on a 33% markup of average wholesale prices in 1991. Generic costs may vary.

techniques and TENS (transcutaneous electrical nerve stimulation) units also are helpful for some patients with problematic pain.

Narcotic Infusions

For pain refractory to oral or transdermal narcotics, a continuous parenteral infusion of morphine is very useful. Administration in the patient's home is possible with the use of a portable pump delivering a continuous subcutaneous infusion of morphine or hydromorphone. The pump is easy to use after "hands-on" instruction to the patient and/or family. Needle placement is also easy and painless. The pumps allow both continuous and bolus drug administration, incorporating the important advantages of consistent analgesia and patient-controlled analgesia. The beginning hourly dose is approximately 25 to 30% of the previous total 24-hour oral dose divided by 24 (usually 5 to 10 mg/hr). Tissue irritation is minimal with hourly volumes of less than 1 to 2 mL of appropriately concentrated narcotic solutions. Any subcutaneous site may be used, but the infraclavicular fossa and chest wall interfere least with ambulation. It is necessary to check the site twice daily for irritation and to change the site weekly.

Patients may also receive continuous intravenous morphine either in the hospital or at home via an intravascular access device. Delivery of continuous intravenous narcotics requires a flow-calibrated infusion device with alarms. Supplemental morphine boluses, possibly by patient-controlled analgesia for appropriate patients, are essential for breakthrough pain. Doses are escalated until pain relief is adequate or side effects become intolerable. There is no ceiling dose, and indeed some patients need hourly doses as high as 500 mg of morphine.

Continuous epidural or intrathecal analgesia approaches pain control via the spinal opioid receptors in the dorsal horn and by suppressing spinothalamic tract neurons. This minimizes distribution of the drug to the brain and consequently reduces systemic central nervous system side effects. Intraspinal narcotic infusion relieves most oncologic pain dramatically and in a highly selective fashion, with an absence of motor, sensory, and sympathetic effects. In properly selected patients, analgesia is often superior to that of narcotics administered by other routes, with fewer side effects because of the significantly lower doses required. Intraspinal infusions frequently relieve opioid-induced mental obtundation and "narcotic bowel syndrome" (pseudo-obstruction). To determine whether patients will respond to intraspinal opioids, the first step is a test dose through a temporary epidural catheter. Those who respond favorably then undergo placement of a Hickman-Broviac–type tunneled catheter to minimize risk of displacement and infection. Central side effects, especially delayed respiratory suppression and autonomic dysfunction, occur rarely in patients previously treated with narcotics. While effective, these approaches remain investigational and are best managed by experienced specialists.

Nerve Blocks and Neurosurgery

Local anesthetic measures, including temporary and permanent nerve blocks, are successful in 22 to 80% of patients. Difficulties arise because multiple sensory nerves serve most painful areas, and thus local treatment is inappropriate for most pain. The choice of nerve block is dependent on the pain location and etiology (Table 25–7). Celiac plexus block, sometimes performed intraoperatively for pancreatic cancer, is usually a transcutaneous procedure that successfully controls mid-abdominal visceral pain in 60 to 80% of patients. Fluoroscopic guidance for needle placement is critical to success. Orthostatic hypotension is a nearly universal but temporary side effect.

Neurosurgical measures for pain relief include cordotomies and placement of epidural, intrathecal, or intraventricular catheters for morphine infusions. Cordotomies, either percutaneous or by open procedure, are most successful for unilateral pain below the waist. Complications include paresis (5%), ataxia (20%), and urinary dysfunction (10%). Since most patients subsequently develop pain in another area, cordotomies have limited value.

ANALGESIA SIDE EFFECTS

Narcotic-induced constipation is sufficiently common that prophylactic treatment is recommended in most cases. Patients benefit from a "sliding scale" bowel regimen that

Table 25–7. **TYPES OF ANESTHETIC PROCEDURES COMMONLY USED FOR CANCER PAIN**

TYPE OF PROCEDURE	MOST COMMON INDICATIONS
Nerve block	
Peripheral	Pain in discrete dermatomes in chest and abdomen
Epidural	Unilateral lumbar or sacral pain Midline perineal pain Bilateral lumbosacral pain
Intrathecal	Midline perineal pain Bilateral lumbosacral pain
Autonomic	
Stellate ganglion	Reflex sympathetic dystrophy Arm pain
Lumbar sympathetic	Reflex sympathetic dystrophy Lumbosacral plexopathy Vascular insufficiency of the lower extremity
Celiac plexus	Midabdominal pain
Continuous epidural infusion with local anesthetics	Unilateral and bilateral lumbosacral pain Midline perineal pain
Trigger-point injection	Focal muscle pain

From Foley KM: The treatment of cancer pain. N Engl J Med 313:84–95, 1985.

provides stronger laxatives (from Colace and Senokot to lactulose and enemas) until a regular bowel habit ensues. It is important to rule out bowel obstruction and fecal impaction when obstipation resists laxative therapy.

For mild narcotic-induced nausea or sedation, it is advisable to reassure patients that these effects are usually transient, resolving spontaneously with tolerance, and to continue the prescribed analgesic regimen. More persistent nausea may decrease with antiemetic treatment (prochlorperazine or metoclopramide). In some cases, psychostimulants such as methylphenidate (Ritalin, 10 mg at 8 AM and 5 mg at noon) or dextroamphetamine will counter narcotic sedation, but agitation is a possible side effect. When side effects are intractable, a trial of a similar, alternative analgesic may be successful, since side effects are often idiosyncratic and may not occur with very similar drugs.

MAINTENANCE AND DISCONTINUATION OF ANALGESIA

Analgesic drug regimens need periodic reassessment. Patients are often reluctant to request more potent analgesia because of fear of addiction. While physical dependence is likely, psychologic addiction and addictive behavior are very rare. If other measures achieve pain relief, provided patients gradually decrease their narcotic intake, significant withdrawal problems are unlikely. Unfortunately, most patients require narcotic analgesia for the duration of their life, and fear of addiction by the patient or physician is inappropriate.

It is important to anticipate increased drug requirements related to progression of disease and the development of physical tolerance. A decreased duration of analgesic efficacy is the most frequent sign of tolerance.

Occasionally a patient inadvertently receives too much narcotic. While this is reversible with naloxone (Narcan), a rapid bolus of naloxone will precipitate an exquisitely painful acute withdrawal. In all but the most life-threatening conditions, a low naloxone infusion will reverse respiratory depression with minimal withdrawal symptoms.

While rarely eliminated altogether, pain is controllable in the vast majority of patients, usually with the careful application of fairly simple pharmacologic measures combined with diagnostic acumen and conscientious follow-up. In the small proportion of patients whose pain is unresponsive to oral analgesics, a variety of alternative measures is available to provide relief of pain.

REFERENCES

Brown DL, Moore DC: The use of neurolytic celiac plexus block for pancreatic cancer: Anatomy and technique. J Pain Symptom Manag 3:206–209, 1988.

Foley KM: Treatment of cancer pain. N Engl J Med 313:84–95, 1985.
Patt R: Interventional analgesia: Epidural and subarachnoid analgesia. Am J Hospice Pall Care 6:11–14, 1989.
Patt R: Nonpharmacologic measures for controlling oncologic pain. Am J Hospice Pall Care 7:30–37, 1990.
Portenoy RK: Practical aspects of pain control in the patient with cancer. CA 38:327–352, 1988.
Swanson G, Smith J, Bulich R, et al: Patient-controlled analgesia for chronic cancer pain in the ambulatory setting: A report of 117 patients. J Clin Oncol 7:1903–1908, 1989.
Twycross RG: The management of pain in cancer: A guide to drugs and dosages. Oncology 2:35–47, 1988.

26
MANAGEMENT OF NAUSEA IN THE CANCER PATIENT

Gary R. Morrow

To complete a potentially curative course of cancer treatment successfully, a patient must be able to tolerate the side effects of therapy. Nausea and vomiting are frequent and troublesome toxicities of many cancer treatments. They reduce the quality of life. These disagreeable side effects may also lead to further treatment difficulties such as dehydration and attendant metabolic imbalance, wound dehiscence, and the psychologic sequelae of depression, anxiety, and "misery." Successful management of these side effects significantly improves compliance with the prescribed chemotherapy regimen.

INCIDENCE OF EMESIS

The incidence of nausea and vomiting varies among patients receiving chemotherapy. In one study, 62% of 1240 consecutive patients reported postchemotherapy nausea and 44% experienced vomiting. Twenty-five percent reported severe, very severe, or intolerable nausea; the description of intolerable nausea increased to 50% in those experiencing emesis. The consistently high prevalence rates persist despite improved antiemetics. One potential explanation is that as patients' tolerance improves, treatment with larger doses of aggressive chemotherapy becomes feasible.

Chemotherapeutic agents differ both in their emetic potential (percent of patients experiencing emesis) and time to peak risk of emesis. Table 26–1 lists these risk of emesis figures for common cytotoxic drugs. A wide range in emetic potential and time to peak emesis is evident. For combination chemotherapy, the emetic potential of the combination is usually additive.

PHYSIOLOGY OF EMESIS

Most information about the physiology of nausea comes from animal research. The emetic center, a topographically distinct area in the lateral reticular formation of the medulla, coordinates vomiting. It receives input from at least four sources: the chemore-

Table 26–1. **EMETIC POTENTIAL AND TIME TO PEAK EMETIC POTENTIAL OF CYTOTOXIC DRUGS**

EMETIC POTENTIAL	DRUGS	TIME TO PEAK POTENTIAL (hr)
"Outstanding" (90%)	Cisplatin	1–6
	DTIC	1–4
	Streptozocin	1–4
"High" (60–90%)	CCNU	2–4
	BCNU	2–6
	Cyclophosphamide	4–12
"Medium" (30–60%)	Adriamycin (doxorubicin)	4–6
	Daunorubicin	2–6
	Actinomycin D	2–6
"Moderate" (10–30%)	Cytarabine	6–12
	Hydroxyurea	6–12
	Methotrexate	4–8
	Etoposide	4–6
"Low" (10%)	5-Fluorouracil	4–8
	Vincristine	4–8
	Tamoxifen	4–8

ceptor trigger zone (CTZ), the periphery, the cortex, and the vestibular apparatus. Figure 26–1 summarizes the paths for pharmacologic stimulation for the first three routes. The location of the CTZ next to the fourth ventricle in the medulla exposes it to both cerebrospinal fluid and the blood circulation. Activated solely by chemical stimuli, the CTZ plays an important role in chemotherapy-induced nausea and vomiting. The periphery responds to chemotherapy through afferents to the emetic center via the vagus nerve and other autonomic nerves. The third important input is from higher cognitive areas within the brain. These areas are close to those associated with long-term memory and imaging. This may be the pathway by which anticipatory side effects take place.

Research efforts continue to improve understanding of the site of emetic action of antineoplastic drugs. Different drugs act at different initiating sites, and a single drug can initiate emesis by stimulation of more than one input source.

PHARMACOLOGIC TREATMENT OF NAUSEA AND VOMITING

Control of nausea and vomiting is often unpredictable in the individual patient. Some patients tolerate highly emetogenic drugs with the aid of simple oral antiemetics, whereas typically well-tolerated antineoplastic drugs can incapacitate other patients. Others find the side effects of the antiemetics to be worse than nausea and vomiting. In clinical practice the initial "preventive" regimen of antiemetics corresponds to the emetic potential of the drugs and the condition of the patient.

Certain patient characteristics are somewhat predictive of the severity of reactive emesis. Patients with a significant daily alcohol ingestion experience less vomiting than those who do not drink. Patients susceptible to motion sickness experience more nausea and vomiting than those who are not susceptible. A third potential factor is age; younger patients report more severe side effects from the same drugs than do older patients. Finally, patients with a prior history of poorly controlled nausea and vomiting are likely to have continued poorly controlled nausea and vomiting with disease recurrence.

With this information concerning expected emesis risk, it is then possible to prescribe antiemetics ranging from low-dose oral phenothiazines to multiple-drug intravenous regimens. Table 26–2 describes commonly used antiemetics along with their doses and schedules.

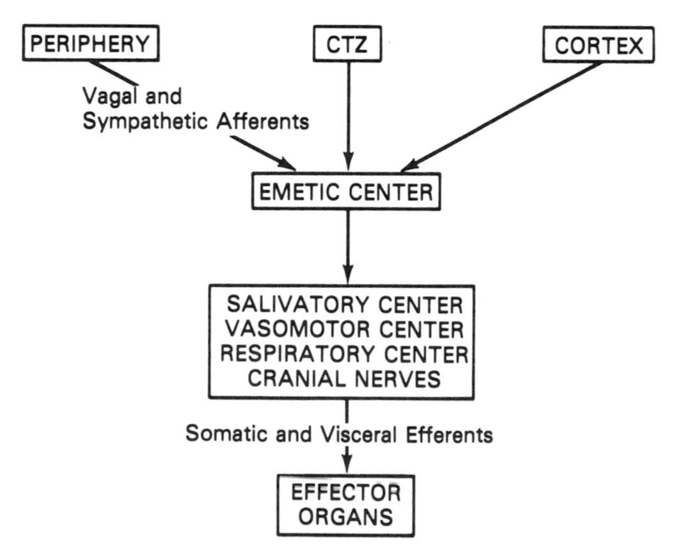

Figure 26–1. Pathways for vomiting initiation. (Reproduced with permission from Siegel LJ, Longo DL: The control of chemotherapy-induced emesis. Ann Intern Med 95:352–359, 1981.)

Table 26–2. **COMMON ANTIEMETIC MEDICATIONS**

AGENT	USUAL DOSE	DOSE INTERVAL (hr)
Prochlorperazine (Compazine)	10 mg orally 25 mg rectally	4–6
Haloperidol (Haldol)	2 mg orally 2 mg IM	4–6
Droperidol (Inapsine)	2–5 mg IM or IV	4–6
Metoclopramide (Reglan)	1–2 mg/kg IV 40–100 mg orally	½ hr before and every 2 hr after chemotherapy for 2–4 doses 2–4
Ondansetron (Zofran)	0.15 mg/kg mg IV or 10 mg	4
Delta-9-tetrahydrocannabinol (THC, Marinol)	5–20 mg orally	2–4
Dexamethasone (Decadron)	10 mg IV or orally	2–4
Lorazepam (Ativan)	1–2 mg IV	6–8

PHENOTHIAZINES

The most commonly used antiemetics for mild chemotherapy-induced nausea are the phenothiazines. They act by depression of dopamine receptors in the CTZ. Among the phenothiazines, prochlorperazine (Compazine) has a greater antiemetic effect and fewer hypotensive side effects but also possibly more extrapyramidal side effects. There are no randomized controlled studies determining the optimal phenothiazine. Other phenothiazines with known antiemetic effect include chlorpromazine (Thorazine), perphenazine (Triavil), and thiethylperazine (Torecan). Phenothiazines produce few side effects. While extrapyramidal side effects occur, especially in young patients, they are rapidly reversible with parenteral diphenhydramine (Benedryl). Phenothiazines are available in oral, rectal, and injectable intramuscular or intravenous preparations. While oral drugs are preferable because of simplicity of administration and low cost, suppositories and injections are helpful for refractory emesis.

BUTYROPHENONES

Haloperidol (Haldol) and droperidol (Inapsine) also inhibit dopamine receptors in the CTZ. At least one study found haloperidol to be superior to prochlorperazine, and another found it only slightly less effective than high-dose metoclopramide. Haloperidol can be administered orally or intramuscularly; droperidol is available only as an intramuscular or intravenous injection. Mild sedation and occasional extrapyramidal reactions are the only significant side effects.

METOCLOPRAMIDE

Metoclopramide (Reglan) is a substituted benzamide that inhibits dopamine receptors in the CTZ; it also inhibits emesis by direct effect on the upper gastrointestinal tract. High-dose metoclopramide has significant antiemetic action. Intravenous doses of 1 or 2 mg/kg, 30 minutes before and 1.5, 3.5, 5.5, and 8.5 hours after cisplatin infusion, are very effective in controlling cisplatin-induced emesis. Metoclopramide is also effective in oral doses of 2 mg/kg (or at least 50 to 100 mg per dose for equivalent effect). The most common side effects are diarrhea, extrapyramidal reactions, and sedation. Extrapyramidal reactions (especially restlessness) occur in 10 to 50% of patients treated with these dose levels;

therefore, preventive treatment with diphenhydramine (Benedryl) or benztropine (Cogentin) is advised. Extrapyramidal reactions are most common in young patients and those receiving high-dose oral metoclopramide.

SEROTONIN ANTAGONISTS

The recent development of serotonin-inhibiting agents, which act by inhibiting the 5-hydroxytryptamine-3 (5-HT-3, a serotonin subtype) receptor, introduced an entirely new class of highly effective antiemetics. Ondansetron (Zofran) is the only agent in this class currently available, but numerous similar compounds are in efficacy trials. Their antiemetic properties against high-dose cisplatin are impressive. These agents also produce less accompanying toxicity than metoclopramide. Unfortunately, ondansetron is extremely expensive and currently available only for intravenous injection. Oral preparations will soon be released; for now, some administer the intravenous preparation orally in juice with apparent antiemetic efficacy. Further research is necessary to establish the efficacy of these agents with other forms of chemotherapy; however, preliminary findings are very promising.

DELTA-9-TETRAHYDROCANNABINOL (THC, MARINOL)

Anecdotal reports of THC antiemetic activity led to confirmatory scientific investigation. However, it is still unclear how THC exerts its antiemetic effect. Some studies found THC to be superior to prochlorperazine (Compazine) for refractory emesis. Others found it active but less effective than metoclopramide for cisplatin-induced emesis. The antiemetic effectiveness of THC requires that patients experience a subjective "high." Young people who previously enjoyed "recreational" marijuana find THC to be more effective and acceptable than older people, who often complain of dysphoria and other mental side effects. THC is available as oral Marinol, which is as effective as the inhaled "street" version, with superior preparation consistency and fewer pulmonary and other toxicities.

CORTICOSTEROIDS

Dexamethasone (Decadron) and methylprednisolone both have antiemetic activity. The physiologic mechanism is unknown. Doses vary significantly among studies. Corticosteroids are typically part of combination antiemetic regimens with phenothiazines, butyrophenones, and metoclopramide. Side effects are very few, but caution is necessary in patients with diabetes or peptic ulcer disease.

OTHER DRUGS

Antihistamines have little antiemetic effect alone, but in combination with a dopamine receptor antagonist they increase the antiemetic effect and prevent extrapyramidal side effects. Anticholinergic drugs, especially transdermal scopolamine, also have mild antiemetic effects. The added antianxiety and amnesic effects of benzodiazepines such as diazepam (Valium) and lorazepam (Ativan) may be useful with some patients. However, sedation poses an added risk of aspiration in patients who vomit.

A PRACTICAL APPROACH TO THE CONTROL OF EMESIS

Figure 26–2 outlines a practical approach to the control of emesis. Patients should eat lightly on the day of treatment, and many take pretreatment antiemetics. For the drugs causing emesis in less than 50% of patients (see Table 26–1), an oral and/or rectal phenothiazine, sometimes with dexamethasone, is advisable before treatment and for 24 to 48 hours after treatment. For patients with refractory emesis despite phenothiazines, a butyrophenone or metoclopramide supplemented by dexamethasone may achieve better symptom control. Patients receiving highly nauseating drugs, such as cisplatin, require treatment before and after chemotherapy with combination antiemetic regimens, including either ondansetron, dexamethasone, and lorazepam or metoclopromide, dexamethasone,

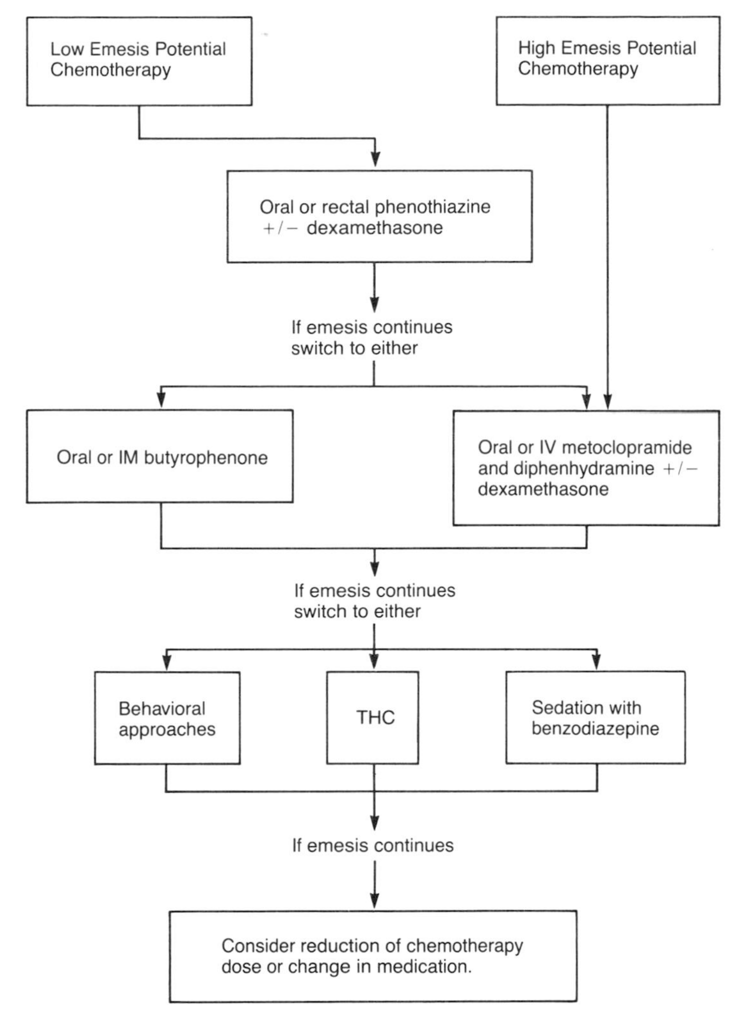

Figure 26–2. A practical approach to antiemetic management.

lorazepam, and diphenhydramine (or Cogentin). For those patients who still find chemotherapy intolerable, remaining options include THC, sedation (with risk of aspiration), or chemotherapy dose reduction (with risk of diminished anticancer effects).

ANTICIPATORY NAUSEA AND VOMITING

In addition to posttreatment nausea and vomiting, many patients undergoing chemotherapy develop nausea and, less frequently, vomiting prior to treatment. This is anticipatory nausea and vomiting. While prevalence rates vary with the number of cycles of treatment and the degree of posttreatment nausea and vomiting, approximately 1 in 4 patients will develop anticipatory nausea and approximately 1 in 10 develops anticipatory vomiting.

Figure 26–3 depicts the mechanism by which anticipatory side effects develop via a conditioning paradigm. The unconditioned stimulus of chemotherapy caused the unconditioned response of nausea and vomiting in the presence of the conditioned stimulus—possibly the sight of the chemotherapy nurse. After repeated exposure to both the

THE FIRST FEW CHEMOTHERAPY TREATMENTS

Conditioned stimulus (Sight of nurse)	No response
Unconditioned stimulus (Chemotherapy drugs)	Unconditioned response (nausea, vomiting)

AFTER SEVERAL CHEMOTHERAPY TREATMENTS

Conditioned stimulus (Sight of nurse)	Conditioned response (nausea, vomiting)

Figure 26–3. Anticipatory nausea conditioning.

unconditioned and conditioned stimulus (drugs and nurse), the presence of the nurse alone can then produce the conditioned response—nausea and vomiting. A variety of indirect data supports this view of development.

DELAYED NAUSEA AND VOMITING

Some patients experience emesis following a 24-hour symptom-free period after chemotherapy. This poorly understood phenomenon is termed delayed nausea and vomiting. Delayed vomiting occurs in approximately 25% of patients following at least one of three successive chemotherapy cycles. Delayed nausea is more common, occurring in approximately one in three patients. Delayed nausea and vomiting are independent; only 5% of patients report both symptoms occurring together. The etiology is unclear, but this problem does seem to occur more commonly with cisplatin chemotherapy.

BEHAVIORAL INTERVENTIONS

Several behavioral approaches are useful for controlling both anticipatory and posttreatment nausea and vomiting in cancer patients. Hypnosis is somewhat effective, with greater benefit for children than for adults. Because of poor patient acceptance and lengthy time commitment, hypnosis is infrequently used for adults. Various relaxation-based techniques are generally effective and increasingly popular.

Systematic desensitization is a successful behavioral approach, which involves the counter-conditioning of those situations likely to elicit anticipatory nausea and vomiting to a response that is incompatible with nausea and vomiting. This new response is deep muscle relaxation. Thus, when the patient sees the previously nauseating stimuli (i.e., the chemotherapy room or nurse), instead of experiencing nausea, the counter-conditioning causes him to experience deep muscle relaxation. Oncologists and oncology nurses can quickly learn and apply this technique with gratifying success.

SUMMARY

A variety of antiemetics is available for the management of nausea and vomiting due to chemotherapy. The ideal antiemetic does not exist, and it may be necessary to try or combine several different antiemetic regimens to derive maximum symptom control. Ease of administration, potential for both physiologic and psychological side effects, and cost are important considerations in choosing a particular agent. Behavioral approaches for control of chemotherapy-induced nausea and vomiting provide an additional nonpharmacologic method to help alleviate this common complication.

REFERENCES

Carey MP, Burish TG, Brenner DE: Delta-9-tetrahydrocannabinol in cancer chemotherapy: Research problems and issues. Ann Intern Med 99:106–114, 1983.

Hesketh PJ, Gandara DR: Serotonin antagonists: A new class of antiemetic agents. J Natl Cancer Inst 83:613–620, 1991.

Kris MG, Gralla RJ, Clark RA, et al: Antiemetic control and prevention of side effects of anticancer therapy with lorazepam or diphenhydramine when used in combination with metoclopramide plus dexamethasone. Cancer 60:2816–2822, 1987.

Lindley CM, Bernard S, Fields SM: Incidence and duration of chemotherapy-induced nausea and vomiting in the outpatient oncology population. J Clin Oncol 7:1142–1149, 1989.

Marty M, Pouillart P, Scholl S, et al: Comparison of the 5-hydroxytryptamine-3 (serotonin) antagonist ondansetron (GR 38032F) with high-dose metoclopramide in the control of cisplatin-induced emesis. N Engl J Med 322:816–820, 1990.

Morrow GR: Chemotherapy-related nausea and vomiting: Etiology and management. CA 39:89–104, 1989.

Morrow GR, Morrell C: Behavioral treatment for the anticipatory nausea and vomiting induced by cancer chemotherapy. N Engl J Med 307:1476–1480, 1982.

27
ONCOLOGIC NURSING

Kathleen S. Doerner

Oncology nurses play a unique role, serving the technical, physical, psychosocial, and educational needs of the cancer patient and the family. Oncology nurses serve as an important resource during all phases of the illness and often bond more closely with their patients than the physicians do. Nursing care focuses on reducing the impact of the disease for both the patient and the family and emphasizes the management of the many side effects associated with various therapies. The attitudes and actions of the nurse influence the way the patient and family cope with the stresses of the disease and its treatment. The goal of nursing a cancer patient is the promotion of well-being in that patient, whether it be physical, psychological, social, or spiritual wellness.

PATIENT AND FAMILY EDUCATION

The diagnosis of cancer can consume much of the patient's (and family's) attention and energies. Adjustment to the disease begins with education. Teaching patients and families about the disease and the therapies planned is an important nursing responsibility. Nurses have the opportunity to develop rapport with patients and families because they have the most consistent contact with them, either during prolonged hospitalizations or during treatments in the outpatient setting. Because of this rapport, patients may find the information explained by the oncology nurse more understandable and less intimidating than that provided by the physician.

Prior to the initiation of any teaching, the nurse must first assess the learning needs and abilities of the patient and family. Teaching about cancer and its treatment is an ongoing process and cannot be completed in a one-time session. Different patients require differing modes of education, and teaching sessions need to be individualized to the specific learner. Patient-family relationships may also play a role in the planning and executing of teaching plans. A lifetime pattern of antagonistic family communications and interrelationships is not likely to improve during illness.

Through effective education the patient and family may regain the ability to take control of their lives. While the nurse teaches about the disease, its treatments, and possible outcomes, the patient and family can start to prepare for the future. Although education is most critical at the time of diagnosis and initial treatment planning, the process must continue throughout the entire cancer experience. Although the specific goals of patient education may change, the need for accurate information is ongoing. The patient and family who are well informed and who have a sense of control over their lives are more likely to be active and successful participants in their care.

NUTRITION

The oncology nurse often takes primary responsibility for managing most nutritional problems in cancer patients. By providing dietary advice, suggestions for symptom management, nutritional supplements, and guidelines for the use of certain pharmacologic agents (e.g., antiemetics, steroids), the oncology nurse can often improve the patient's nutritional status without resort to invasive procedures.

Anorexia and taste alteration represent two of the major causes of malnutrition in cancer patients. These problems may occur in response to the disease itself, the treatment of the disease with chemotherapy or radiation therapy, or as a consequence of the psychologic or social implications associated with a diagnosis of cancer. The nurse must complete a thorough nutritional assessment and thus be able to advise the patient and family about methods to improve nutritional status. Patients who are already maintaining good food intake should be reassurred that elaborate or unusual diets are not necessary and have no proven benefit. Anorexic patients may need to change their eating habits from the usual three meals a day to a schedule of smaller, more frequent meals. Patients may also be able to maintain a desired weight as well as regain lost weight by supplementing their diet with high-calorie, vitamin-enriched supplements such as Ensure, Citrotein, or Carnation Instant Breakfast. Patients with head and neck or esophageal malignancies may require nutritional support via feeding tubes (nasogastric or gastrostomy) because of mechanical barriers to adequate oral intake. Total parenteral nutrition has little value in most cancer patients. Parenteral hyperalimentation may be useful during the perioperative period or in those patients with nonremediable bowel obstruction who could maintain good physical condition with nutritional support. Although oncology nurses handle the everyday nutritional problems of cancer patients, a therapeutic dietitian can address the more complex dietary problems and represents an asset to any oncology team.

ADMINISTRATION OF CHEMOTHERAPY

A major role of the oncology nurse consists of the administration of antineoplastic agents. This is a specialized skill performed by expertly trained nurses with an emphasis on safety and accuracy. Oncology nurses may also be responsible for the preparation of these agents. Nurses who perform these tasks must be aware of the pharmacology and the handling and delivery of the drugs, as well as their toxicities. Along with a knowledge of the drugs themselves, the nurse must possess expertise in venipuncture and intravenous therapy. Most chemotherapeutic agents have a narrow range between the therapeutic dose and that which causes severe toxicity. Therefore, good nursing practice demands careful checking of all chemotherapy orders as well as the patient's laboratory values prior to drug administration.

Cancer chemotherapeutic agents can be administered by many different routes, including the oral route, topical application, or parenteral administration. Some cancers respond better to chemotherapy delivered directly into the tumor or into a specific body cavity. Hospitalization is usually required for intra-arterial or intracavity chemotherapy, since invasive procedures are required to establish direct access to the site of administration. However, patients receiving infusions by means of implantable pumps or those receiving direct intraventricular injections via an Omaya reservoir can be treated on an outpatient basis. The nurse's role in the administration of chemotherapy by these methods varies from institution to institution.

INTRAVENOUS CHEMOTHERAPY

The majority of chemotherapeutic agents are administered intravenously. Safe administration of these drugs requires that the nurse establish an intravenous line and ensure its patency throughout the treatment. Existing peripheral intravenous lines should be avoided, since their patency and the condition of the vein are often questionable. Scalp vein needles (butterflies) are often used because of their ease of manipulation and minimal trauma to small, fragile veins. Jelco catheters may be used for patients receiving a chemotherapy infusion or for those patients who receive concurrent hydration or antiemetic therapy. This allows the patient more freedom and mobility during the treatment period, which may last several hours to several days. Small-gauge needles (23 or 25) appear to cause less phlebitis and less scar formation—an important consideration for patients subject to repeated venipuncture for ongoing therapy.

Once venous access has been established, one of four different modes of intravenous administration may be chosen. Intravenous push delivers the chemotherapeutic agent directly into a vein. This method is best for drugs given in small volume over 1 to 5 minutes. Slow administration from a syringe via a needle into the sideport of a free-flowing IV is similar to the intravenous push method. This technique allows rapid dilution of the medication through mixture with the IV fluids. Intravenous piggyback infusions may be given if the drugs must be diluted in larger volumes (usually 50 to 100 mL) of fluid for safe administration. The piggyback medication is infused through the sideport of a primary intravenous line. Drugs given by piggyback infusion are usually administered over 15 minutes to 1 hour. Chemotherapy can also be delivered intravenously as a primary infusion over a period of hours to days. Here the chemotherapeutic agent is diluted in larger volumes, usually 250 to 1000 mL of IV fluid.

The method for intravenous administration of chemotherapy depends on the drug and dose ordered and also on the condition of the patient's veins. Patients may experience a variety of sensations during the infusion of chemotherapy; the nurse must note these sensations and allieviate any discomfort. This may require slowing the infusion, changing from an IV push to an IV piggyback, or changing the IV site all together.

VESICANT DRUGS AND EXTRAVASATION

A vesicant drug is defined as an agent that can cause severe tissue destruction if infiltrated. Vesicants should be administered either IV push or through the sideport of a running IV. This minimizes the duration of exposure to the drug and also ensures that the nurse is present throughout the entire procedure. When administering a known vesicant (Table 27–1), it is imperative to check for patency of the vein by drawing back on the syringe to check for blood return. If a flashback of blood does not follow, the site must be thoroughly examined for signs of infiltration. The occurrence of pain, erythema, or swelling suggests extravasation, whether or not a blood return is observed, and mandates that the infusion be stopped.

Whenever suspicion of vesicant extravasation arises, the effects of the drugs on the surrounding tissue and underlying structures must be minimized. The institutional policy for extravasation management should be implemented immediately. The treatment of extravasation is controversial, and no treatment has definite efficacy. Prior to removal of the needle, the nurse should attempt to aspirate any residual blood and drug from the site of infiltration. The needle should then be withdrawn and minimal pressure applied to the area. Usually either heat or cold is then applied to the site. The choice of heat or cold depends on the drug, institutional preferences, and the drug manufacturer's recommendations. Heat increases drug dispersal and minimizes local concentration of the drug. Heat is usually applied to extravasation of plant alkaloids such as vincristine or vinblastine. Cold decreases blood flow and can minimize the exposed area. Cold is usually applied to extravasation of antibiotics such as Adriamycin (doxorubicin) or daunomycin. Both have theoretical advantages, but cold has the additional benefit of decreasing pain associated with vesicant infiltration. Warm or cold compresses are generally applied for up to 50 minutes per hour for a 24-hour period.

Controversy surrounds the use of local antidotes such as thiosulfate, hyaluronidase, sodium bicarbonate, and hydrocortisone for chemotherapy extravasation. Topical dimethyl sulfoxide (DMSO) has proven effective in the treatment of anthracycline extravasation in some clinical trials. Any patient with an extravasation or even a suspected extravasation should receive close follow-up. Telephone follow-up 24 and 48 hours after the incident is considered good practice, with prompt medical evaluation if the area worsens. Signs and symptoms of an extravasation may first appear many hours or even days after the event. Thorough documentation of the incident and follow-up should be completed by the nurse. Any evidence of local tissue necrosis such as continued redness, pain, or ulceration requires immediate referral to a plastic surgeon with experience in the management of chemotherapy extravasations.

VENOUS ACCESS DEVICES

Many patients who are receiving chemotherapy lose their peripheral venous access with repeated treatments, or lack adequate venous access at the outset, and require alternate

Table 27–1. **VESICANT/IRRITANT CHEMOTHERAPEUTIC AGENTS**

VESICANTS	IRRITANTS
Dactinomycin	Carmustine
Daunomycin	Dacarbazine
Doxorubicin	Etoposide
Idarubicin	Streptozocin
Mechlorethamine	
Mithramycin	
Mitomycin C	
Vinblastine	
Vincristine	

Table 27–2. **MAINTENANCE OF SILASTIC RIGHT ATRIAL (HICKMAN/BROVIAC) CATHETERS**

1. Irrigate daily with 3 mL heparinized saline solution (100 units/mL)
2. Apply occlusive dressing with aseptic technique every other day
3. Change catheter cap every 7 days
4. Tape catheter to patient to prevent undue tension on catheter
5. Clamp over protective covering when clamping catheter
6. Showering and bathing permitted

routes for intravenous administration of medications, fluids, and blood products. Under these circumstances, implanted venous access devices permitting drug delivery directly into a central vein represent the best solution. Four different types of venous access devices are available: cuffed, tunneled Silastic atrial catheters; small-gauge, nontunneled central venous catheters; implanted vascular ports; and peripherally inserted central catheters.

The Silastic right atrial catheters (Hickman or Broviac) are extremely versatile, with single- and multiple-lumen models that allow rapid, reliable, and durable venous access for infusion of medications, intravenous fluids, blood products, and other supportive therapies as well as blood sampling. Hickman/Broviac catheters are particularly well suited to the needs of patients who require frequent, intensive multilumen access; i.e., patients with acute leukemia, those undergoing bone marrow transplantation, and those requiring long-term nutritional support. The ports on these catheters are external and require daily maintenance with aseptic technique. Table 27–2 lists instructions for routine care. Small-gauge nontunneled central venous catheters function primarily as temporary measures until a more durable vascular access device can be placed.

The totally implanted vascular ports are inserted surgically under local anesthesia and have a permanently attached Silastic catheter tunneled from the subcutaneous port to a central vein. Patients often prefer the ports because they are completely subcutaneous, causing little or no alteration in appearance or lifestyle and requiring no daily maintenance (unlike the Hickman/Broviac catheters). Monthly flushes with a heparin solution suffice to maintain patency. Implanted ports should be accessed with special noncoring (Huber) needles. Right-angle Huber needles with extension tubing allow greater ease in administration of medications and continuous infusions. If the patient is receiving a continuous infusion, the Huber needle can remain in place for 3 to 5 days before replacement is necessary. Intra-arterial and intraperitoneal placement of implanted ports allows for direct administration of chemotherapy via these routes. Maintenance of vascular access ports is outlined in Table 27–3.

The peripherally inserted central catheter (PICC line) is usually inserted through an antecubital vein and advanced to a central venous location; no surgery is required. The PICC lines can be inserted by trained, certified nurses. The catheter can remain in place for long periods. Blood sampling through these catheters is not recommended. The hub of the catheter is external and requires a daily heparin flush. Weekly dressing changes are recommended. The catheter can be discontinued at the completion of treatment.

All of the vascular access devices discussed above are subject to complications, particularly infection and thrombosis. Guidelines are available for management of these problems and for determining when removal of the device is necessary.

AMBULATORY INFUSION PUMPS

Venous access devices combined with ambulatory infusion pumps enable even those patients receiving prolonged infusional chemotherapy to remain outpatients during treat-

Table 27–3. **MAINTENANCE OF IMPLANTED VASCULAR ACCESS DEVICES**

1. Heparinize every 4 weeks with 5 mL heparinized saline (100 units/mL) when not in use.
2. Heparinize after each use
3. Flush with 20–30 mL saline following blood drawing
4. Showering/bathing not recommended while port is accessed
5. No restrictions on patient activities when port is not accessed

ment. These pumps are small and light, allowing patients to wear them comfortably on their belts. Pumps such as the CADD or Infumed deliver medication from an external reservoir bag. The medication bags can be changed in the home or in the oncology clinic. Narcotic analgesics can also be infused by this method, either subcutaneously or intravenously. Patient motivation and the ability to partcipate in the care of the pump are required to make this form of therapy successful. Patients and families must be instructed in the recognition and management of pump failure, needle displacement, local infection, and other complications.

SAFE HANDLING OF ANTINEOPLASTIC AGENTS

The actual health risk to professionals handling antineoplastic agents remains undefined. Since these agents have mutagenic, teratogenic, carcinogenic, and local irritant properties, precautions to minimize secondary exposure through aerosol inhalation or skin contact seem prudent. Guidelines for the preparation, administration, and disposal of antineoplastic agents have been established to minimize risk. Only properly trained personnel should prepare these agents for administration. Preparation should take place in an externally vented Class II biological safety cabinet. Personnel should wear impermeable latex gloves and protective gowns. During drug administration nurses should wear protective gowns and gloves. Careful hand washing after drug handling is mandatory. Syringes with Luer-Lok fittings should be used to prevent leakage. All items that come in contact with the antineoplastic agents during preparation and administration should be treated as hazardous waste and placed in leakproof, punctureproof containers for proper disposal.

NURSING MANAGEMENT OF ONCOLOGY PROBLEMS

Oncology nurses are routinely called upon to offer advice for various oncologic problems. Many times the nurse is the first person the patient calls with questions, concerns, or problems regarding symptom management, pain control, and psychosocial issues. Thorough training, experience, and continuing education provide the nurse with the information and judgment to deal with these issues properly.

A difficult nursing problem in cancer patients is the care and management of various skin conditions. Edema, pruritus, cutaneous metastases, and secondary infections are common. The effects of chemotherapy, radiation therapy, steroids, and malnutrition alter skin integrity and affect wound healing. Three principal factors influence wound healing: the condition of the patient, the location of the wound, and the presence of infection. A thorough nursing assessment of the patient's overall condition, nutritional status, and treatment history determines which factors may contribute to the problem. The location of the lesion should be assessed for adequate blood supply and lymphatic drainage. Nursing decisions can then be made concerning which dressings and local measures will promote optimal wound healing. If infection is present, antiseptic solutions or isotonic irrigations may be of benefit.

Cutaneous metastases from cancers of the breast, lung, head and neck, and malignant melanoma often develop into draining, necrotic lesions and present a real challenge to the oncology nurse. It is essential to cleanse these wounds thoroughly by irrigation with sterile water or normal saline and by nonsurgical debridement with wet to dry dressings. Continuously wet dressings should be avoided, since fragile skin can easily be macerated and bacterial growth enhanced.

Unpleasant odors from cutaneous tumors distress the patient and family. Innovative dressing techniques can improve the situation. Irrigation with a mild soap or acetic acid solution is the initial step. Deodorizing agents such as baking soda applied to the top layer of an occlusive dressing may help to decrease odor. Dressings with a charcoal filter are also effective but expensive and are ineffective if soiled or wet. The choice of dressing will vary from patient to patient and depends on the need for debridement, protection, and absorption. The layer of dressing in contact with the wound should be sterile and should allow drainage to pass through to the absorbent layer of the dressing. The middle layer should collect the drainage while allowing the outer layer to remain dry. Synthetic dressings (OpSite and Tegaderm) and absorption dressings (Bard Absorption Dressing, Debrisan) are available but should not be used on infected wounds.

REFERENCES

Brager BL, Yasko J: Care of the Client Receiving Chemotherapy. Reston, VA, Reston Publishing, 1984.

Cuzyell JZ: Wound care forum: Artful solutions to chronic problems. Am J Nurs 85:162–169, 1985.

Foltz AT: Nursing care of ulcerating metastatic lesions. Oncol Nurs Forum 7:8–13, 1980.

Goodman MS, Wickman R: Venous access devices: An overview. Oncol Nurs Forum 11:16–23, 1984.

Hubbard SM, Seipp CA: Administering cancer treatment: The role of the oncology nurse. Hosp Pract 20:167–174, 1985.

Johnson BL, Gross J: Handbook of Oncology Nursing. New York, John Wiley & Sons, 1985.

Masoorli S, Angeles T: PICC lines: The latest home care challenge. RN 53:44–51, 1990.

McNally JC, Stair JC, Somerville ET: Guidelines for Cancer Nursing Practice. New York, Grune & Stratton, 1985.

Oncology Nursing Society: Access Device Guidelines. Pittsburgh, Oncology Nursing Society, 1989.

Oncology Nursing Society: Cancer Chemotherapy Guidelines. Pittsburgh, Oncology Nursing Society, 1988.

Tenebaum L: Cancer Chemotherapy: A Reference Guide. Philadelphia, WB Saunders, 1989.

Thompson S: Front line antiseptics. Geriatr Nurs 10:235–236, 1989.

Yasko J: Guidelines for Cancer Care: Symptom Management. Reston, VA, Reston Publishing, 1983.

28
INFECTIONS IN THE CANCER PATIENT

H. Reid Mattison

Patients with neoplastic diseases are at increased risk of infection due to the immune suppression caused by the underlying disease and its treatment. As the cancer treatment becomes more intensive, the immunosuppression becomes more profound and prolonged. Subsequent infections are a major source of morbidity and mortality in cancer patients.

DEFECTS IN THE CANCER PATIENT'S DEFENSES

The immunologic impairment of the cancer patient is dependent upon the specific lesion in the immune system and the degree of immune suppression. Infection arises when microbial pathogens overcome local and systemic immune defenses. Table 28–1 lists factors associated with immunocompromise and infection in the cancer patient.

Granulocytopenia due to bone marrow malignancy or myelosuppressive therapy is the single most important risk factor for infection in cancer patients. The incidence and severity of infection are inversely related to the absolute granulocyte count. The rate of granulocyte decline and duration of neutropenia also correlate with the risk of infection. Impaired granulocyte function, associated with myeloproliferative disorders and corticosteroids, additionally increases the infection risk. Granulocytopenic patients most commonly develop infections caused by gram-positive and gram-negative bacteria, and in prolonged granulocytopenia, with fungi.

Impaired cell-mediated immunity occurs as a consequence of malignancy (Hodgkin's disease, some chronic and acute leukemias), immunosuppressive and cytotoxic therapy, and certain viral infections (cytomegalovirus, herpes simplex virus, human immunodeficiency virus). These defects predispose to infections with intracellular pathogens, including bacteria (*Listeria, Legionella, Salmonella*), fungi (*Candida, Cryptococcus, Aspergillus*), parasites/protozoa (*Pneumocystis, Toxoplasma, Strongyloides*), and viruses (herpes simplex, cytomegalovirus, varicella-zoster).

Defective humoral immunity results from reduced or defective antibody production, associated with multiple myeloma and acute and chronic lymphocytic leukemia, or as a consequence of immunosuppressive or cytotoxic therapy. The spleen produces antibody and clears opsonized bacteria from the blood, so asplenic patients share the infection risks of impaired humoral immunity. Patients with defective humoral immunity are particularly susceptible to pyogenic infections with encapsulated organisms (*Streptococcus pneumoniae, Haemophilus influenzae, Neisseria meningitidis, Klebsiella pneumoniae).*

Cancer patients also suffer from disruption of the natural anatomic barriers to infection. The tumor or its therapy can cause skin or mucosal erosion or mass effect, which may lead to abscess, fistula, perforation, or obstruction. Secondary infections of the lungs, kidneys, and peritoneum commonly follow obstruction. Access devices, including vascular, endotracheal, nasogastric, CNS-ventricular, and urinary catheters, reduce barrier defenses and provide an entry portal for pathogenic organisms. Prolonged immunosuppression and treatment with broad-spectrum antibiotics may eliminate naturally protective endogenous bacteria and promote colonization with highly resistant pathogens. Reactivation of latent infections (tuberculosis, *Toxoplasma,* herpes simplex, varicella-zoster, *Strongyloides*) is another potential consequence of the immune suppression produced by the cancer and its treatment.

CLINICAL APPROACH TO THE CANCER PATIENT WITH AN INFECTION

Initial evaluation of the patient with cancer and suspected infection involves a careful history and meticulous physical examination. It is important to define the type and extent of the cancer as well as the past and current treatments. Noninfectious causes such as

Table 28–1. **IMMUNE DEFECTS, CAUSES, AND ASSOCIATED INFECTIONS IN CANCER PATIENTS**

IMMUNE DEFECT	CAUSES	INFECTIONS
Granulocyte-related 1. Granulocytopenia 2. Impaired granulocyte function	Acute leukemia Myelosuppression Cytotoxic therapy Radiation Therapy Myeloproliferative disorders AML, CML Myeloid metaplasia Immunosuppressive agents Corticosteroids	Bacteria *Pseudomonas* *Klebsiella* *E. coli* *S. aureus* *S. epidermidis* *S. viridans* *Enterococcus* Fungi *Candida* *Aspergillus*
Cellular immune system	Malignancy Hodgkin's disease ALL, AML CLL Hairy cell leukemia Immunosuppressives Corticosteroids Cyclosporine Cytotoxic therapy HIV or CMV infection	Bacteria *Listeria* *Legionella* *Nocardia* *Mycobacterium* *Brucella* *Salmonella* Fungi *Cryptococcus* *Candida* *Aspergillus* *Histoplasma* *Coccidiodes* Viruses CMV Herpes simplex Varicella-zoster Parasites *Pneumocystis* *Toxoplasma gondii*
Humoral immune system	Malignancy Multiple myeloma CLL, ALL Hodgkin's disease Immunosuppressives Corticosteroids Splenectomy	Bacteria *Pneumococcus* *Haemophilus influenzae* *Neisseria meningitidis* *Klebsiella* Virus Echovirus Parasites Malaria *Giardia*

Abbreviations: HIV: Human immunodeficiency virus; ALL: acute lymphocytic leukemia; CMV: cytomegalovirus; AML: acute myelocytic leukemia; CLL: chronic lymphocytic leukemia.

"tumor fever" and reactions to antibiotics, chemotherapy drugs, and transfusions should be part of the differential diagnosis. The physical examination must be especially thorough because the usual signs of inflammation or infection may be absent or subtle in the granulocytopenic patient. The oral mucosa, venous access sites, lungs, abdomen, and perirectal area require particular attention because of the frequency of infections in these areas.

Laboratory tests indicated for the immunocompromised patient with suspected infection depend on the history and physical assessment. However, all patients require blood counts with differentials; blood, urine, sputum, and possibly wound Gram stains and cultures; serum chemistries; and chest x-rays. If central venous access devices are present, it is important to obtain and label central and peripheral blood cultures. Communication with the microbiology laboratory facilitates the evaluation; the laboratory can provide special cultures and closer attention to organisms that might otherwise be considered unimportant contaminants.

FEVER AND NEUTROPENIA

Fever in the granulocytopenic patient usually indicates infection, which may be difficult to detect yet rapidly progressive. The risk of infection significantly increases when the granulocyte count is below 500/mm^3 and even more dramatically when it is under 100/mm^3. The rate of decline of the granulocyte count and the duration of granulocytopenia also significantly contribute to the infection risk. The arbitrary but accepted definition of a significant fever is one measurement above 38.3°C or two measurements above 38°C in association with a granulocyte count below 1000/mm^3.

ETIOLOGY

In febrile neutropenic patients the etiology of the fever is infection in 60 to 75% of cases reported in the literature. The most common sources of infection are the respiratory, genitourinary, and alimentary tracts, particularly if they are already injured by either cancer or cancer therapy. The most common infecting organisms are gram-negative bacilli (*Escherichia coli, Klebsiella, Pseudomonas*), gram-positive cocci (*Staphylococcus aureus*, coagulase-negative *Staphylococcus, Streptococcus*), and fungi (*Candida, Aspergillus*). The most frequent organisms involved vary regionally and from hospital to hospital.

DIAGNOSIS

Fever is usually the first and often the only sign of infection in the neutropenic patient. However, it is important to heed all potential signs and symptoms of infection. Clinical consideration needs to include the possibilities of sinusitis, gingivitis, pharyngitis, esophagitis, meningitis, pneumonia, cellulitis, vascular access device infection, colitis, cystitis, pyelonephritis, and perirectal infection. Complete cultures of all suspicious sites determine the cause of infection in only 30 to 50% of febrile neutropenic patients. Less than half of bacteremic neutropenic patients display any specific physical findings. In one study of neutropenia only 8% of patients with pneumonia had purulent sputum; only 11% with urinary tract infections had pyuria, and 38% with gram-negative pneumonia had initially normal chest x-rays.

THERAPY

Fever in the neutropenic patient is due to infection unless proven otherwise and warrants prompt initiation of empiric antibiotic therapy. The precipitous mortality of gram-negative bacteremia in the neutropenic patient underlies the urgency for empiric therapy. In one study of neutropenic patients with pseudomonal sepsis who did not receive immediate empiric therapy, the mortality was 15% at 12 hours, 57% at 24 hours, and 70% at 48 hours. Patients treated with appropriate empiric antibiotics had a 74% recovery rate.

The optimal empiric antibiotic regimen remains controversial. Because of varying bacterial flora and patterns of antibiotic resistance, each hospital should determine its own preferred regimens based on microbial prevalence and sensitivity. The selected antibiotics should be intravenous, broad-spectrum, bactericidal, synergistic, and administered at maximal doses. Cost, toxicity, and ease of administration are also important considerations. Most centers use a combination of an aminoglycoside (gentamicin, tobramycin, or amikacin) and an antipseudomonal beta-lactam (piperacillin, mezlocillin, azlocillin, or cefotaxime, ceftazidime, cefoperazone). No particular combination is superior (Table 28–2).

Initial use of single-agent, extended-spectrum antibiotic therapy for empiric management of the febrile neutropenic patient remains investigational. Studies with ceftazidime and moxalactam indicate reasonable efficacy and feasibility in small numbers of selected patients who required compulsive observation and immediate modification in antibiotic therapy for any clinical deterioration. Concern exists that gram-positive organisms may be inadequately covered by monotherapy and that resistance (especially of *Pseudomonas*) may develop, so standard therapy remains a two-drug combination. Single-agent antibiotic therapy is an option for the closely monitored patient with preexisting renal disease or concomitant nephrotoxic treatments (cisplatin or amphotericin) with granulocyte counts less than 100/mm^3 and expected recovery from granulocytopenia within 1 week.

Table 28–2. **ANTIBIOTIC MANAGEMENT OF THE FEBRILE NEUTROPENIC PATIENT**

INITIAL TREATMENT			
Aminoglycoside plus beta-lactam antipseudomonal penicillin or *plus* third-generation cephalosporin	*Two* beta-lactam antibiotics (antipseudomonal penicillin *and* third-generation cephalosporin)	Monotherapy with ceftazidime, moxalactam, or imipenem	Any of the other empiric regimens *plus* vancomycin
REEVALUATE TREATMENT (after 48–72 hr)			
Afebrile Neutropenic	**Afebrile Neutrophils >500**	**Febrile Neutropenic**	**Febrile Neutrophils >500**
1. If clinically well, stop antibiotic regimen after 7 afebrile days 2. If not clinically well, continue antibiotic regimen until recovery	1. Without infection, stop antibiotic regimen when neutrophils >500 2. With infection, stop antibiotic regimen when appropriate for treatment	1. If clinically well, continue original antibiotic regimen, add amphotericin B for fever >7 days 2. If patient deteriorates, add vancomycin, or if already receiving vancomycin switch to monotherapy at day 4 or 5 and add amphotericin B at day 7	Stop antibiotic regimen after 4 or 5 days of neutrophils >500 and search for cause of fever

Modified from Hughes WT, Armstrong D, Bodey GP, et al: Guidelines for the use of antimicrobial agents in neutropenic patients with unexplained fever. J Infect Dis 161:381–396, 1990.

With the increase in vascular access devices and related infections, some centers use vancomycin as part of their initial empiric regimen. Some recent studies indicate that initial vancomycin reduces the morbidity of gram-positive infections and the use of empiric amphotericin. Other studies show no improvement in morbidity or mortality. While empiric vancomycin remains controversial, patients presenting with signs or symptoms of vascular access device infection may benefit.

TREATMENT COURSE

The clinical course and duration of neutropenia determine the course of antibiotic therapy. Patients with solid tumors with expected resolution of granulocytopenia within a week usually receive their empiric regimen for the duration of the neutropenia. Provided that all cultures and lab tests were normal, the antibiotics stop when the granulocyte count is above 500/mm^3, and the patients are discharged if they remain afebrile for 24 hours. Patients with clinical evidence of infection receive a course of antibiotics appropriate for the etiologic organism and type of infection.

Patients with prolonged neutropenia who defervesce and appear clinically well without identifiable infection receive treatment for 7 days with the initial empiric regimen. In 40% of these patients fever will recur. Thus, after discontinuation of antibiotics in a neutropenic patient, close observation and rapid reinstitution of antibiotics for fever are mandatory. Patients with prolonged neutropenia who defervesce but are *not* clinically well with persisting mucositis, granulocytes less than 100/mm^3, or unstable vital signs should remain on their empiric regimen until clinical or granulocyte recovery.

Persistence of fever despite empiric antibiotic therapy raises concern about drug resistance, subtherapeutic antibiotic concentrations, abscess, fungal infection, and nonbacterial and noninfectious causes such as tumor or drug fever. If fever and neutropenia persist after 4 to 7 days and reassessment for infection is unrevealing, the empiric regimen changes with the addition of vancomycin and/or amphotericin B.

Granulocyte transfusions remain a controversial modality for febrile neutropenic patients with persisting fever and documented infection who do not respond to appropriate antibiotic therapy. No controlled data indicate improvement in short- or long-term survival for the persistingly febrile neutropenic patient treated with granulocyte transfusions.

Additional factors discouraging their use include high cost, pulmonary toxicity, and alloimmunization.

PNEUMONIA

PATHOGENESIS

Pneumonia is the most common form of serious infection in the cancer patient. The etiologic agents vary depending on the type of cancer and treatment, the associated immune defects, and whether the infection is acquired at home or in the hospital.

Patients with humoral immune defects from multiple myeloma and hypoglobulinemia are more susceptible to pneumonia caused by encapsulated bacteria such as *Streptococcus pneumoniae* and *Haemophilus influenzae*. Patients with the cellular immune defects of Hodgkin's disease are predisposed to infections with intracellular pathogens, including bacteria (*Listeria, Nocardia, Mycobacterium*), fungi (*Candida, Cryptococcus, Aspergillus*), viruses (cytomegalovirus, herpes simplex, varicella-zoster), and parasites (*Pneumocystis carinii, Toxoplasma, Strongyloides*). Splenectomized Hodgkin's disease patients are also at risk for pneumonia due to *S. pneumoniae, H. influenzae, E. coli, Staphylococcus aureus,* and *Neisseria meningitidis*.

The etiologic agents for community-acquired pneumonias include the common respiratory pathogens (*S. pneumoniae, H. influenzae*, influenza virus), ubiquitous opportunistic agents (*Legionella, Nocardia*, cytomegalovirus, *Cryptococcus*), and reactivated latent pathogens (tuberculosis, herpes simplex virus, *Pneumocystis*). Hospital-acquired infections differ because the hospital endogenous flora has variable and decreased antibiotic sensitivity. They commonly include gram-negative bacilli, *Staphylococcus aureus*, and fungi (*Candida, Aspergillus*). Recently, *Legionella* has become a more common opportunistic hospital pathogen. Infections of mixed etiology occur up to 20% of the time, and prolonged antibiotic therapy in granulocytopenic patients predisposes to secondary fungal pneumonias. Table 28–3 gives a differential diagnosis of pneumonia in the cancer patient according to the type of infiltrate and the granulocyte count.

DIAGNOSIS

The diagnosis of pneumonia is easily made when fever, leukocytosis, and pulmonary infiltrates are present. However, in neutropenic patients hypothermia may substitute for fever, and the white count is depressed. With neutropenia the chest x-ray may be normal and sputum absent. The only clinical clues may be dry cough, pleuritic pain, or tachypnea. Serial examinations and x-rays may be necessary to establish the diagnosis of pneumonia.

Noninfectious causes need to be part of the differential diagnosis of pulmonary infiltrates in the cancer patient. Cancer progression, radiation and chemotherapy-induced pneumonitis, aspiration, hemorrhage, pulmonary edema, and pulmonary emboli can closely resemble infectious pneumonia.

Extrapulmonary findings may focus attention on potential pathogens. Skin lesions such as ecthyma gangrenosum suggest *Pseudomonas*, whereas *S. aureus* can cause abscesses and pneumonia. Mycobacteria and fungi may also cause concomitant skin lesions and pneumonia. Coexistent pulmonary and central nervous system infections suggest involvement by bacteria (gram-negative bacilli, *S. aureus, Nocardia*), fungi (*Aspergillus, Cryptococcus*), and mycobacteria. Pulmonary infiltrates associated with diarrhea suggest the possibility of infections by *Legionella*, herpes simplex virus, cytomegalovirus, and *Strongyloides*.

The pace of the onset of the pneumonia may be helpful. A pneumonia rapidly evolving over 24 hours is probably of bacterial origin. Cavitary pneumonia can occur with infection by common bacteria, Mycobacterium tuberculosis, *Nocardia*, fungi (*Aspergillus, Cryptococcus*), and rarely *Legionella*. Active tuberculosis occurs in 1% of cancer patients.

CULTURES

Sputum assessment includes Gram stain and culture for bacteria, potassium hydroxide evaluation and culture for fungi, and acid-fast stain and culture for mycobacteria. Additionally, direct fluorescent antibody (DFA) testing and culture for *Legionella*, modified

Table 28–3. **DIFFERENTIAL DIAGNOSIS OF PNEUMONIA IN CANCER PATIENTS**

LOCALIZED INFILTRATE	DIFFUSE INFILTRATE
Nonneutropenic Patients Bacteria: *Pneumococcus, Haemophilus, Mycobacterium* Fungi: *Cryptococcus, Histoplasma, Coccidiodes* Virus: RSV*, adenovirus Underlying tumor Drugs: Busulfan, bleomycin, cyclophosphamide, methotrexate, cytosine arabinoside Radiation	**Nonneutropenic patients** Parasites: *Pneumocystis, Toxoplasma, Strongyloides* Bacteria: *Mycobacterium, Nocardia, Legionella, Chlamydia* *Mycoplasma* Virus: Herpes simplex, varicella-zoster, cytomegalovirus, measles, influenza, adenovirus Fungi: *Aspergillus, Candida,* Zygomycetes, *Cryptococcus* Radiation Drugs
Neutropenic Patients Bacteria: Any gram-positive or gram-negative, *Mycobacterium, Nocardia* Fungi: *Aspergillus,* Zygomycetes, *Candida, Cryptococcus, Histoplasma* Virus: Herpes simplex, varicella-zoster Drugs Radiation	**Neutropenic Patients** Bacteria: Any gram-positive or gram-negative, *Mycobacterium, Nocardia, Legionella, Chlamydia, Mycoplasma* Fungi: *Candida, Aspergillus,* Zygomycetes, *Cryptococcus, Histoplasma* Parasites: *Pneumocystis, Toxoplasma, Strongyloides* Virus: Herpes simplex, varicella-zoster, cytomegalovirus, measles, influenza, adenovirus, RSV* Radiation Drugs

From Pizzo PA, Meyers J: Infections in the Cancer Patient. In DeVita VT, Hellman S, Rosenberg SA (eds): Cancer: Principles and Practice of Oncology. Philadelphia, JB Lippincott, 1989.
*RSV: respiratory syncitial virus.

acid-fast stain for *Nocardia,* silver stain for *Pneumocystis,* and cultures for viruses and *Chlamydia* may be appropriate in certain cases. The results of sputum evaluations may be misleading because of the possibility of colonization of the upper respiratory tract by many of the potential pathogenic organisms. *Legionella, Mycobacterium* tuberculosis, and dimorphic fungi (*Histoplasma capsulatum, Coccidiodes immitis*) are pathogenic when isolated from the sputum.

In selected patients with localizing abnormalities, cultures of pleural fluid, urine, bone marrow, skin lesions, cerebrospinal fluid, and stool can provide the etiologic agent for the pneumonia.

TREATMENT

Figure 28–1 outlines an approach to the cancer patient with a pulmonary infiltrate. Localized pulmonary infiltrates are usually bacterial infections, and appropriate treatment is broad-spectrum antibiotics with reassessment for response at 48 to 72 hours. A lack of response or clinical deterioration leads to consideration of bronchoscopy with endobronchial lavage and biopsy or open lung biopsy. Diffuse interstitial pneumonias indicate that an "atypical" pneumonia may be present, caused by *Legionella, Cytomegalovirus, Chlamydia,* or *Pneumocystis.* Accordingly, the empiric treatment is trimethoprim-sulfamethoxazole and erythromycin (with or without additional broad-spectrum antibiotics). Lack of response to 72 to 96 hours of this treatment suggests the need for bronchoscopy or open lung biopsy to look for fungal, viral, or noninfectious etiologies, depending on the patient's condition and prognosis. Multiple, coexistent pathogens and secondary superinfections may complicate diagnosis and treatment.

GASTROINTESTINAL TRACT INFECTIONS

The alimentary tract is a reservoir of microorganisms that also serves as an entry portal for local and systemic infections in the immunocompromised host.

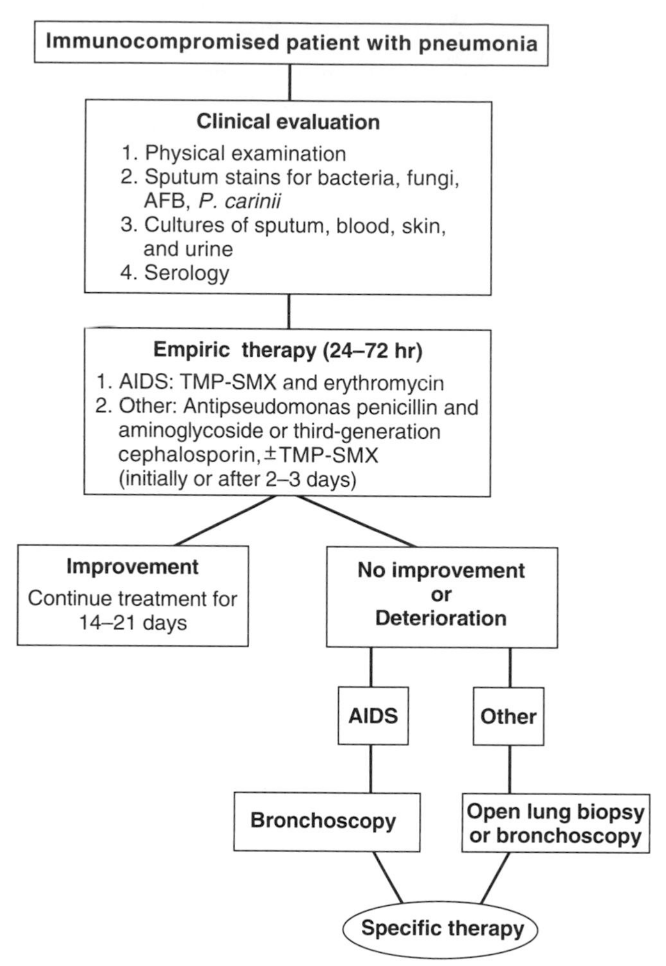

Figure 28–1. Clinical approach to the immunocompromised patient with pneumonia. (*Adapted from* Wilson WR, Cockerill FR III, Rosenow EC III: Pulmonary disease in the immunocompromised host. Mayo Clin Proc 60:610–631, 1985.)

OROPHARYNGEAL INFECTION

The oropharyngeal cavity is populated by large numbers of aerobic and anaerobic bacteria. Oropharyngeal infection is frequently a first sign of acute leukemia. Pharyngitis may be caused by bacteria, fungi, viruses, or treatment. Oropharyngeal mucositis commonly complicates chemotherapy and local radiation therapy, predisposing to local infection and allowing systemic entry to pathogens. Patients derive symptomatic improvement with diphenhydramine, nystatin, or Maalox and viscous lidocaine mouthwashes. Oral candidiasis (thrush) is a common, painful infection in the neutropenic patient. Although it is usually superficial, it may allow *Candida* systemic entry. Oral candidiasis usually responds to nystatin, clotrimazole, ketoconazole, or fluconazole. Resistant or life-threatening infections may require amphotericin B.

Reactivation infection with oral herpes simplex virus is common. Lesions may present with an atypical appearance and may be indistinguishable from other causes of oral ulceration. Viral culture or immunofluorescence may be necessary for diagnosis. Oral or intravenous acyclovir is effective treatment.

ESOPHAGITIS

Esophagitis is common in cancer patients and may have infectious (bacterial, fungal, viral) or noninfectious (radiation, chemotherapy, emesis, reflux) origins. Infectious esophagitis occurs most commonly in the granulocytopenic or AIDS patient. Symptomatic (retrosternal pain, odynophagia), radiographic (barium swallow), and endoscopic findings are not distinctive. Diagnosis requires biopsy, culture, and histologic examination. *Candida* is the most common cause of infectious esophagitis in neutropenic patients, followed by herpes simplex virus and gram-negative bacilli. Thrombocytopenia frequently contraindicates endoscopy with biopsy, so it is reasonable to initiate an empiric trial with antifungal therapy. Failure to respond to antifungal therapy in 48 to 96 hours leads to reconsideration of endoscopy and biopsy versus an empiric trial of acyclovir.

INTRA-ABDOMINAL INFECTIONS

Cancer patients can develop all the common intra-abdominal infections but the clinical presentation may be subtle or unusual because of the cancer and its treatment. Granulocytopenia and corticosteroids may greatly diminish the signs and symptoms associated with intra-abdominal infection and inflammation. Infectious enteritis in the compromised host may be a manifestation of bacterial, viral, fungal, or parasitic disease. Necrotizing enterocolitis (typhlitis) is an inflammation of the cecum caused by gram-negative bacilli and anaerobes, which occurs occasionally in patients with prolonged granulocytopenia receiving broad-spectrum antibiotics. Presenting with subacute or acute right lower quadrant pain, it may be accompanied by fever, diarrhea, and prostration, and it is treated supportively and with antibiotics, though surgery may be required.

Antibiotics and some forms of chemotherapy (5-fluorouracil and leucovorin) may result in colitis due to *Clostridium difficile* toxin. Diarrhea, abdominal pain, fever, and leukocytosis (occasionally as high as 50,000/mm^3) are the presenting symptoms; most patients demonstrate fecal leukocytes. Treatment is supportive hydration and either metronidazole or oral vancomycin.

Hepatitis is more common in the immunocompromised patient and may be a primary infection or secondary to a disseminated infection. Frequent transfusions lead to the increased incidence of hepatitis B and C. Disseminated infections involving the liver include bacterial, fungal (*Candida*), viral (cytomegalovirus, herpes simplex virus, Epstein-Barr virus, coxsackievirus, adenovirus), and parasitic (*Toxoplasma*) diseases.

In the granulocytopenic leukemic patient, perirectal cellulitis is a common and painful infection, which may lead to bacteremia. Actual abscess formation is less common. Predisposing factors to perirectal cellulitis include rectal mucositis from treatment, hemorrhoids, anal fissures, and manipulation (rectal examinations, sigmoidoscopy). Bowel anaerobes (*Bacteroides*), aerobic gram-negative bacilli (*Pseudomonas, Klebsiella, E. coli*), and group D streptococci are frequently causative organisms. Intervention includes antibiotics and surgical incision and debridement as necessary. Herpes simplex virus may also cause perirectal cellulitis indistinguishable from bacterial infection. Viral cultures will disclose herpes simplex infection, which is treatable with acyclovir.

CATHETER-RELATED INFECTION

Infections related to indwelling venous access devices (IVADs) such as Hickmans, Broviacs, and Port-a-caths are increasing in incidence. The infectious complications of these devices include exit-site infections, blood stream infections, tunnel infections, and septic thrombophlebitis. The manifestations may be local tenderness, erythema, increased warmth, line occlusion, and purulent drainage. Gram-positive cocci, predominantly *Staphylococcus epidermidis* and *Staphylococcus aureus*, account for most catheter-associated infections. Other causative organisms include gram-negative bacilli, corynebacteria, and *Candida*.

Quantitative blood cultures from all catheter lumens and the peripheral blood are important to diagnose catheter-related infection. The IVAD lumen pathogen colony counts are usually significantly higher than peripheral site counts in catheter-associated infections. Antibiotic treatment is usually successful for bacteremia and exit-site infections without removal of the device. Tunnel infections and catheter-associated septic thrombophlebitis are less responsive to antibiotic treatment and usually require catheter removal. Some experts feel that catheters infected with *Candida, Corynebacterium* JK, and *Bacillus* sp. require removal. If other catheter-related infections do not respond to 48 hours of antibiotic treatment, catheter removal may be necessary.

CENTRAL NERVOUS SYSTEM INFECTION

Central nervous system (CNS) infections (meningitis, encephalitis, and brain abscess) occur relatively infrequently in cancer patients, representing less than 1% of admissions to large cancer centers. Meningitis occurs most frequently with cell-mediated immune defects and is frequently caused by *Cryptococcus neoformans* and *Listeria monocytogenes.* The course is often atypically indolent. Splenectomized patients have an increased risk of meningitis due to encapsulated organisms *(Streptococcus pneumoniae, Neisseria meningitidis).* Caused by the age-appropriate bacteria, meningitis in the granulocytopenic patient may be very subtle at presentation even when due to organisms usually associated with a fulminant course.

Encephalitis, a diffuse parenchymal invasion of the brain, is most commonly due to viral (herpes simplex, varicella-zoster, measles virus) or *Toxoplasma gondii* infection. Definitive diagnosis requires brain biopsy; however, many opt for a therapeutic trial of acyclovir first.

The differential diagnosis of a focal mass lesion in the brain of a cancer patient focuses primarily on metastasis versus abscess. Most brain abscesses have an identifiable cause in either a contiguous (otitis media, sinusitis, dental) or distant (pulmonary) infection. Causes of brain abscesses in the cancer patient include expected aerobic and anaerobic bacteria, plus *Nocardia* and fungi (*Aspergillus, Cryptococcus, Candida, Mucor*). Pulmonary infection leading to brain abscess suggests possible infection with *Nocardia, Aspergillus, Mucor, Cryptococcus*, or *Candida.*

REFERENCES

Anaissie EJ, Fainstein V, Bodey GP, et al: Randomized trial of beta-lactam regimens in febrile neutropenic cancer patients. Am J Med 84:581–589, 1988.

Armstrong D: Problems in management of opportunistic fungal diseases. Rev Infect Dis 11(Suppl 7):S1591–S1599, 1989.

Bodey GP: Evolution of antibiotic therapy for infection in neutropenic patients: Studies at MD Anderson Hospital. Rev Infect Dis 11 (Suppl 7):S1582–S1590, 1989.

Bodey GP, Fainstein V, Elting LS, et al: Beta-lactam regimens for the febrile neutropenic patient. Cancer 65:9–16, 1990.

The EORTC International Antimicrobial Therapy Cooperative Group: Ceftazidime combined with a short or long course of amikacin for empirical therapy of gram-negative bacteremia in cancer patients with granulocytopenia. N Engl J Med 317:1692–1698, 1987.

Hughes WT, Armstrong D, Bodey GP, et al: Guidelines for the use of antimicrobial agents in neutropenic patients with unexplained fever. J Infect Dis 161:381–396, 1990.

Karp JE, Dick JD, Angelopulos C, et al: Empiric use of vancomycin during prolonged treatment-induced granulocytopenia. Am J Med 81:237–242, 1986.

Maurier F: Fluconazole treatment of fungal infections in the immunocompromised host. Semin Oncol 17 (3 Suppl 6):19–23, 1990.

Pizzo PA: Considerations for the prevention of infectious complications in patients with cancer. Rev Infect Dis 11(Suppl 7):S1551–S1563, 1989.

Pizzo PA, Hathorn JW, Hiemenz J, et al: A randomized trial comparing ceftazidime alone with combination antibiotic therapy in cancer patients with fever and neutropenia. N Engl J Med 315:552–558, 1986.

29
AIDS-ASSOCIATED MALIGNANCIES

Deepak Sahasrabudhe

Certain cancers occur more frequently in primary immunodeficiency disorders and with iatrogenic immunosuppression. The same spectrum of malignancies develops in patients with the acquired immunodeficiency syndrome (AIDS). These include Kaposi's sarcoma, non-Hodgkin's lymphomas, Hodgkin's disease, cancers of the anogenital region, and squamous cell carcinomas of the head and neck. There are also case reports of virtually all histologic types of cancers in patients with AIDS. AIDS-associated malignancies are usually disseminated at presentation, aggressive in their clinical course, and refractory to treatment. Treatment of AIDS-associated cancer is evolving, and minimizing toxicity is critical. Therefore, if possible, patients with AIDS-associated malignancies should be referred to an AIDS Clinical Trials Group (ACTG) center for follow-up and treatment.

NON-HODGKIN'S LYMPHOMA

EPIDEMIOLOGY

Soon after the description of AIDS, the significantly increased incidence of Burkitt's lymphoma in the same populations-at-risk resulted in a revision of the AIDS diagnostic criteria to include intermediate- and high-grade non-Hodgkin's lymphoma (NHL). The age-adjusted incidence of NHL in never-married males increased from 12.3 to 31.8 per 100,000 from 1980 to 1984 in New York City, and in San Francisco the incidence of NHL increased fivefold compared to the pre-AIDS epidemic rates. NHL occurs in 4 to 10% of AIDS patients, and unlike Kaposi's sarcoma, all subgroups of patients with AIDS are at risk.

In human immunodeficiency virus (HIV)–infected patients treated with zidovudine-containing regimens,14.5% developed high-grade B-cell NHL after a median follow-up of 23.8 months. The estimated probability of developing NHL was 28.6% by 30 months and 46.4% by 36 months. The degree of immunosuppression, predicted by the number of CD4+ (T-helper) cells in the peripheral blood, correlated with early development of NHL. With an estimated 1 to 1.2 million people infected with the AIDS virus in the United States, the number of cases of AIDS-associated NHL is expected to increase greatly. By 1992, 8 to 27% of all NHL in the United States will result from HIV infection.

PATHOGENESIS

Surface marker and immunoglobulin gene rearrangement studies reveal that AIDS-associated lymphadenopathy and AIDS-associated NHL contain oligoclonal B cells. Epstein-Barr virus (EBV) has been found in some AIDS-associated NHL; EBV infection and other similar infections may predispose patients to the development of NHL by causing a polyclonal B-cell proliferation. After another infection or genetic event causes c-*myc* oncogene rearrangement (similar to that in endemic Burkitt's lymphoma), a true malignant B-cell lymphoma may arise.

PATHOLOGY

Virtually all AIDS-associated NHL are B-cell lymphomas. The majority are either high-grade immunoblastic lymphomas, small noncleaved cell lymphomas, or intermediate-grade large cell lymphomas. Occasional case reports exist of AIDS-related T-cell lymphoma, indolent lymphoma, and chronic lymphocytic leukemia.

CLINICAL FEATURES

Extranodal involvement of nearly any organ occurs in 87% of AIDS-associated NHL at diagnosis. The most common sites of extranodal involvement are the gastrointestinal tract,

22%; central nervous system, 17%; bone marrow, 17%; and liver, 12%. Most patients present with advanced-stage disease. The distribution according to stage in one study was stage I, 6%; stage IE, 17%; stage II, 7%; stage III, 9%; and stage IV, 42%.

The symptoms of NHL depend on the site of involvement. Lymphomatous "B symptoms" are difficult to distinguish from symptoms of the underlying HIV infection. Gastrointestinal lesions may be asymptomatic or cause pain and bleeding. Liver involvement may cause abnormal liver function studies, pain, or signs of biliary obstruction. Central nervous system (CNS) lymphomas present with memory loss, lethargy, mental status changes, hemiparesis, seizures, cranial nerve palsies, and headaches. Computed tomography (CT) or magnetic resonance imaging (MRI) brain scanning reveals single or multiple enhancing lesions. To differentiate CNS lymphoma from toxoplasmosis, toxoplasma serology may be helpful; biopsy is usually required.

Prognostic factors including performance status (Karnofsky score of >70), absence of a prior diagnosis of AIDS, CD4+ lymphocyte count of >100/mm^3, absence of extranodal involvement, polyclonality, and morphologic subtype (low-grade, intermediate-grade large cell, small noncleaved cell) correlate with longer median survival. Progressive NHL is the cause of death in 37 to 50% of patients, underscoring the potential importance of antineoplastic treatment.

TREATMENT

Increased susceptibility to opportunistic infections and excess hematologic toxicity complicate systemic chemotherapy of NHL. Using standard combination chemotherapy regimens, the complete response rate is only 33 to 50%. The median survival is 5 to 6 months. Dose-intensive chemotherapy regimens result in a formidably high incidence of opportunistic infections. Recently, the ACTG completed a study of low-dose m-BACOD chemotherapy (Chap. 10), achieving a complete response rate of 46% with reduced hematologic toxicity. The ACTG current randomized trial compares low-dose versus standard dose m-BACOD with recombinant human granulocyte-macrophage colony-stimulating factor (rGM-CSF). Prophylaxis for meningeal lymphoma and for *Pneumocystis carinii* pneumonia is included, and all patients receive antiretroviral therapy.

CNS lymphomas are often diagnosed postmortem. Ninety percent are high grade. While the response rate to cranial irradiation approaches 70%, the prognosis is poor. Median survival is only 2 to 5 months. Decisions about diagnostic brain biopsy and treatment should be individualized.

REFERENCES

DeVita VT, Hellman S, Rosenberg SA (eds): AIDS. Philadelphia, JB Lippincott, 1988.

Formenti SC, Gill PS, Lean E, et al: Primary central nervous system lymphoma in AIDS. Results of radiation therapy. Cancer 63:1101–1107, 1989.

Gail MH, Pluda JM, Rabkin CS, et al: Projections of the incidence of non-Hodgkin's lymphoma related to acquired immunodeficiency syndrome. J Natl Cancer Inst 83:695–701, 1991.

Pluda JM, Yarchoan R, Jaffe ES, et al: Development of non-Hodgkin's lymphoma in a cohort of patients with severe human immunodeficiency virus (HIV) infection on long-term antiretroviral therapy. Ann Intern Med 113:276–282, 1990.

Raphael BG, Knowles DM: Acquired immunodeficiency syndrome-associated non-Hodgkin's lymphoma. Semin Oncol 17:361–366, 1990.

KAPOSI'S SARCOMA

AIDS-associated Kaposi's sarcoma (KS) is distinct from the classic and the endemic forms of this disease. Classic KS is rare, occurring predominantly in older men of Mediterranean heritage and involving the skin of the lower extremities. The indolent course of classic KS lasts 10 to 15 years. Thirty-seven percent of patients with classic KS develop NHL. Endemic KS occurs in central Africa. The patients are males 25 to 40 years old. Endemic KS causes diffuse nodular lesions. The course is indolent with survivals of 5 to 8 years. Another form of KS occurs in iatrogenically immunosuppressed renal transplant recipients. The distribution of lesions and clinical course is variable. Lesions may regress after discontinuation of immunosuppresssion. Epidemic KS occurs in HIV-infected patients. There is involvement of the skin, lymph nodes, and viscera. The course is fulminant with death due to complications of the underlying immunodeficiency or the KS by 2 years.

INCIDENCE

The risk of developing KS increases 100-fold in patients with AIDS. KS is eight times more common in homosexual and bisexual men than in other groups with AIDS. The actual cause for this predominance in homosexuals is unknown, but proposed predisposing cofactors include cytomegalovirus (CMV) infection, inhaled nitrites, and receptive anal intercourse. The incidence of epidemic KS in AIDS patients declined in the New York City area from 43% in 1983 to 26% in 1986, and to 19% in 1989. Possibly, altered sexual practices and/or underreporting of cases contributed to this decline.

PATHOGENESIS

KS originates from lymphatic or vascular endothelial cells. HIV-derived DNA is not found in KS lesions, ruling out a direct role for HIV in the pathogenesis. KS cells in cell culture secrete both autocrine and paracrine growth factors that stimulate angiogenesis in mice. Theoretically, KS is a multiclonal neoplastic proliferation of abnormal blood vessels, resulting from secretion of angiogenic growth factors due to the HIV infection rather than a true monoclonal malignancy. This theory is supported clinically by the course of AIDS-associated KS, which parallels the course of the HIV infection.

PATHOLOGY

The histologic appearance of the different forms of KS is similar. Early KS lesions demonstrate proliferation of vessels in the reticular dermis. There is perivascular infiltration of lymphocytes, plasma cells, neutrophils, and macrophages. Nodular lesions exhibit palisading pleomorphic spindle-shaped cells. Extravasation of red blood cells into slitlike spaces between spindle-shaped cells is characteristic.

CLINICAL MANIFESTATIONS

While any organ can be involved by KS, common sites are the skin, lymph nodes, gastrointestinal (GI) tract, oral mucosa, conjunctivae, and lungs. Skin lesions are usually the first manifestation, and their distribution can be widespread. Beginning as pink to purple patches, they rapidly progress to plaques and nodules that will often coalesce. Initially, the lesions are asymptomatic. Pain, disfiguration, and lymphedema occur with progression. The incidence of lymph node involvement is difficult to ascertain owing to concomitant AIDS-related adenopathy.

In patients with cutaneous KS, 33% have involvement of the oral mucosa and 50% have involvement of the GI tract. The GI tract may be extensively involved despite minimal skin disease. Symptoms include abdominal pain and occult or overt symptomatic blood loss. Endoscopy is preferred to diagnose GI KS and any coexisting infections. Contrast radiographic studies result in a high incidence of false negatives. Pulmonary KS causes cough and dyspnea. Chest x-rays show bilateral infiltrates, nodules, and mediastinal and hilar lymphadenopathy. Pleural effusions are uncommon. Bronchoscopy for visualization of characteristic lesions and for culture and silver staining is helpful in differentiating between KS and *Pneumocystis carinii* pneumonia. Open lung biopsies are sometimes required. The median survival of patients with pulmonary KS is 3 months.

TREATMENT

The purpose of treatment is palliation. Therefore, treatment choices depend on the extent of disease, symptoms, the immunologic status of the patient, and other AIDS-related problems. The AIDS-KS staging system (Table 29–1) divides patients into good-risk and poor-risk categories and is useful in the selection of treatment.

Local treatments for symptomatic cutaneous KS include radiation, intralesional che-

Table 29–1. **STAGING OF AIDS-ASSOCIATED KAPOSI'S SARCOMA**

	GOOD RISK (All of the Following)	POOR RISK (Any of the Following)
Tumor	Confined to skin and/or lymph nodes and/or minimal oral disease*	Tumor-associated edema or ulceration Extensive oral KS Gastrointestinal KS Other visceral KS
Immune system	CD4+ cells ≥200	CD4+ cells <200
Systemic illness	No history of opportunistic infections or thrush No "B" symptoms† Performance status ≥70 (Karnofsky)	History of opportunistic infections or thrush "B" symptoms Performance status <70 Other HIV-related illness (lymphoma, neurologic disease)

From Krown SE, Metroka C, Wernz JC: Kaposi's sarcoma in the acquired immune deficiency syndrome: A proposal for uniform evaluation, response, and staging criteria. J Clin Oncol 7:1201–1207, 1989.

*Minimal oral disease is nonnodular KS confined to the palate.

†"B" symptoms are unexplained fever, night sweats, >10% involuntary weight loss, or diarrhea persisting more than 2 weeks.

motherapy with vinca alkaloids, and cryotherapy with liquid nitrogen. For skin lesions, a total dose of 2000 cGy delivered in 200- to 400-cGy daily fractions produces relief of pain in 2 weeks and reduction in the size of tumors in up to 80% of patients. However, the duration of response is short. While radiation therapy is effective for oral mucosal KS, radiation mucositis detracts from its benefit.

Alpha interferon (IFNα) is active treatment for epidemic KS with antiviral, antiproliferative, and immunomodulatory activity. There is a decline in HIV titers in patients receiving INFα. The overall response rate is 25 to 50% (Table 29–2) depending on the CD4+ cell count and the presence or absence of concurrent B symptoms. High-dose treatment is more effective than low-dose treatment. Maximal response occurs after 4 to 12 weeks. Maintenance therapy is required for continued response. Beta and gamma interferons are ineffective.

Combination biological therapy with INFα and zidovudine results in overall response rates of 33 to 46%. The maximum tolerated doses of INFα and zidovudine are 4.5 million

Table 29–2. **SYSTEMIC TREATMENT OF KAPOSI'S SARCOMA**

TREATMENT	RESPONSE RATE (%)
Chemotherapy	
Vinblastine (VBL)	26
Etoposide	76
Vincristine (VCR)	61
Bleomycin (Bleo)	77
VCR + VBL	45
Bleo + VBL	62
Adriamycin + Bleo + VBL or VCR	66–86
Biologic Therapies	
IFNα 2a	38
IFNα 2b	40
+ etoposide	21
+ VBL	29–60
+ VCR	15
IFN beta	5
IFN gamma	0
Interleukin 2 + IFN beta	0–6
Retroviral Therapies	
Zidovudine	0
+ IFNα	42

From Krigel RL, Friedman-Kien AE: Epidemic Kaposi's sarcoma. Semin Oncol 17:350–360, 1990.

U/day and 200 mg every 4 hours or 18 million U/day and 100 mg every 4 hours, respectively. Toxicity consists of neutropenia, thrombocytopenia, anemia, increased transaminase levels, a flulike syndrome, and fatigue. HIV cultures become negative in up to 50% of patients. The combination of INFα and etoposide achieved a 21% response rate but a 33% incidence of opportunistic infections.

Many chemotherapeutic agents have activity against epidemic KS, as shown in Table 29–2. Hematologic toxicity is dose limiting. The nonmyelosuppressive combination of vincristine and bleomycin is generally well tolerated. Combination chemotherapy with Adriamycin (doxorubicin), bleomycin, and vinblastine (ABV) produces responses in over 80% of patients. However, bone marrow suppression and opportunistic infections are prohibitive. Currently, the ACTG is conducting a phase II study of oral etoposide administered once weekly.

The recently released hemopoietic colony-stimulating factors are being combined with chemotherapy, antiretroviral agents, and interferons in an attempt to reduce toxicity while maintaining a high response rate.

REFERENCES

Chak LY, Gill PS, Levine AM, et al: Radiation therapy for acquired immunodeficiency syndrome–related Kaposi's sarcoma. J Clin Oncol 6:863–867, 1988.

Ensoli B, Nakamura S, Salahuddin SZ, et al: AIDS-Kaposi's sarcoma-derived cells express cytokines with autocrine and paracrine growth effects. Science 243:223–226, 1990.

Krigel RL, Friedman-Kien AE: Epidemic Kaposi's sarcoma. Semin Oncol 17:350–360, 1990.

Krown SE, Metroka C, Wernz JC: Kaposi's sarcoma in acquired immune deficiency syndrome: A proposal for uniform evaluation, response, and staging criteria. J Clin Oncol 7:1201–1207, 1989.

Krown SE, Gold JWM, Niedzwiecki D, et al: Interferon-alpha with zidovudine: Safety, tolerance, and clinical and virologic effects in patients with Kaposi's sarcoma associated with the acquired immunodeficiency syndrome (AIDS). Ann Intern Med 112:812–821, 1990.

OTHER CANCERS ASSOCIATED WITH AIDS

No convincing epidemiologic evidence suggests an increase in the incidence of Hodgkin's disease since the onset of the AIDS epidemic. Case reports indicate that AIDS patients with Hodgkin's disease usually have B symptoms, and 77% have stage III or stage IV disease at diagnosis. Lymphocyte-depleted and mixed cellularity subtypes are much more common. Tolerance of standard Hodgkin's disease chemotherapy (Chap. 9) is poor, and the complete response rate (31%) is low. It is conceivable that the immunodeficiency state contributes to these differences.

Squamous cell carcinomas of the anogenital region are increased 25- to 50-fold in the AIDS population. Cervical carcinoma risk also increases with HIV infection. Concurrent papillomavirus infection possibly contributes to the pathogenesis of these frequently very aggressive lesions. These malignancies may also be promoted by other venereal diseases and high-risk sexual activity.

REFERENCES

Biggar RJ: Cancer in the acquired immunodeficiency syndrome: An epidemiologic assessment. Semin Oncol 17:251–260, 1990.

Levine AM: Miscellaneous cancers associated with HIV infection. Curr Opin Oncol 2:1172–1174, 1990.

30
HOSPICE CARE

Julia L. Smith

The words *hospice* and *hospital* come from the Latin *hospes*, meaning guest or stranger. Both are hospitable, that is, providing welcome and kindness to strangers. Modern hospitals are institutions dedicated to providing life-prolonging care if not cure of disease. Modern hospices, on the other hand, are dedicated to the provision of comfort care to people with terminal illnesses. The modern roots of the hospice movement developed in England at St. Christopher's Hospice, founded by Dame Cicely Saunders. The concept has spread to the United States only over the past 15 to 20 years.

Hospice programs emphasize patient comfort, avoid prolonging the dying process, and involve a team of caregivers to support both the patient and the family. Cancer patients predominate in most hospices because of their relatively predictable course. However, this type of care is applicable to anyone in the terminal stages of a fatal illness, with an estimated prognosis of 6 months or less. Patients with end-stage pulmonary or cardiac disease, progressive neurologic illnesses such as amyotrophic lateral sclerosis, acquired immunodeficiency syndrome (AIDS), and those who elect to discontinue or refuse dialysis for uremia can all benefit from the symptomatic hospice approach. Fortunately, most health insurers cover care on certified hospice programs.

Physicians often perceive a need to actively diagnose and treat diseases. Comfort care of dying individuals seems more closely related to nursing or counseling than to medicine. In fact, however, continuing involvement with dying patients can be immensely rewarding to the physician as well as to the patient and family. Comfort care involves adjusting medications to obtain relief of symptoms, providing explanations of likely causes of symptoms, and reassuring families that the constellations of symptoms they witness are expected. Thus, hospice care requires flexibility, knowledge of pharmacologic agents, physical measures, interpersonal skills, and an understanding of the dying process.

TEAM APPROACH

Hospice care involves symptom management and support for the patient's psychosocial and spiritual needs, as well as support for the grief of the family, and therefore the work demands an interdisciplinary group of caregivers. These individuals are responsible for educating the family and making available the necessary tools to provide care at home or in an inpatient setting. The physician is in charge of the medical aspects. A community health nurse oversees the care of the patient at home, carrying out medical orders and coordinating access to social work, spiritual counseling, and home health aide services. Other services, such as nutritional counseling and physical and occupational therapy, are provided as needed. Volunteer help can be enlisted for companionship or errand running. Care provided to the family does not end with the patient's death, but rather extends into the period after the death to support the bereavement process.

The interdisciplinary team meets weekly to facilitate communication about patient and family needs and progress. Twenty-four-hour on-call coverage is available, usually with home visits when necessary. Although the family carries the major responsibilty for providing hands-on care, the team must be sure assistance is available and may recommend respite inpatient care if the family becomes fatigued. Both the availability of respite care and the ability to care for terminally ill people in the chronic phase distinguish hospice care from other home nursing care programs.

SYMPTOM CONTROL

The relief of physical symptoms is of primary importance in terminal care. Not only is it good medicine to provide comfort when curative or life-prolonging treatment is no longer available, but as long as the patient and family are absorbed with distressing physical problems, the important communications associated with saying good-bye cannot go forward.

Early in the course of the disease a cancer patient may be highly functional, and by treating the underlying illness and other intercurrent problems, good-quality life may be prolonged. This is especially true of the responsive tumors such as breast cancer, small cell lung cancer, lymphomas, leukemias, and prostate cancer. As the disease progresses, treatment options dwindle and symptoms increase. Each patient must consider whether continuation of treatments directed against the malignancy is still justified. Since all but a few cancers are incurable once metastasis has occurred, most antineoplastic therapy is actually palliative and not curative. It can be difficult to distinguish between chemotherapy and radiation therapy intended to control disease progression and the use of either modality purely to palliate symptoms. A useful rule of thumb is to ask whether the side effects of treatment, including transportation to the treating facility, are outweighed by the benefit achieved. When the goal is comfort, diagnostic tests and parenteral treatments become onerous and burdensome. Good patient management at this point no longer requires the measurement of tumor size and the follow-up of abnormal laboratory tests. Good care can usually be given empirically based on careful history taking and physical assessment. However, anticipation and explanation of changes in the patient's condition remain important so that both the patient and family are prepared mentally for new developments and appropriate treatment alternatives for changing physical status. For instance, many patients lose the ability to swallow but continue to need analgesics. Frantic phone calls and delays in relieving symptoms can be avoided if suppositories are prescribed in advance. A family may be comforted to have suction equipment available in the home in order to clear oral secretions, even if its use is never required. Families who remain more concerned about the patient's physical symptoms than the patient himself or herself may benefit from discussions with the nurse and physician and by a chance to explore their feelings with a social worker, clergyman, or counselor.

PAIN

Pain is the most common symptom encountered in cancer patients. The elements of pain control are presented in Chapter 25, but several special aspects of pain control deserve mention in a discussion of terminal care. Since the goal of hospice is usually to provide care in the home until death, the routes of choice for administration of narcotic analgesics are oral and rectal. There is no dose ceiling for narcotics except the limits imposed by the physical volume of medication or by uncontrollable side effects. Volume limitations are encountered less frequently since the introduction of concentrated oral solutions of morphine (20 mg/mL) and sustained-release morphine tablets (15, 30, 60, and 100 mg). The sustained-release tablets are well absorbed rectally when the oral route is lost. Another option is the use of fentanyl (Duragesic) transdermal patches, which provide 72 hours of continuous medication. In selected patients for whom the enteral route is unavailable or inadequate, continuous subcutaneous infusions are often effective and well tolerated.

An invariable consequence of narcotic analgesic use is constipation. This symptom requires both preventive and therapeutic measures (see below and Table 30–1).

NAUSEA

Nausea and vomiting are discussed in Chapter 26 but also deserve comment here. These symptoms are not only distressing by themselves, but they also may interfere with adequate pain management. Since injectable medications are best avoided in the terminal patient, the physician must gain familiarity with the use of antiemetics in the form of rectal suppositories and even by the transdermal route with scopolamine patches. Glucocorticoids may help reduce nausea in some patients. Occasionally, continuous subcutaneous infusion of a drug such as metoclopramide or haloperidol is necessary in order to regain control of the symptom; once this is accomplished, then a noninjectable route may be successful.

ANOREXIA AND DEHYDRATION

Anorexia is commonly associated with advanced cancer. During the terminal phase, eating often becomes a focus of contention within the family: the family subconsciously

Table 30–1. **USEFUL TREATMENTS FOR SPECIFIC SYMPTOMS**

SYMPTOM	TREATMENT
Sore or dry mouth	Hydration, mouthwash, mouth swabs, artificial saliva Chewing gum, if patient is alert Petroleum jelly to lips Viscous lidocaine solution—"swish and swallow" Nystatin, ketoconazole, or clotrimazole if candidal infection present
Anorexia	Explanation, reassurance Small meals, food choices, cheerful environment Treat sore mouth Prednisone, 10–20 mg/day Megace (megestrol), 120–360 mg/day
Dyspnea	Treat easily reversible causes Conserve energy Calming presence, relaxation Increased airflow (fan or window) Anxiolytic (diazepam, lorazepam) Morphine, 5 mg PO or 3 mg SC every 4–8 hr Oxygen Scopolamine patch for "death rattle"
Terminal restlessness	Haloperidol, 2–10 mg/day Chlorpromazine suppositories, 50–100 mg Ensure adequate pain control Check for constipation, wet sheets, etc.
Constipation	Maximize activity and fluid intake Preventive stool softeners Cathartics as needed Rule out impaction Lactulose, 30–60 mL/day

identifies failure to eat with the reality of dying, and the refusal of food as the refusal of love. When pain and nausea are controlled and poor appetite persists, the physician should explain the normalcy of this symptom to the family and educate them in catering to the small appetite. The patient may also need the doctor's permission to turn down foods he or she does not want and to have foods that were previously prohibited due to diabetes, heart disease, hypertension, or elevated cholesterol. Small meals served in a cheerful environment, allowing the patient to select favorite items, and providing concentrated calories such as milk shakes or dietary supplements are useful strategies. It may also help to point out that if the patient is not hungry, he or she is not suffering from starvation. The nutritionist can serve as a valuable resource to the physician and family.

As patients become more debilitated, they may desire only fluids. Eventually, many patients completely lose the ability to swallow; at this point, intravenous hydration is often considered. Fully alert patients must choose whether to accept intravenous hydration after the pros and cons have been explained by the physician. When the patient is obtunded or comatose, intravenous fluids offer no advantage over gentle cleansing of the mouth, frequent ice chips or moist swabs, and frequent lubrication of the lips. In fact, withholding intravenous fluids leads to *greater* comfort in several ways: resorption of edema fluid, decreased pulmonary congestion, and decreased urinary output and therefore less incontinence and less need for urinary catheters. Furthermore, intravenous lines can become objects of torture and frustration to family and professionals as well. Agitated patients often either pull the IV out or require restraints. Venous access becomes increasingly difficult, necessitating multiple attempts and frequent replacement of lines. Well-intentioned attempts to improve comfort with intravenous hydration often backfire. The time and effort expended on intravenous hydration can be applied in more useful ways such as quiet bedside chats and simple "pillow fluffing" care.

BOWEL OBSTRUCTION

Bowel obstruction represents a similar dilemma in the terminal patient. Surgery is generally not indicated when large or multiple tumor masses cause obstruction, as in advanced ovarian cancer, or when bowel obstruction is recurrent, or in very debilitated patients. Continuous suction and hydration are uncomfortable and difficult to do at home. Occasional vomiting each day may be less uncomfortable, as long as the associated symptoms of nausea, colic, and pain are relieved. When the obstruction is partial, oral feedings with low-bulk purees and oral medications can continue as the patient tolerates. In some cases, metoclopramide may enhance peristaltic emptying, but it can aggravate colic. Constipation should be prevented with docusate rather than stimulant laxatives such as senna or Dulcolax (bisacodyl) in order to minimize cramping. Dexamethasone may reduce edema in the bowel wall and improve obstructive symptoms as a result. Antispasmodics can relieve colic, and H_2 blockers can decrease gastric secretions. Suppository medications should be available, and if repeated vomiting or complete obstruction occurs, continuous subcutaneous infusions of analgesics and/or antiemetics by portable pump may be required. Frequent oral hygiene should be provided.

DYSPNEA

Dyspnea is a frightening symptom present in many patients with advanced cancer. It is a frequent end-stage problem in lung cancer and in patients with metastatic disease to the pleura or lungs. When reversible causes of dyspnea (e.g., pneumonia, pleural or pericardial effusion, bronchoconstriction, congestive heart failure) have been corrected, or if the patient is too ill for procedures like thoracentesis, a multifaceted approach to managing this symptom should be instituted. The soothing presence of staff and family coupled with increased room air circulation will help. Medication to relieve anxiety and low-dose morphine to reduce tachypnea and the sense of suffocation are often remarkably helpful. If the patient is already on morphine for pain control, the morphine dose should be increased by 50%. Nasal oxygen may or may not provide relief. The majority of cancer patients with dyspnea are not hypoxemic.

A related problem is the "death rattle" of a patient in the last days or hours of life. While the patient is usually too obtunded to be troubled by this sound, the family often becomes quite anxious. Oral suctioning is intrusive and not always available, but scopolamine patches will decrease the oral secretions responsible for the noise.

RESTLESSNESS

Restlessness is another common problem as death approaches and is often disconcerting to the patient and especially for observers. Assurance that pain is controlled is the first step in evaluation and treatment. Discomfort associated with constipation, wet sheets, dyspnea, and other problems should be corrected. Haloperidol orally, buccally with concentrated solution, or parenterally is a readily available drug treatment. Less commonly used agents are chlorpromazine suppositories and methotrimeprazine (Levoprome), which is available only by injection in the United States.

GENERAL MEASURES

During the last days of life it is helpful to reduce the polypharmacy of medications. As oral intake declines, the need for antidiabetic medications decreases. As activity is restricted, the need for cardiac medications declines. Similarly, any other medications not directly contributing to patient comfort should be reevaluated and discontinuation considered. Doses and side effects of the primary symptomatic treatments should be reevaluated to ensure proper route, schedule, and effect. At times, it is possible to use one agent for more than one purpose. For example, haloperidol is a good antiemetic and anxiolytic and helps control terminal agitation and restlessness. Morphine, the drug of choice for pain, also relieves dyspnea and may help reduce anxiety and restlessness as well.

SUMMARY

It is not an easy task to determine a patient's prognosis or to define the point where palliation of symptoms takes precedence over control of the disease. Life expectancy is

Table 30–2. **QUESTIONS REGARDING PROPOSED INTERVENTIONS IN HOSPICE PATIENTS**

Will clarification of the exact diagnosis with laboratory or imaging tests alter the treatment?
Is the patient's general condition and stamina sufficient to permit him or her to undergo the treatment recommended?
Will reversal of the problem provide lasting benefit?
Are the symptoms severe enough to justify the intervention?
Do the patient and family understand what is involved and desire the treatment?

more often overestimated than underestimated by physicians, and patients are often referred late to hospice programs. Despite the requirement of an estimated 6-month survival, the average length of hospice care nationally is only 5 to 6 weeks. With such short lengths of participation in the hospice program, symptom management may occupy the patient, family, and staff to the extent that spiritual and psychological issues are not adequately addressed.

Generally, care for dying patients requires the involvement of a team of professionals. Patients should be allowed to call the shots as much as they are able and should therefore be included in compassionate explanations of the disease process and of the options open to them. Support and education of the family members empower them to participate actively in the care planning and giving. Useful guidelines to discuss with the patient and family whenever a problem arises are shown in Table 30–2. These questions should be asked (and answered) regarding aggressive intravenous treatment of hypercalcemia, nephrostomy for ureteral obstruction, surgery for bowel obstruction, and even for the simpler, and medically less complicated, procedures such as transfusion, antibiotics, para- and thoracentesis, and of course for parenteral fluids in the dying period. When patients have unremitting and distressful symptoms and are very near death, not interacting with the people around them, and unable to swallow medicines, then withholding even life-sustaining treatments is appropriate.

REFERENCES

Billings A: Outpatient Management of Advanced Cancer. Philadelphia, J.B. Lippincott, 1985.

Forster LE, Lynn J: Predicting life span for applicants to inpatient hospice. Arch Intern Med 148:2540–2543,1988.

Hermann JF: Psychosocial support: Interventions for the physician. Semin Oncol 12:466–471, 1985.

Levy M, Catalano RB: Control of common physical symptoms other than pain in patients with terminal disease. Semin Oncol 12:411–430, 1985.

Miller RJ: The role of chemotherapy in the hospice patient: A problem of definition. Am J Hospice Care 6:19–26, 1989.

Pearlman R: Inaccurate predictions of life expectancy: Dilemmas and opportunities. Arch Intern Med 148:1586–1591, 1988.

Saunders C, Baines M: Living with Dying—The Management of Terminal Disease, 2nd ed. New York, Oxford University Press, 1989.

Sergi-Swinehart P: Hospice home care: How to get patients home and help them stay there. Semin Oncol 12:461–465, 1985.

Twycross R, Lack S: Therapeutics in Terminal Cancer. New York, Churchill Livingstone, 1990.

31
BONE MARROW TRANSPLANTATION

Jane L. Liesveld

Bone marrow transplantation is being used increasingly for a number of indications, including many hematologic, neoplastic, immune deficiency, and congenital disorders (Table 31–1). In 1989, approximately 4000 patients received allogeneic marrow transplants and a comparable number received autologous transplants for the treatment of leukemia and various solid tumors.

Marrow transplantation involves the intravenous infusion of marrow cells, usually obtained from the posterior iliac crests of the donor, into the recipient host. The marrow cells reach the marrow cavity and lodge there by mechanisms that are poorly understood. In the host marrow cavities the donor cells begin to replicate and eventually repopulate the marrow and blood with functional hemopoietic elements of all lineages. Marrow sources for transplantation are of three general types: (1) syngeneic, from a genetically indentical individual (usually a monozygotic twin); (2) allogeneic, from a genetically different individual of the same species; and (3) autologous, from the patient himself or herself.

Most patients are referred to marrow transplantation centers by hematologists/oncologists. The patient's primary care physician plays a vital role in helping the patient understand the rationale and indications for marrow transplantation and in assisting in the diagnosis and management of posttransplant problems, in consultation with the transplant team.

REFERENCES

Champlin R (ed): Bone marrow transplantation. Boston, Kluwer Academic Publishers, 1990.
Deeg HJ, Klingemann H-G, Phillips GL: A Guide to Bone Marrow Transplantation. New York, Springer-Verlag, 1988.

PROCEDURAL TECHNIQUES INVOLVED IN MARROW TRANSPLANTATION

DONOR

Marrow donors, after giving informed consent for operation, undergo multiple (150–250) marrow aspirations under general or spinal anesthesia, usually from the posterior iliac crests. The anterior iliac crests may also be utilized, if necessary. The marrow is collected in heparin and filtered to remove particulate material. For autologous harvests, 1 to 3 ×

Table 31–1. **PARTIAL LISTING OF DISEASES TREATED WITH BONE MARROW TRANSPLANTATION**

MALIGNANT	NONMALIGNANT
Acute nonlymphocytic leukemia	Aplastic anemia
Acute lymphocytic leukemia	Paroxysmal nocturnal hemoglobinuria
Chronic myelogenous leukemia	Hemoglobinopathies
Hodgkin's disease	Thalassemias
Non-Hodgkin's lymphomas	Congenital immunodeficiencies
Multiple myeloma	Osteopetrosis
Myelodysplastic syndromes	Storage diseases
Selected solid tumors	
Neuroblastoma	
Breast cancer	
Small cell lung cancer	
Testicular carcinoma	
Ewing's sarcoma	

10^8 mononuclear cells per kilogram donor body weight are harvested. For allogeneic transplants, this number is 2 to 10 × 10^8/kg. The average volume of marrow collected is about 750 to 1000 mL for an adult. The major risks of the procedure to the donor are those of general anesthesia. The donor often has local discomfort for a few days after the procedure. The aspirated marrow is replenished quickly. Infectious and cardiovascular complications are rare.

RECIPIENT

Most recipients of marrow infusion require what is termed "preparation." Only patients transplanted for severe combined immune deficiencies require no special preparation. In other cases, immediately before transplantation, chemoradiotherapy or chemotherapy alone is administered. Radiation is usually given as total body irradiation (TBI). The choice of preparative regimen depends on the disease and on the type of marrow used, i.e., allogeneic or autologous. The regimens are usually administered as combinations of agents and modalities. They are given to immunosuppress the host to prevent the host from rejecting the graft, to eliminate residual malignant cells in the host, and to create space in the marrow for the infused graft. Table 31–2 lists some typical preparative regimens for various transplantation indications. Numerous variations of these exist.

The main side effects of total body irradiation include nausea, emesis, alopecia, skin rash, and liver function test abnormalities. Use of cyclophosphamide at these dosages can result in hemorrhagic cystitis, cardiomyopathy, and veno-occlusive disease of the liver. High-dose busulfan can result in seizures, and prophylactic phenytoin is utilized. After the preparative regimen is completed, the marrow product is infused through a large-bore central line, usually a Hickman catheter, over a 2- to 4-hour period. Tachycardia and hemolysis with hematuria may be noted during marrow reinfusion, which is usually quite well tolerated.

In cases of autologous transplantation, marrow is harvested and stored for future use at −197°C in a cryopreservative such as 10% dimethyl sulfoxide (DMSO). Such marrow can be stored for more than 5 years. When needed, it is rapidly thawed at 37°C and reinfused. Flushing, cramps, nausea, cardiac arrhythmias, and hemoglobinuria may occur during the reinfusion of a product previously frozen in DMSO.

ALLOGENEIC TRANSPLANTATION

DONOR SELECTION AND HLA TYPING

In allogeneic marrow transplantation, a decision must be made regarding the optimal donor. An identical twin (syngeneic) donor genetically identical to the host is an ideal but rare source of marrow. Donors and hosts submit to histocompatibility typing by serologic and mixed leukocyte culture techniques to determine the alleles at the HLA-A, B, DR, and D loci. Such techniques allow determination of the major histocompatibility antigens, which are located on the short arm of chromosome 6. Minor histocompatibility antigens are more diffucult to detect. HLA loci are transmitted as a haplotype. Thus, each person

Table 31–2. **EXAMPLES OF CONDITIONING REGIMENS**

REGIMEN	SCHEDULE	PRIMARY INDICATIONS
Cyclophosphamide plus fractionated TBI	60 mg/kg × 2 days 200 cGy daily × 6	Acute leukemias/some lymphomas
Bu/CY		
Busulfan	1 mg/kg q 6 hr × 16 doses	Acute leukemia/CML
Cyclophosphamide	60 mg/kg x 2 days	
CBV		
Cyclophosphamide	6 g/m² days 1, 2, 3, 4	Hodgkin's (autologous BMT)
Carmustine	300 mg/m² x 1 day, day 1	
Etoposide	600 mg/m² days 1, 2, 3	

possesses two HLA haplotypes, one from each parent. Approximately 40% of Caucasian patients who have siblings will have a sibling identical at the major HLA loci.

Since the majority of people do not have a histocompatible sibling, other less perfectly matched donors must be found. These may include parents, offspring, or siblings who share one haplotype with the recipient host. Patients transplanted from a donor who differs for only one HLA antigen have a prognosis comparable to completely matched HLA individuals. The results become less optimal as the extent of mismatch increases. Other potential marrow sources are unrelated phenotypically matched donors located through donor banks and registries. Experience with these transplants is limited, but successful long-term engraftments without significant graft versus host disease have been reported.

REFERENCES

Anasetti C, Amos D, Beatty PG, et al: Effect of HLA compatibility on engraftment of bone marrow transplants in patients with leukemia or lymphoma. N Engl J Med 320:197–204, 1989.

Bach FH, Sachs DH: Current concepts: Transplantation immunology. N Engl J Med 317:489–492, 1987.

Hansen JA, Choo SY, Geraghty DE, et al: The HLA system in clinical bone marrow transplantation. Hematol Oncol Clin North Am 4:507–511, 1990.

SIDE EFFECTS OF CONDITIONING REGIMENS

Patients are usually cytopenic by the day of marrow infusion, and during the time before engraftment they are subject to infectious and hemorrhagic complications of the cytopenic state. Many early toxicities are multifactorial, so it is often difficult to determine the direct contribution of the preparative conditioning regimen. Oral mucositis is often seen with use of TBI, etoposide, and melphalan, and may be worsened by methotrexate given for graft versus host disease prophylaxis. Severe mucositis usually necessitates parenteral nutrition, analgesia, and treatment with topical mycostatin to prevent fungal infection and systemic acyclovir to prevent herpes simplex lesions. As mentioned previously, high-dose cyclophosphamide can result in cardiomyopathy and hemorrhagic cystitis. To prevent the latter, hydration and diuretics are prescribed during the preparative regimen administration. Veno-occlusive disease is an often fatal disorder seen after administration of high-dose chemotherapy, which results in fluid retention, tender hepatomegaly, and jaundice. It occurs more often in allogeneic than in autologous transplants. Histologically, fibrosis of the small hepatic venules is seen. Veno-occlusive disease usually appears within 30 days of transplantation, which may help to differentiate it from hepatic graft versus host disease, which may not appear until later. Since infections, hepatotoxic medications, and hyperalimentation can also result in liver dysfunction posttransplant, the clinical picture is not always clear-cut. Treatment is largely supportive.

INFECTIOUS COMPLICATIONS

Infections that occur posttransplantation are usually grouped by time of occurrence after the transplant. Most transplant recipients will remain cytopenic for the first 2 to 4 weeks after marrow infusion prior to engraftment. Engraftment is characterized by declining transfusion requirements indicating active hematopoiesis, and in allogeneic transplants, by a state of chimerism wherein cytogenetics, red cell antigen markers, or DNA studies such as restriction fragment–linked polymorphisms (RFLPs) show the presence of donor-type cells within the host. During the immediate posttransplant period, patients are susceptible to all infections associated with neutropenia. Commonly involved infectious sites include the lungs, perirectal area, skin, mouth, and sinuses. Predisposition to these infections persists until the absolute neutrophil count reaches greater than 500/mm^3.

Infections commonly seen during this time include gram-negative bacterial infections and fungal infections. Patients with indwelling central catheters are also at risk for gram-positive septicemias. As in all neutropenic patients who develop fever, transplant patients are treated empirically with broad-spectrum antibiotic coverage. If fever persists, empiric antifungal therapy (amphotericin B) is also begun. Many transplant centers employ laminar airflow systems, but these have not been shown to improve outcomes except in the case of allogeneic transplants for aplastic anemia. During the immediate posttransplant period patients are also at risk for viral infections such as herpes simplex virus and varicella-zoster viruses. Prophylactic acyclovir is usually given during this period.

From 30 to 100 days posttransplantation, recipients are at risk for interstitial pneumonitis, which is associated with use of TBI during conditioning. In some cases, cytomegalovirus (CMV) or *Pneumocystis carinii* are causative, but 40% of cases are idiopathic. Prophylactic intravenous immune globulin decreases the incidence of CMV-related interstitial pneumonitis. Documented cases of CMV pneumonitis can be treated with ganciclovir. Use of CMV-negative blood products and IV immune globulin in CMV seronegative donor-recipient pairs also decreases the incidence of CMV infections.

Infections after day 100 posttransplant are often related to the presence of chronic graft versus host disease that delays the return of immune function. Encapsulated bacterial pathogens and varicella-zoster virus cause many of these infections. Figure 31–1 illustrates the time course for viral and bacterial complications of bone marrow transplantation.

Immune reconstitution posttransplantation depends upon many factors, among which are immunosuppressive medications such as those used for graft versus host disease prophylaxis (cyclosporin A, methotrexate), the presence and severity of graft versus host disease, and the presence of onging infection. The helper:suppressor (CD4:CD8) T-cell ratio is often reversed after transplantation, even briefly following autologous transplantation. T-cell function and B-cell function are also decreased and may remain suboptimal for months to a year or more, especially in the presence of chronic graft versus host disease.

GRAFT VERSUS HOST DISEASE

Graft versus host disease (GVHD) represents a state wherein immunocompetent donor lymphocytes recognize and react to so-called "minor" host histocompatibility antigens that are not detected by current tissue typing techniques, or in the case of mismatched transplants, to major histocompatibility antigens.

Acute Graft Versus Host Disease

Acute GVHD occurs within the first 100 days posttransplantation and in anywhere from 35 to 60% of allogeneic transplants. Manifestations of acute GVHD involve the skin, liver,

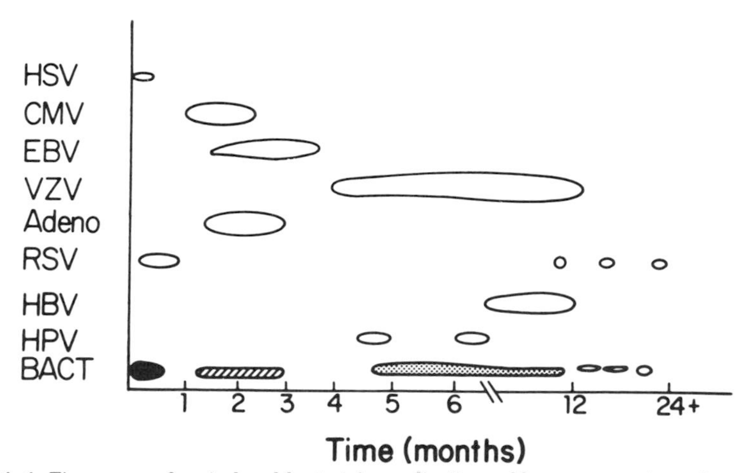

Figure 31–1. Time course for viral and bacterial complications of bone marrow transplantation. The time-line maps the occurrence of infection with herpes simplex virus (HSV), human cytomegalovirus (CMV), varicella-zoster virus (VZV), Epstein-Barr virus (EBV), adenovirus (Adeno), respiratory syncytial virus (RSV), hepatitis B virus (HBV), and human papillomavirus (HPV). Bacterial infections are shown during initial neutropenia (black), acute graft-versus-host disease (dark grid), and chronic graft-versus-host disease (stipple). (*From* Zaia JA: Viral infection associated with bone marrow transplantation. Hematol Clin North Am 4:603–623, 1990.)

and gastrointestinal tract (Table 31–3). Skin involvement occurs primarily as a maculopapular skin rash involving the face, palms, and soles. Gastrointestinal involvement is usually manifest as diarrhea. Patients with acute GVHD are also more prone to infectious complications of immune deficiency. Severe acute GVHD can be treated with steroids, antithymocyte globulin, or anti-CD5 (pan–T-cell) monoclonal antibody infusions.

To prevent the occurrence of acute GVHD, allogeneic transplant recipients are given immunosuppressive medications such as methotrexate, cyclosporin A, or combinations of these agents. Cyclosporin A is usually started 1 day before transplant and continued for 3 to 12 months thereafter. Since acute GVHD is thought to be mediated by donor T lymphocytes, attempts to prevent GVHD using T-cell depletion with monoclonal antibodies and lectin agglutination have been undertaken. While effective depletion of T lymphocytes results in a reduced incidence of GVHD, the incidence of both graft failure and leukemic relapse is increased.

Chronic Graft Versus Host Disease

Chronic GVHD is estimated to occur in 20 to 40% of allogeneic transplant recipients and begins between 100 and 450 days posttransplantation. Its clinical manifestations are like those of autoimmune diseases, with involvement of the skin, oral mucosa, lacrimal glands, esophagus, and somtimes muscles and serosal membranes. Chronic GVHD has been classified by its relationship to acute GVHD as progressive (continued GVHD throughout course), quiescent (acute GVHD followed by absence of GVHD followed by chronic GVHD), or de novo chronic GVHD. The progressive type of chronic GVHD has the worst prognosis. The presence of acute GVHD and increasing recipient age are positive risk factors for developing chronic GVHD. Patients who have thrombocytopenia concurrent with chronic GVHD are thought to also have a worse prognosis.

Skin involvement occurs in more than 90% of patients with chronic GVHD and is characterized by a spectrum ranging from dryness, itching, and anhidrosis to tightness and contractures. The oral mucosa is usually affected in chronic GVHD with pain, dryness, and lichen planus–type changes that may be mistaken for thrush. Xerostomia often leads to development of dental caries. The eyes may become affected with a siccalike syndrome with keratitis and scarring, which can be treated with artificial tears. Patients who have received TBI are also at risk for cataract development. A sicca-type syndrome can involve the pulmonary and genital tracts. Obstructive lung disease may occur in 5 to 10% of patients post–allogeneic transplantation and is probably multifactorial in origin. The esophagus may develop webs, and many patients (approximately 90%) with chronic GVHD have abnormal liver function tests.

Chronic GVHD patients have decreased B- and T-cell function and decreased secretory forms of IgA, which leads to sinobronchial infections. They are also at risk for infection with varicella-zoster virus and with encapsulated bacteria such as *Pneumococcus pneumoniae*. Patients with chronic GVHD are given trimethoprim-sulfamethoxazole antibacterial prophylaxis (one double-strength tablet twice per week), and some centers use prophylactic intravenous immune globulin.

Chronic GVHD is usually diagnosed at day 100 posttransplantation by skin biopsy, oral mucosal biopsy, Schirmer's test for tear secretion, and chemical tests of liver function. Extreme cases of chronic GVHD require treatment with prednisone alone for standard-risk patients and with a combination of agents such as prednisone and azathioprine for high-risk patients. Patients who progress despite high-dose steroid therapy are often placed on a combination of alternate-day prednisone and cyclosporine A.

Supportive care remains very important in the management of chronic GVHD and

Table 31–3. **CLINICAL STAGES OF ACUTE GRAFT VERSUS HOST DISEASE**

STAGE	SKIN	LIVER (bili)	GUT (mL diarrhea)
I	Rash <25%	2.0–3.5	500–1000
II	Rash 25–50%	3.5–8.0	1000–1500
III	Erythroderma	8–15	1500–2500
IV	Bullae, desquamation	>15	>2500

From Vogelsang GB, Wagner JE: Graft-versus-host disease. Hematol Clin North Am 4:625–639, 1990.

includes prompt treatment of infections with antibiotics, attention to oral hygiene, use of artificial tears and saliva, skin protection with sun-block creams, and application of topical estrogens to the vagina if involved with a sicca-type syndrome.

REFERENCES

Storb R, Deeg HJ, Pepe M, et al: Methotrexate and cyclosporine versus cyclosporine alone for prophylaxis of graft-versus-host disease in patients given HLA-identical marrow grafts for leukemia: Long-term followup of a controlled trial. Blood 73:1729–1734, 1989.

Sullivan KM, Witherspoon RP, Storb R, et al: Alternating-day cyclosporine and prednisone for treatment of high-risk chronic graft-v-host disease. Blood 72:555–561, 1988.

Vogelsang GB, Wagner JE: Graft-versus-host disease. Hematol Oncol Clin North Am 4:625–639, 1990.

GRAFT FAILURE

Graft failure may appear as primary failure of engraftment or as initial engraftment followed by loss of the graft. In allogeneic transplantation, graft rejection may occur. In autologous transplantation, graft failure may result from a deficiency or defect in repopulating stem cells or a defect in the marrow microenvironment. Three allogeneic transplant situations in which graft failure is most commonly seen include patients with aplastic anemia previously sensitized by blood product transfusions, histoincompatible grafts, and T-cell–depleted grafts in which the incidence of graft failure may be as high as 45%. If aplastic anemia patients must be transfused before marrow transplantation, white cell–poor, irradiated blood products should be used.

SECONDARY MALIGNANCIES

Some evidence suggests that recipients of marrow transplantation have a higher incidence of secondary leukemias and solid tumors compared to matched cohort controls. Whether this relates to the transplant process itself, the underlying disease for which the transplant was performed, or a genetic predisposition to malignancy in these patients remains undetermined.

REFERENCES

Nemunaitis J, Singer JW, Buckner CD, et al: Use of recombinant human granulocyte-macrophage colony-stimulating factor in graft failure after bone marrow transplantation. Blood 76:245–253, 1990.

Witherspoon RP, Fisher LD, Schoch G, et al: Secondary cancers after bone marrow transplantation for leukemia or aplastic anemia. N Engl J Med 321:784–789, 1989.

USE OF TRANSPLANTATION AND OUTCOMES IN MALIGNANCIES

While marrow transplantation has been used frequently for aplastic anemia and many other nonmalignant disorders, this chapter will review only malignant diseases for which transplantation has found widespread use.

ACUTE MYELOGENOUS LEUKEMIA

Allogeneic Transplantation

All patients with acute myelogenous leukemia (AML) are first treated with chemotherapy for remission induction. Use of conventional chemotherapy with daunorubicin and cytosine arabinoside results in 70 to 80% complete remission and 20 to 30% long-term survival when followed by standard consolidation with chemotherapy. Patients who receive allogeneic transplants in first complete remission have long-term disease-free survival rates of approximately 50–60%. Figure 31–2 shows disease-free survival and overall

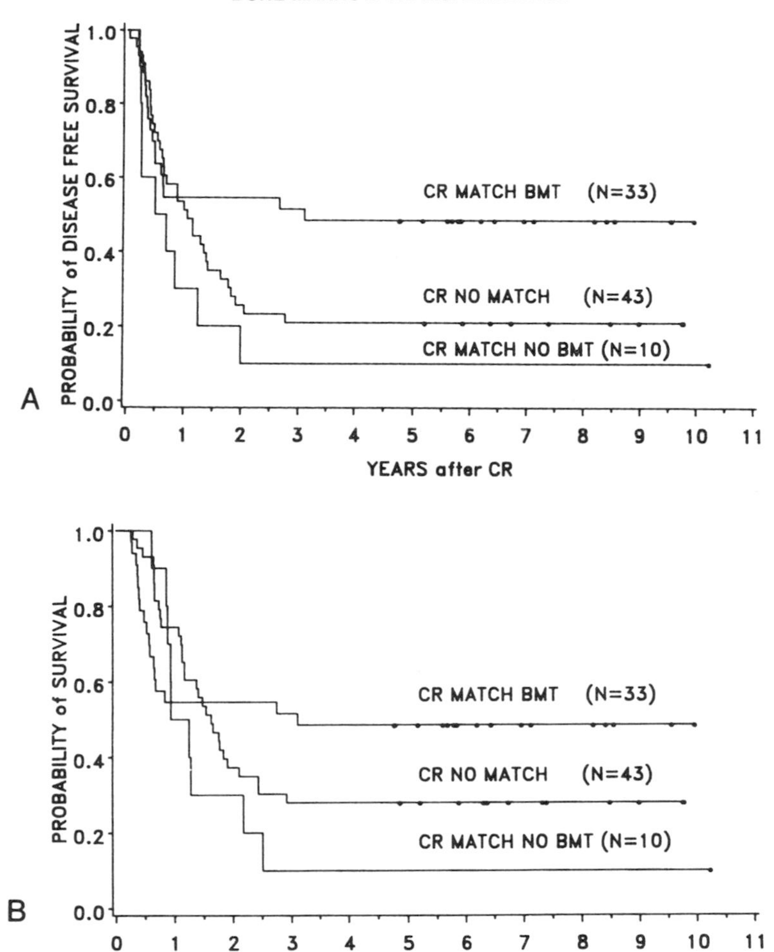

Figure 31–2. Kaplan-Meier product limit estimates of the probability of disease-free survival *(A)* and survival *(B)* of patients who achieved a complete remission and had no matched family donor (n = 43), had a matched donor but were not transplanted (n = 10), or had a matched donor and later received a transplant (n = 33). (*From* Appelbaum FR, Fisher LD, Thomas ED, et al: Chemotherapy versus marrow transplantation for adults with acute nonlymphocytic leukemia: A five-year follow-up. Blood 72:179–184, 1988.

survival of leukemia patients in first complete remission who are transplanted versus those who received chemotherapy alone due to lack of a matched sibling donor.

Patients with AML who receive allogeneic transplantation have a lower relapse rate as a consequence of a possible graft versus leukemia effect and owing to the intensity of the conditioning regimen (usually cyclophosphamide 60 mg/kg for 2 days followed by 9 to 15 Gy total body irradiation, generally given with dose fractionation to avoid nonhematopoietic toxicities). Long-term survival after allogeneic transplantation is only 50 to 60% owing to early deaths from such causes as GVHD and interstitial pneumonitis. Centers with large transplantation experience such as the University of Washington (Seattle) favor transplantation for patients less than 45 years old who have a histocompatible donor, whereas older patients are treated with chemotherapy alone and observed for relapse. For younger patients without a sibling match, consideration can be given to alternate donors or to autologous transplantation (see below).

For patients who never enter a complete remission or who relapse following chemotherapy, allogeneic transplantation is superior to chemotherapy and represents the only chance for long-term disease-free survival. It is generally believed that if a patient has a histocompatible donor, transplantation in first relapse may actually be preferable to transplantation in second complete remission, because toxicities from prior chemotherapy are less. When patients are transplanted early in relapse, approximately 25% long-term disease-free survival may be achieved. Most relapses (75%) will occur in the first 2 years and will be of host origin.

Autologous Transplantation

The rationale for autologous transplantation is that for most chemotherapeutic agents: myelosuppression is dose-limiting. If myelosuppression can be "rescued" with marrow harvested before chemotherapy is given, then one can give more chemotherapy to maximum doses allowed by nonmarrow toxicity in the hope of improving long-term outcomes. The use of autologous transplantation for diseases like acute myelogenous leukemia that involve the marrow has raised several issues. Even if the the patient is transplanted in a clinical first remission, might not undetectable leukemia cells be reinfused with the autologous marrow product? Should such marrow be treated in vitro ("purged")? Also, is the benefit of transplantation versus chemotherapy due to the intensity of the preparative regimen alone or due to a graft versus leukemia effect that would be present only in allogeneic and not in autologous transplantation? These questions remain largely unanswered. Some centers purge autologous transplant products with cyclophosphamide derivatives or with antibody and complement. Whether this improves results has never been demonstrated in a prospective, randomized fashion. One retrospective study from a European cooperative group suggested a slight advantage for those autologous infusions purged with maphosphamide (a cyclophosphamide derivative). Much evidence also exists, however, that relapses are often the result of inadequacy of available preparative regimens as opposed to reinfusion of undetectable leukemic cells.

When autotransplants have been performed for AML in first complete remission, disease-free survivals of 30%, and up to 70% with double transplants, have been reported in various small nonrandomized series. Recurrence is rare after 1 year, and treatment-related mortality is usually 5 to 10%. The longer the complete remission before autotransplant is performed, the better the disease-free survival after transplant. Autotransplants have also been performed in second complete remission with 5-year disease-free survival rates of 30% reported by some centers. Outcomes for autotransplantation have been poor for secondary leukemias or cases antedated by a preleukemic state. The rate of performance of autologous transplants for AML is increasing, and its place in the overall treatment of AML is evolving.

REFERENCES

Appelbaum FR, Dahlberg S, Thomas ED, et al: Bone marrow transplantation or chemotherapy after remission induction for adults with acute nonlymphoblastic leukemia: A prospective comparison. Ann Intern Med 101:581–588, 1984.

Geller RB, Saral R, Piantadosi S, et al: Allogeneic bone marrow transplantation after high-dose busulfan and cyclophosphamide in patients with acute nonlymphocytic leukemia. Blood 73:2209–2218, 1989.

Gorin NC, Aegerter P, Auvert B: Autologous bone marrow transplantation for acute myelocytic leukemia in first remision: A European survey of the role of marrow purging. Blood 75:1606–1614, 1990.

Korbling M, Hunstein W, Fliedner T, et al: Disease-free survival after autologous bone marrow transplantation in patients with acute myelogenous leukemia. Blood 74:1898–1904, 1989.

McGlave PB, Haake RJ, Bostrom BC, et al: Allogeneic bone marrow transplantation for acute nonlymphocytic leukemia in first remission. Blood 72:1512–1517, 1988.

ACUTE LYMPHOCYTIC LEUKEMIA

Owing to the favorable results with chemotherapy alone in children with low- or average-risk acute lymphocytic leukemia (ALL), transplantation for this type of leukemia is not recommended in first complete remission. For adults with ALL with high-risk factors such as high blast counts, a mediastinal mass, null cell leukemia, age >35, or chromosomal abnormalities such as the Philadelphia chromosome, transplant is recommended in first complete remission.

For patients considered poor risk with chemotherapy alone and transplanted in first complete remission, with allogeneic transplants disease-free survival is approximately 35 to 60% and with autologous transplants it is 25 to 50%. For adults in second complete remission, 5-year survival with chemotherapy alone is less than 10%. With allogeneic transplantation, this may increase to 25 to 50% and with autologous transplantation to 20 to 30%. For patients transplanted in higher remission number, the risk of relapse becomes greater.

REFERENCES

Blume KG, Forman SJ, Snyder DS et al: Allogeneic bone marrow transplantation for acute lymphoblastic leukemia during first complete remission. Transplantation 43:389–392, 1987.

Carey PJ, Proctor SJ, Taylor P: Autologous bone marrow transplantation for high-grade lymphoid malignancy using melphalan/irradiation conditioning without marrow purging or cryopreservation. Blood 77:1593–1598, 1991.

CHRONIC MYELOGENOUS LEUKEMIA

Allogeneic transplantation represents a potentially curative treatment for chronic myelogenous leukemia (CML), and a donor search is recommended for all CML patients less than 50 years old. The use of hydroxyurea rather than busulfan in the chronic phase may lead to less pulmonary toxicity after transplantation.

The question of when transplantation should be performed in this disease remains an important issue. Those transplanted in chronic phase within 1 year of diagnosis have the best prognosis, but whether this is the best timing remains controversial owing to early transplant-related mortality. The median duration of chronic phase CML is 4 years and of blast crisis 2 to 5 months. When patients are transplanted in the so-called accelerated phase or in blast crisis, rates of relapse and graft failure are high and there is little prolongation of disease-free survival (Fig. 31–3).

Those less than 20 years of age at the time of transplantation have the best prognosis. When transplantation is performed in chronic phase, the long-term survival rate is 50 to 70%; in accelerated phase, this falls to 15 to 40%; and in blast crisis, to less than 15%. Patients with massive splenomegaly at the time of transplant may have delayed engraftment, but the role for splenectomy is not clear-cut. There is also some suggestion that those with severe myelofibrosis have worse prognoses.

The role of autologous transplantation in chronic myelogenous leukemia is also in evolution. Some patients may have prolongation of the chronic phase by reinfusion of marrow harvested in early chronic phase after high-dose marrow ablative therapy, but this remains a controversial mode of treatment.

REFERENCES

Goldman JM, Gale RP, Horowitz MM, et al: Bone marrow transplantation for chronic myelogenous leukemia in chronic phase. Increased risk for relapse associated with T-cell depletion. Ann Intern Med 108:806–814, 1988.

Martin PJ, Clift RA, Fisher LD, et al: HLA identical marrow transplantation during accelerated-phase chronic myelogenous leukemia. Analysis of survival and remission duration. Blood 72:1978–1984, 1988.

Thomas ED, Clift RA: Indications for marrow transplantation in chronic myelogenous leukemia. Blood 73:861–864, 1989.

HODGKIN'S DISEASE

Hodgkin's disease is sensitive to chemotherapy and radiotherapy, and long-term disease-free survivals and cures are achieved in approximately 50% of patients. For patients who relapse or who are partially treatment resistant at presentation, high-dose chemotherapy

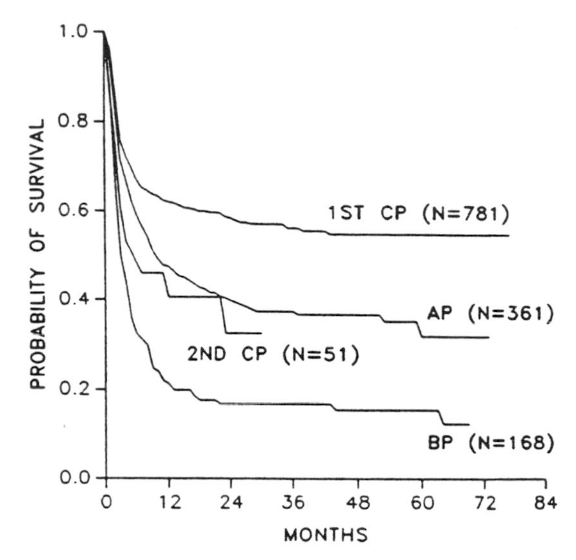

Figure 31–3. Results of life table analyses demonstrating that CML recipients of HLA-identical sibling bone marrow transplant in first chronic phase (1st CP) have a significantly higher probability of survival (55%) than patients transplanted in either accelerated phase (AP) (32%) or in second chronic phase (2nd CP) (33%). Patients transplanted in the blastic phase (BP) have a significantly poorer probability of survival (16%) than any other group. (*From* McGlave PB: Therapy of chronic myelogenous leukemia with bone marrow transplantation. *In* Champlin R (ed): Bone Marrow Transplantation. Boston, Kluwer Academic, 1990.)

with bone marrow rescue offers a better chance for long-term disease-free survival than traditional salvage chemotherapy regimens. Some patients with relapsed Hodgkin's disease have been treated with allogeneic transplantation, but these numbers are small. Whether the marrow rescue product is from an allogeneic or autologous source most likely does not matter in terms of either disease-free survival or probability of relapse after transplant in Hodgkin's disease. Since many Hodgkin's disease patients have no marrow involvement, an autologous graft is the most readily available and circumvents GVHD-related toxicities. The best prognosis is seen in patients with early disease with minimal pretreatment and small tumor burden.

Preparative regimens used in cases of Hodgkin's disease often contain cyclophosphamide, bleomycin, carmustine, and etoposide. In one large series, 118 patients treated with a similar preparative regimen had a complete remission rate of 47%. Some preparative regimens have employed TBI with an improvement in complete remission rates but a concomitant increase in toxic deaths, resulting in no overall survival benefit. Patients with significant marrow contamination or prior pelvic irradiation at sites of usual bone marrow harvest may have autografting with peripheral blood stem cells.

NON-HODGKIN'S LYMPHOMA

For non-Hodgkin's lymphoma of intermediate or high grade, second-line or salvage chemotherapy usually has no long-term effectiveness. Such patients may benefit at relapse from high-dose myeloablative therapy and marrow rescue. Tumor sensitivity to salvage chemotherapy at relapse is the best predictor of continuous disease-free survival after autologous transplant. Prospective randomized studies to compare conventional salvage treatments to high-dose chemotherapy/autologous bone marrow transplantation are now in progress. Interest has also been generated for using high-dose chemotherapy/autologous bone marrow transplantation as early consolidation or even as initial treatment for patients with high-risk disease. Small series of patients transplanted for indolent non-Hodgkin's lymphomas have also been published. In these diseases in which median survivals are long but conventional therapies have no curative potential, long-term follow-up will be needed to assess the impact of high-dose chemotherapy followed by autologous bone marrow transplantation.

MULTIPLE MYELOMA

Many patients with multiple myeloma are older than 60 years at diagnosis and are consequently not good candidates for allogeneic transplantation. Autologous bone marrow transplantation is questionable in this setting because of almost universal marrow involvement. Autologous bone marrow transplantation has been performed for refractory, advanced cases, especially in younger patients. Marrow purging is usually utilized. Long-term follow-up data are not yet available in these patients, who have often been heavily pretreated. Small series of allogeneic transplants for multiple myeloma, again especially in younger patients, have also been reported.

REFERENCES

Armitage JO: Bone marrow transplantation in the treatment of patients with lymphomas. Blood 73:1749–1758, 1989.

Gribben JG, Linch DC, Singer CRJ, et al: Successful treatment of refractory Hodgkin's disease by high-dose combination chemotherapy and autologous bone marrow transplantation. Blood 73:340–344, 1989.

Kessinger A, Armitage JO, Landmark JD, et al: Autologous peripheral hematopoietic stem cell transplantation restores hematopoietic function following marrow ablative therapy. Blood 71:73–77, 1988.

AUTOLOGOUS BONE MARROW TRANSPLANTATION FOR SOLID TUMORS

Autologous bone marrow transplantation has been employed for numerous solid tumors (see Table 31–1). Different cytoreductive regimens are used at different centers. Results published to date indicate promising complete remission rates, but long-term follow-up data in larger numbers of patients are not yet available. Autologous bone marrow infusion allows dose-escalation of chemotherapeutic agents in the hope of overcoming drug resistance. In small cell lung cancer, early results of high-dose chemotherapy followed by autologous bone marrow transplantation do not appear superior to those obtained with conventional therapy alone. Autologous bone marrow transplantation in metastatic breast cancer achieves the best results in those patients with minimal disease, little prior chemotherapy, and good performance status.

REFERENCES

Antman K, Gale RP: Advanced breast cancer: High-dose chemotherapy and bone marrow autotransplants. Ann Intern Med 108:570–574, 1988.

Cheson BD, Lacerna L, Leyland-Jones B, et al: Autologous bone marrow transplantation: current status and future directions. Ann Intern Med 110:51–65, 1989.

Humblet Y, Symann M, Bosly A, et al: Late intensification chemotherapy with autologous bone marrow transplantation in selected small-cell carcinomas of the lung; a randomized study. J Clin Oncol 5:1864–1873, 1987.

FOLLOW-UP OF THE POSTTRANSPLANT PATIENT

Many primary care physicians will become involved in the follow-up of transplant patients after they return home from their transplant centers. During the first few months after allogeneic transplantation, patients are instructed to avoid exposure to measles, rubella, chickenpox, and varicella-zoster. For those exposed to herpes zoster, zoster immune globulin is recommended. For those who develop herpes zoster infection, early intravenous acyclovir is recommended. Most allogeneic transplant patients are maintained on trimethoprim-sulfamethoxazole twice per week as bacterial infection prophylaxis. GVHD prophylaxis is usually continued until 6 to 12 months after transplant. Blood products should be irradiated for 6 months after both autologous and allogeneic transplantation. Booster immunization with attenuated *Haemophilus influenzae,* diphtheria tetanus (dT), and *dead* polio and pneumovax vaccines is recommended 12 months post–allogeneic transplant by many centers. Contacts of allogeneic marrow transplant recipients should not receive live polio vaccine during the immediate posttransplant period. Patients usually return to work 6 to 9 months after transplantation.

32
HEMATOPOIETIC GROWTH FACTORS

Elizabeth M. Cyran

ERYTHROPOIETIN

Erythropoietin is the hormone responsible for regulating red cell production. It is produced primarily in the kidney, with another 10 to 15% being produced in the liver. In response to local tissue hypoxia, the peritubular interstitial cells in the kidney release erythropoietin into the blood stream. Erythropoietin then binds to specific receptors on bone marrow erythroid progenitor cells, the burst-forming unit–erythroid (BFU-E), and colony-forming unit–erythroid (CFU-E). This stimulation of the BFU-E and CFU-E to proliferate and differentiate causes increased production of erythroblasts, increases the rate at which erythroid cell divisions occur, and promotes release of reticulocytes into the peripheral blood. An accurate radioimmunoassay can now measure erythropoietin levels, with normal ranging approximately 9 to 26 mU/mL. This low level of erythropoietin may reflect the basal rate of red cell production. An inverse relationship exists between the red cell mass and the erythropoietin level. Anemia triggers increased production of erythropoietin when the hemoglobin is less than 11 g/dL. When the red cell mass is above normal, erythropoietin production is suppressed. The erythropoietin response to anemia may be blunted, however, in cancer patients.

Erythropoietin, first isolated and purified in 1977, is a 166 amino acid glycoprotein with a molecular weight of 30,000 daltons. The gene, located on chromosome 7, has been cloned, and recombinant technology now produces sufficient amounts of erythropoietin for investigational and clinical use. Erythropoietin can be given either by the intravenous or subcutaneous route. The subcutaneous route is associated with a lower peak level but longer half-life than the intravenous route and has similar hematologic efficacy; thus it is ideal for patient self-administration at home.

Initial trials of erythropoietin were conducted in renal dialysis patients with anemia. A large multi-institutional study demonstrated a dose-dependent rise in hematocrit by 2 to 3 weeks in over 90% of patients. Erythropoietin also appears to be helpful in patients with acquired immunodeficiency syndrome (AIDS)–related anemia who have erythropoietin levels less than 500 mU/mL. It has been approved for use in these two conditions and is commercially available. Erythropoietin is safe, effective, and well tolerated. Starting doses of 50 to 150 U/kg three times a week subcutaneously or intravenously are recommended, although some patients need up to 250 to 500 U/kg two to three times per week for response. Blood pressure may rise during treatment and should be monitored. The rate of rise in hematocrit has been found to be an important factor in elevating blood pressure. The rate of rise should not exceed 3% every 2 weeks. If a target hematocrit of 35% has been reached, the dose of erythropoietin can be tapered by 25 U/kg every 2 weeks to a maintenance level.

Patients who respond to erythropoietin may develop an absolute or relative iron deficiency due to increased utilization of iron in erythropoiesis. Iron deficiency can interfere with response to erythropoietin treatment; thus serum iron levels should be monitored prior to and during therapy, particularly if the hematocrit rise is less than expected or the reticulocyte index falls. Oral iron supplementation can be started if the iron saturation is $<$20%, even with high ferritin levels.

Preliminary results suggest erythropoietin may be effective in patients with myeloma or bone marrow infiltration, especially in patients who have suboptimal erythropoietin levels for their degree of anemia. It also may be effective in cancer patients receiving cyclic cisplatin-containing chemotherapy. However, the indications for and efficacy of erythropoietin in these settings await results of controlled clinical trials.

The use of erythropoietin in myelodysplasia has not been promising; most patients have high endogenous levels and fail to respond. Erythropoietin therapy can be considered in patients with erythropoietin levels less than 500 mU/ml.

Whether treatment with erythropoietin will be cost effective is another consideration. However, there are significant benefits over red cell transfusion, including decreased viral transmission, decreased patient treatment time and inconvenience, and avoidance of transfusion reactions and iron overload.

REFERENCES

Erslev AJ: Erythropoietin titers in health and disease. Semin Hematol 28(Suppl 3):2–8, 1991.
Ludwig H, Fritz E, Kotzmann H, et al: Erythropoietin treatment of anemia associated with multiple myeloma. N Engl J Med 322:1693–1699, 1990.
Miller CB, Jones RJ, Piantadosi S, et al: Decreased erythropoietin response in patients with the anemia of cancer. N Engl J Med 322:1689–1692, 1990.
Oster W, Herrmann R, Gamm H, et al: Erythropoietin for the treatment of anemia of malignancy associated with neoplastic bone marrow infiltration. J Clin Oncol 8:956–962, 1990.

COLONY-STIMULATING FACTORS

The colony-stimulating factors (CSFs) are glycoproteins that support the production, differentiation, and function of hematopoietic cells. They were discovered in the mid-1960s during observations on the in vitro growth of murine bone marrow progenitor cells on semisolid culture media. Researchers noted that growth was not supported unless the cultures contained added tissue or tissue products. This led to the hypothesis that a specific growth factor might be present in tissue that stimulated the formation of colonies of macrophages and granulocytes, and this was termed a colony-stimulating factor (CSF). Multiple different CSFs acting at various levels of cell maturation were found, but their isolation and purification were slow. By the late 1970s and early 1980s, four factors had been identified (named for the mature cells produced): granulocyte-macrophage colony-stimulating factor (GM-CSF), granulocyte colony-stimulating factor (G-CSF), macrophage colony-stimulating factor (M-CSF), and multipotential colony-stimulating factor (better known as interleukin 3, or IL-3). However, available amounts of these growth factors were too small to permit study until molecular biology techniques were developed to clone the gene sequences and produce the proteins by recombinant technology in mammalian cells, yeast, and bacteria. These recombinant products were then shown in animal studies to be active in vivo, by causing elevated peripheral blood counts and increased marrow cellularity. At least 11 growth factors have now been identified, some through culture systems studying lymphocyte proliferation and differentiation and thus labeled as interleukins. However, only the original four growth factors have been tested in clinical trials so far. This chapter will focus on their biology and application to cancer treatment.

Each growth factor is a glycoprotein of 14,000 to 90,000 daltons molecular weight encoded by a single gene. Growth factors are produced by endothelial cells, fibroblasts, monocytes, and activated T lymphocytes. Low circulating levels of G-CSF and M-CSF can be detected, suggesting that there is some basal production; however, GM-CSF and IL-3 are produced only by activated cells in response to endotoxin, antigenic challenge, tumor necrosis factor, or IL-1. The function of CSFs in the steady-state regulation of hematopoiesis is not known; they may be more important in responses to inflammation and stress. The genes that code for GM-CSF, IL-3, and M-CSF are located on the long arm of chromosome 5, and deletion of this is the most common chromosomal abnormality in the acute nonlymphoid leukemias and myelodysplasias. Additionally, the gene for G-CSF is on chromosome 17, the translocation of which is associated with promyelocytic leukemia. Whether and how these relationships impact on clinical disease is not known, but they have led to further interest in this area.

Hematopoietic cells carry specific membrane receptors for each CSF on their surfaces, and the interaction of the growth factors with the receptors has a variety of influences on the cell. In general, all promote progenitor cell proliferation by stimulating them to enter the S phase of the cell cyle; they promote cell differentiation and maturation; and they prolong survival and enhanced functional activity of mature cells, including enhanced phagocytosis and antibody-dependent cytotoxicity.

Growth factors may show effects on multiple lineages. Many are synergistic or additive with each other. G-CSF and GM-CSF receptors have been identified on nonhematopoietic cells such as breast, small cell, and colon carcinomas, although no in vivo solid tumor growth in their presence has been demonstrated thus far.

The actions of CSFs in increasing marrow cellularity and peripheral cell counts, in inducing cells into S phase, and in enhancing cell function such as antibody-dependent cytotoxicity have led to many different uses in oncology, hematology, and infectious diseases that are now being tested in clinical trials (Table 32–1).

Table 32–1. **POTENTIAL APPLICATIONS OF COLONY-STIMULATING FACTORS**

Prevention of chemotherapy-induced neutropenia and infection
Myelodysplasia
Leukemia
Bone marrow transplantation
Graft failure
Peripheral stem cell harvesting
Neutropenia due to bone marrow infiltration
Cyclic neutropenia
Idiopathic/congenital neutropenia
Aplastic anemia
AIDS-related neutropenia

GRANULOCYTE-MACROPHAGE COLONY-STIMULATING FACTOR (GM-CSF)

Source and Activity

GM-CSF, produced by monocytes, fibroblasts, endothelial cells, and activated T lymphocytes, has multilineage actions, including increasing formation of granulocyte and macrophage colonies at lower concentrations and stimulating eosinophil and megakaryocyte colonies at higher concentrations. It also works synergistically with erythropoietin and IL-3 to increase early erythroid production. These actions suggest an effect on an early or immature progenitor cell, but GM-CSF primarily affects the granulocyte-macrophage lineage. Increased peripheral blood granulocytes, monocytes, and eosinophils are seen after administration of GM-CSF. Other important effects include enhanced function of mature cells, including increased chemotaxis, phagocytosis, oxidative metabolism, adhesion, and cytotoxicity. Interestingly, GM-CSF decreases neutrophil migration into skin windows, perhaps preventing neutrophils from leaving an area of inflammation. GM-CSF can induce monocytes to release tumor necrosis factor (TNF) and interleukin 1. Leukemic blasts possess receptors to GM-CSF.

Administration

GM-CSF (as well as the other growth factors) can be given intravenously or subcutaneously. Intravenous bolus administration has a short half-life of only 1 to 3 hours, whereas the subcutaneous route and slower intravenous infusions are associated with more sustained effects. There is a dose-dependent effect on periperhal blood counts, but the optimal dose has not been determined; however, doses of 250 $\mu g/m^2$/day have been recommended. Toxicities include rash, bone pain, fever, malaise, myalgias, anorexia, and elevated liver function tests. These side effects may be due to the release of TNF or IL-1 stimulated by GM-CSF and are usually mild to moderate in severity. They often improve with repeated administration and respond to antipyretics or analgesics. Doses higher than 20 to 30 μg/kg/day have been associated with capillary leak syndrome, edema, weight gain, pleural/pericardial effusions, atrial arrhythmias, and phlebitis or thrombosis around central lines. Effects of GM-CSF given daily are seen within 3 to 4 days after initiation of treatment. GM-CSF has been approved for use in accelerating myeloid recovery after bone marrow transplantation.

GRANULOCYTE COLONY-STIMULATING FACTOR (G-CSF)

Source and Activity

G-CSF, produced by monocytes, fibroblasts, and endothelial cells, binds to receptors on mature, committed granulocytic progenitor cells, causing increased numbers and function of mature neutrophils; thus G-CSF is considered to be lineage specific. However, it may also act in synergy with IL-3 on other lineages, particularly megakaryocyte precursors. Effects on mature neutrophil function are similar to those of GM-CSF except that G-CSF does not inhibit neutrophil migration. Most myeloid leukemic blast cells also have receptors to and proliferate in response to G-CSF, raising the potential that G-CSF could be used to cycle leukemic cells into the S phase of the cell cycle where they might be more sensitive to phase-specific chemotherapeutic agents.

Administration

Treatment with G-CSF in clinical trials has been in a dose range of 1 to 60 μg/kg/day. It has most commonly been given as an IV infusion over 30 minutes but also appears effective when given in small doses as a subcutaneous injection. G-CSF does not cause fever, and no maximal tolerated dose has been defined. Transient bone pain is common and thought to be related to marrow expansion from hematopoiesis. G-CSF has been approved for use in patients receiving myelosuppressive chemotherapy at starting doses of 5 μg/kg/day.

MACROPHAGE COLONY-STIMULATING FACTOR (M-CSF)

Source and Activity

M-CSF, produced by monocytes, fibroblasts, endothelial cells, and B lymphocytes, increases the number of mature monocytes and macrophages and thus is lineage specific, acting on a mature, committed progenitor cell. M-CSF enhances monocyte antibody-dependent cell cytotoxity, macrophage antimicrobial activity, and antitumor activity. It may be indirectly myelostimulatory by promoting the release of G-CSF, GM-CSF, and other cytokines by monocytes and macrophages. M-CSF stimulates monocyte antibody-dependent cell cytotoxicity against human melanoma and neuroblastoma cell lines, suggesting a role for it in antitumor treatment, perhaps with the addition of tumor-specific monoclonal antibodies.

Administration

Clinical testing with M-CSF has been limited. It is given intravenously in doses ranging from 10 to 80 μg/kg/day. Reported side effects include fever, diaphoresis, pruritus, hypotension, and thrombocytopenia.

INTERLEUKIN 3 (IL-3)

Source and Activity

IL-3, produced by T lymphocytes, appears to act on early multipotent progenitor cells, with responses seen in neutrophilic, erythroid, monocytic, and megakaryocytic lines. IL-3 also acts as a growth factor for mast cells and basophils. Peripheral blood effects are not seen until the second to fourth week after initiation of therapy, suggesting that IL-3 acts on an even earlier stage of progenitor cells than G-CSF or GM-CSF. Current interest centers around combining IL-3 with G-CSF or GM-CSF for a multilineage effect with more rapid improvement in neutrophil counts.

Administration

The optimal dose and route of delivery of IL-3 are not defined, but recommended doses range from 30 to 500 μg/m^2, and it appears effective both intravenously and subcutaneously. Side effects include fever, headache, flushing, and erythema at the injection site.

CLINICAL USES OF THE COLONY-STIMULATING FACTORS

USAGE WITH CHEMOTHERAPY

The ability of CSFs to ameliorate the toxicities of chemotherapy through accelerated recovery of neutrophil counts has been demonstrated in several trials. Studies have shown that growth factors can be used safely in patients undergoing chemotherapy and are effective in improving neutrophil counts and decreasing febrile eipsodes, although no reduction in overall mortality is achieved. G-CSF has now been approved for prevention of chemotherapy-related neutropenia. Whether its use will permit higher and more frequent dosing of chemotherapy, and whether this will in turn affect response rate or survival remain to be established.

USAGE IN LEUKEMIA

The use of CSFs in leukemia is being investigated. Growth factors are being used to induce leukemic blasts to enter the S phase of the cell cycle, where they may be more sensitive to cell cycle–specific chemotherapeutic agents. Another use is to ameliorate the neutropenia due to intensive induction chemotherapy, particularly in older patients with acute leukemia. A potential concern is that growth factors may accelerate the course of leukemia or contribute to relapse of disease. One recent study suggested that leukemic cells were being cycled by GM-CSF without any detrimental effect on initial remission rate.

USAGE IN MYELODYSPLASIA

Infection is a common cause of morbidity and mortality in neutropenic patients with myelodysplasia. Growth factors have been tested to see if peripheral neutrophil counts can be improved without stimulating leukemic blasts and causing progression of disease. A large multicenter trial used GM-CSF versus placebo in a crossover design. Patients were treated with 3 μg/kg/day of GM-CSF given subcutaneously for 3 months versus placebo. Patients receiving placebo were crossed over to the treatment arm if they had persistent fever in spite of intravenous antibiotics. There was a statistically significant increase in the absolute neutrophil count in the treatment group as well as a significant decrease in infectious episodes. Although GM-CSF has multilineage effects, there was no statistically significant difference in the platelet counts, hemoglobin levels, or number of platelet and red cell transfusions required in either group. Increases in peripheral blood eosinophils, monocytes, and lymphocytes were seen. GM-CSF did not promote an increase in bone marrow leukemic blasts compared with the observation group, although other studies have suggested that growth factors can increase leukemic blast counts, particularly if excess marrow blasts (>15%) are present initially. Toxicities in this study included bone pain, injection site reactions, fever, and fatigue in less than 20% of patients.

USAGE IN BONE MARROW TRANSPLANTATION

CSFs have been used in patients undergoing autologous bone marrow transplantation for a variety of malignancies, including lymphomas, breast cancer, and other solid tumors. Several studies using GM-CSF have shown a shorter duration of low neutrophil counts compared with historical controls and in some studies a significant decrease in the number of febrile days and hospital admission days. Additional benefits of lower peak bilirubin and creatinine levels posttransplant as well as a decrease in total units of platelets transfused have also been reported. Most studies suggest that the time to first appearance of neutrophils is unchanged, but that once neutrophils appear, a more rapid increase in counts follows, with shorter durations to absolute neutrophil counts of 500/μL and 1000/μL and higher neutrophil counts by day 14 posttransplant. GM-CSF is approved for use in bone marrow transplants to accelerate myeloid recovery.

CSFs have also been used successfully in treating graft failure after autologous or allogeneic bone marrow transplantation. Approximately 10% of patients fail to engraft or develop graft failure (ANC <100/μL by day 28 or a decrease in ANC to <500/μL after initial engraftment was achieved). This is a serious complication with survival at 1 year of only 23%. Treatment previously consisted of supportive care or repeat marrow infusions. A nonrandomized study of patients with graft failure treated with GM-CSF showed improved survival rates compared with historical controls, without any increase in graft-versus-host disease or increase in relapse rate of myeloid leukemia.

Another use of growth factors is to treat cytomegalovirus (CMV)–induced myelosuppression in the posttransplant setting. CMV infections may cause myelosuppression and graft failure in allogeneic transplant recipients, and ganciclovir treatment for CMV is also potentially myelosuppressive. Growth factors such as GM-CSF may help preserve neutrophil counts during this treatment.

USAGE IN PERIPHERAL STEM CELL HARVESTING

Although most stem cells reside in the marrow cavity, a small number circulate in the peripheral blood. A significant number of these may be harvested through repeated leukaphoresis procedures, after which they may be used for autologous transplants. This method of collecting stem cells is especially attractive in patients who have bone marrow involvement by tumor or extensive prior irradiation, making traditional iliac crest harvesting less desirable. The collection of peripheral blood stem cells is greatly enhanced by pretreating the patient with GM-CSF.

SUMMARY

The use of growth factors in the treatment of patients with cancer is one of the most exciting areas of clinical research in oncology today. Clinical trials suggest they are effective in shortening the duration of neutropenia after chemotherapy and marrow transplantation, with a corresponding decrease in the number of febrile episodes, days of antibiotic use, and hospital days. How broadly they should be applied to cancer chemotherapy programs and their cost effectiveness remain to be determined. Whether the use of growth factors will support an increase in intensity of treatment and whether this will result in improved response rates and overall survival is a focus of active investigation.

REFERENCES

Bettelheim P, Valent P, Andreeff M, et al: Recombinant human granulocyte-macrophage colony-stimulating factor in combination with standard induction chemotherapy in de novo acute myeloid leukemia. Blood 77:700–711, 1991.

Crawford J, Ozer H, Stoller R, et al: Reduction by granulocyte colony-stimulating factor of fever and neutropenia induced by chemotherapy in patients with small cell lung cancer. N Engl J Med 325:164–170, 1991.

Groopman JE, Molina JM, Scadden DT: Hematopoietic growth factors: Biology and clinical applications. N Engl J Med 321:1449–1459, 1990.

Metcalf D: The colony stimulating factors: Discovery, development and clinical applications. Cancer 65:2185–2195, 1990.

Nemunaitus J, Singer JW, Buckner CD, et al: Use of recombinant human granulocyte-macrophage colony-stimulating factor in graft failure after bone marrow transplantation. Blood 76:245–253, 1990.

INDEX

Note: Page numbers in *italics* refer to illustrations; page numbers followed by (t) refer to tables.